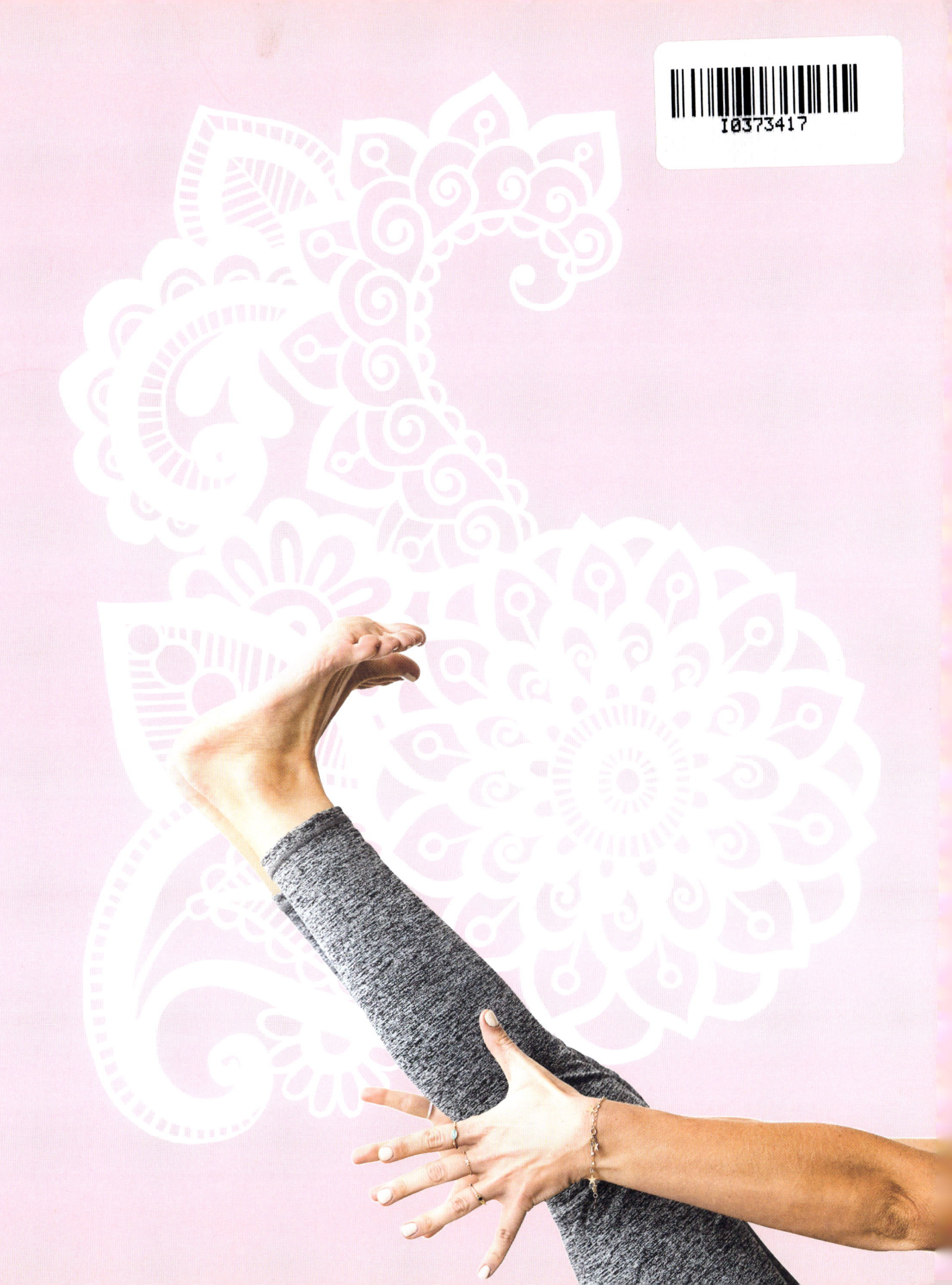

Pippa Shaw, you inspire me more than you know. I've never had a trainer like you; you challenge me, make me laugh, support me, empower me, and you are one of the strongest and yet gentle souls I've met. You've been there when I've felt alone and when I've felt on top of the world, with unwavering kindness and genuine care. You've not only helped me achieve my physical goals, but you've taught me loads about self-worth and doing what feels right for me. I'm very grateful to not only train with you, but to call you a friend.

Thank you, Pippy.

We advise that the information contained in this book does not negate personal responsibility on the part of the reader for their own health and safety. It is recommended that individually tailored advice is sought from your healthcare or medical professional. The publishers and their respective employees, agents and authors are not liable for injuries or damage occasioned to any person as a result of reading or following the information contained in this book.

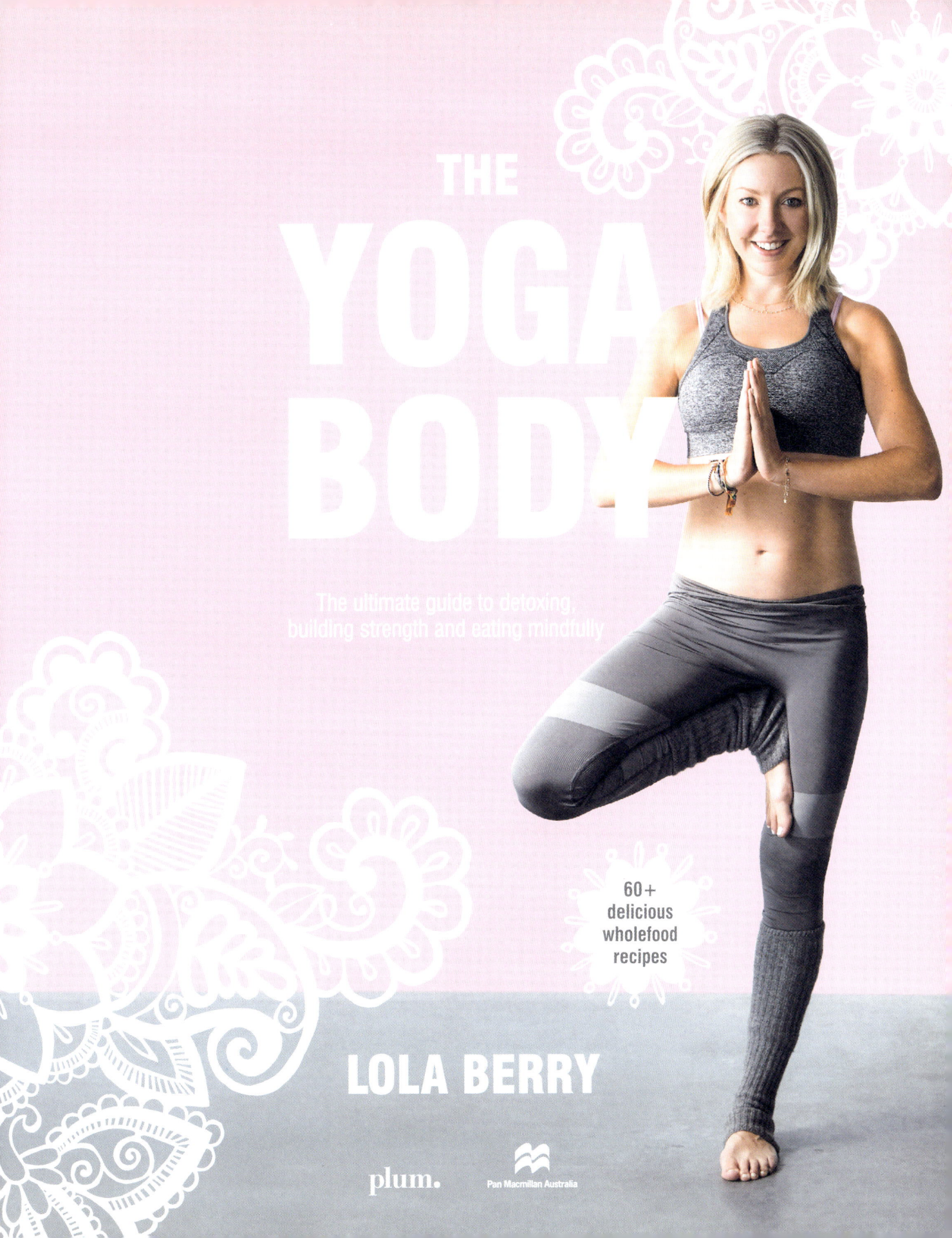

THE YOGA BODY

The ultimate guide to detoxing, building strength and eating mindfully

60+ delicious wholefood recipes

LOLA BERRY

plum.   Pan Macmillan Australia

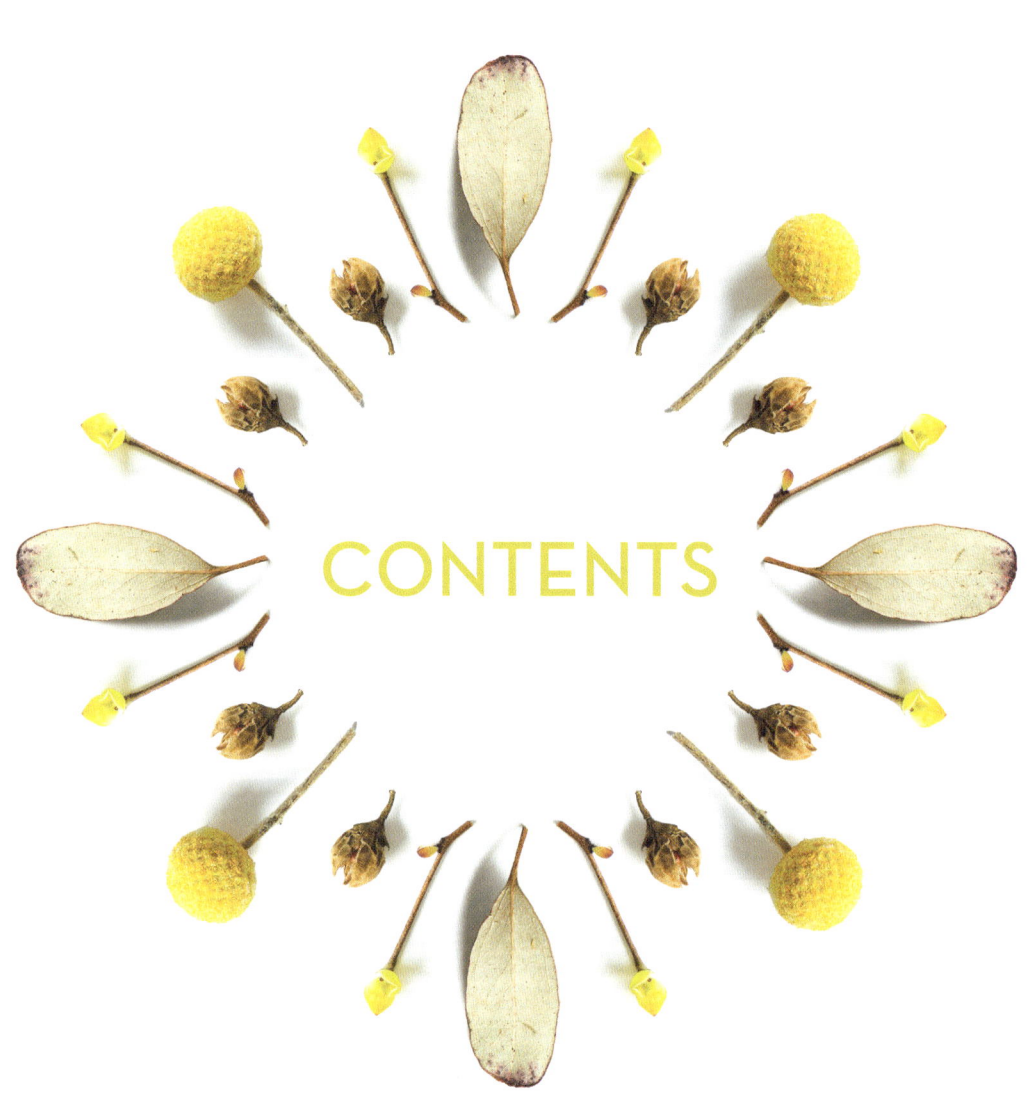

Introduction _ 6

PART 1
YOGA PRACTICE

Why yoga is so amazing _ 14
Styles of yoga _ 20
Choosing a yoga studio _ 26
Your first class _ 30
Awesome yoga sequences _ 35

PART 2
YOGA FOOD

Tips for clean eating _ 65
Seven-day vegan cleanse _ 83
The yoga body recipes _ 103

Drinks _ 111
Breakfast _ 129
Savoury _ 151
Sweet _ 195

PART 3
YOGA MIND

The eight limbs of yoga _ 222
Things we can learn from yoga _ 226

Thanks _ 230
Index _ 232

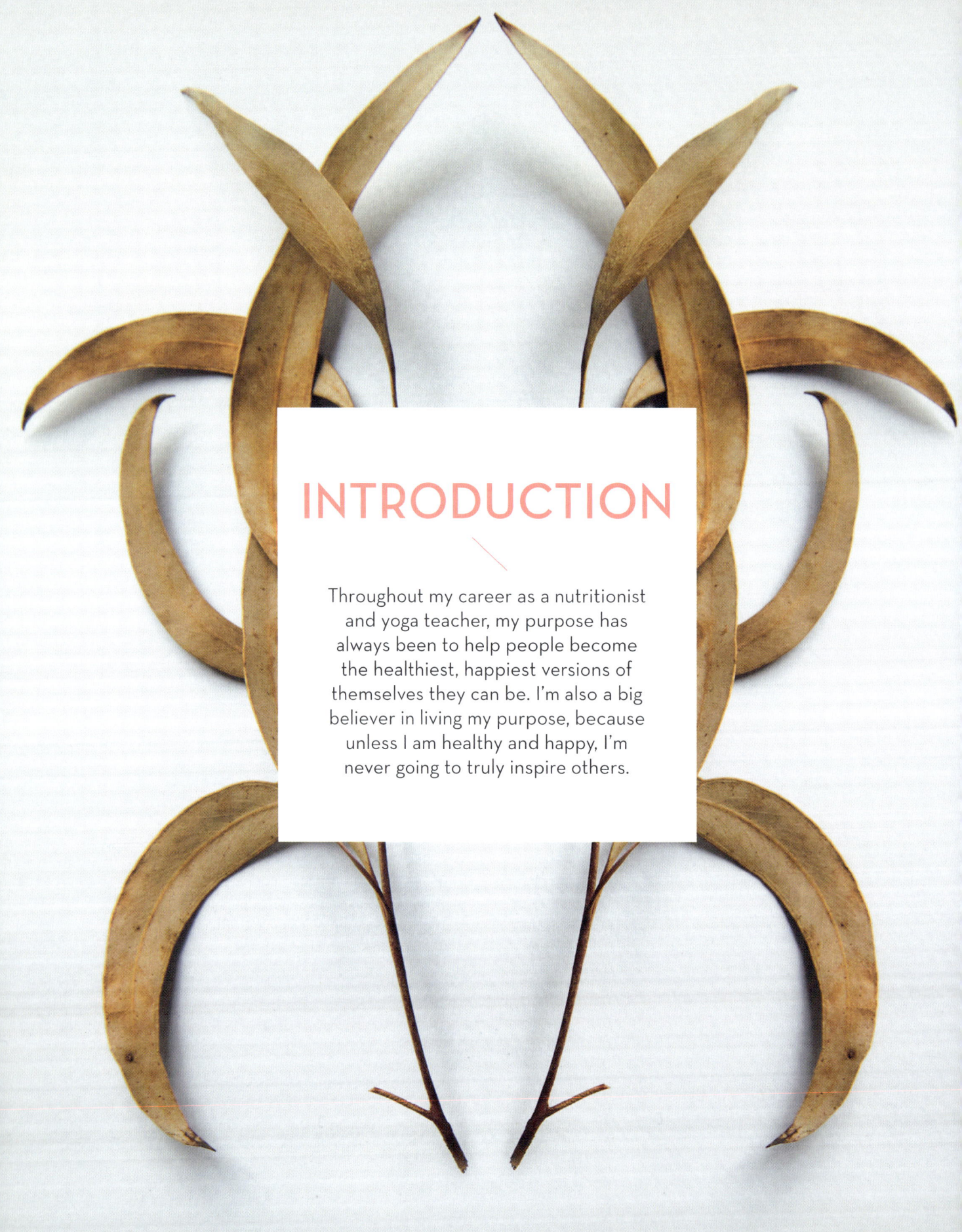

INTRODUCTION

Throughout my career as a nutritionist and yoga teacher, my purpose has always been to help people become the healthiest, happiest versions of themselves they can be. I'm also a big believer in living my purpose, because unless I am healthy and happy, I'm never going to truly inspire others.

> I tend to live by the mantra 'the harder you work, the luckier you get', so at times it can be a challenge for me to slow down.

At twenty-three I'd published my first book, was practising as a nutritionist and had just been signed to a morning TV gig. I'd also started working with a personal trainer who kept saying, 'Lola, you'd love yoga', but I said, 'No way. Too slow for me. I'd rather do boxing.' Then one night I was working at a smoothie bar and one of the regular customers convinced me to attend her Bikram class the next morning. I'll never forget it. The room was heated to 40°C and about 45 per cent humidity and I remember not being allowed to drink water for the first half hour (this was one of the rules). I thought I was going to vomit for all but ten minutes of the 90-minute class! But the teacher was awesome, and since I'd bought a ten-day pass, I thought I might as well use it so I found myself back on the mat the following morning. By the third session I was hooked. I loved the poses, I loved the sweat and I loved the deep relaxation I felt after every class. I was really starting to feel the benefits.

If you haven't tried yoga before you might think it's lots of meditating and hippy jazz, but if you practise the asanas (the yoga poses) it does wonderful things for your body – it improves posture, flexibility, strength and even aids weight management. Now, I have to confess that when I first started, it was the physical stuff that drew me in, but the more I practised, the more I became fascinated with yoga's philosophical and spiritual roots. I wanted to learn how to be more present, to calm my mind-chatter and to change the way I spoke to myself. More importantly, I wanted to learn about my ego and how to let go of it, or at the very least decrease it. Let me explain.

I'd been practising yoga for a while when I was asked to do a TV segment advising women on the kind of diet required to become a lingerie model. I remember being so hypnotised by the whole idea of working on television that I didn't stop to ask myself if this was the right thing for me to do. Anyway, I got home after doing the segment and I started crying. I felt horrible, as if I had let everyone down. Encouraging women to pursue such an unrealistic body image was way out of alignment with my values and I was inspiring no one, least of all myself.

Then I caught up with a friend who said, 'Lola, you're fake, you're in this for the fame.' I was mortified and I didn't want to believe her. But you know what? She was spot on. I wasn't doing this to help others, I was doing it to raise my media profile so I'd be booked for more TV gigs. It was wrong on so many levels. So I decided to let go of TV and focus on becoming more connected to myself – I wanted to be clear in my mind and to feel happier. I wanted to act with integrity. And I knew that yoga had a deeper, spiritual side that would encourage the kind of self-inquiry I needed.

> I'm here to tell you that *anyone* can do yoga. If you can breathe, you can do yoga. There are many different styles, and it's just a matter of finding one that feels right for you.

About three years after I'd started Bikram, a friend took me to my very first vinyasa class, and I remember thinking that I could do this forever – it was challenging and strengthening but at the same time felt very nourishing. I loved it so much that I decided to train as a vinyasa teacher. Yet despite all my practice, I still felt I wasn't learning to calm my mind. I still tended to live in 'yang' (fiery, passionate, right-brained, fast-paced) so I decided to try yin yoga. This is where you hold the poses for a long time (anywhere from four to ten minutes) and are encouraged to shut your eyes as you slowly melt into them. Boy was it hard to slow down! But I persevered, and the benefits were amazing. After every class I felt deeply relaxed (I call it 'yoga stoned'), plus I'd sleep really well and wake up feeling super refreshed. So I trained to become a yin yoga teacher as well, and it turns out that yin yoga is the perfect partner for vinyasa.

Now, some people I teach have confessed that they were scared to try yoga in case they weren't flexible enough. Others worried that they wouldn't be fit enough to hold the poses and still others said that they felt self-conscious about their bodies. I'm here to tell you that *anyone* can do yoga. If you can breathe, you can do yoga. There are many different styles, and it's just a matter of finding one that feels right for you. Even if you have an injury or physical challenge, a good teacher will be able to modify poses to suit your needs.

In any case, I've learned that yoga isn't just about making your body strong, flexible and healthy – it's also about making your *mind* strong, flexible and healthy. The word yoga itself comes from the Sanskrit word *yuj*, which means to join or unite. (Sanskrit is the language of ancient India and is still one of India's twenty-two official languages.) Yoga, then, is about the connection between mind, body and spirit.

When we think of yoga here in the West, we almost always think of the physical practice (the asanas or poses), yet according to the ancient teachings, the asanas are just one step on the eight-fold path to purifying the body and mind and attaining bliss. The others include the yamas (ethical principles that guide how we relate to other people), niyamas (the principles that guide how we take care of ourselves) and pranayama (breath control). More about these later on.

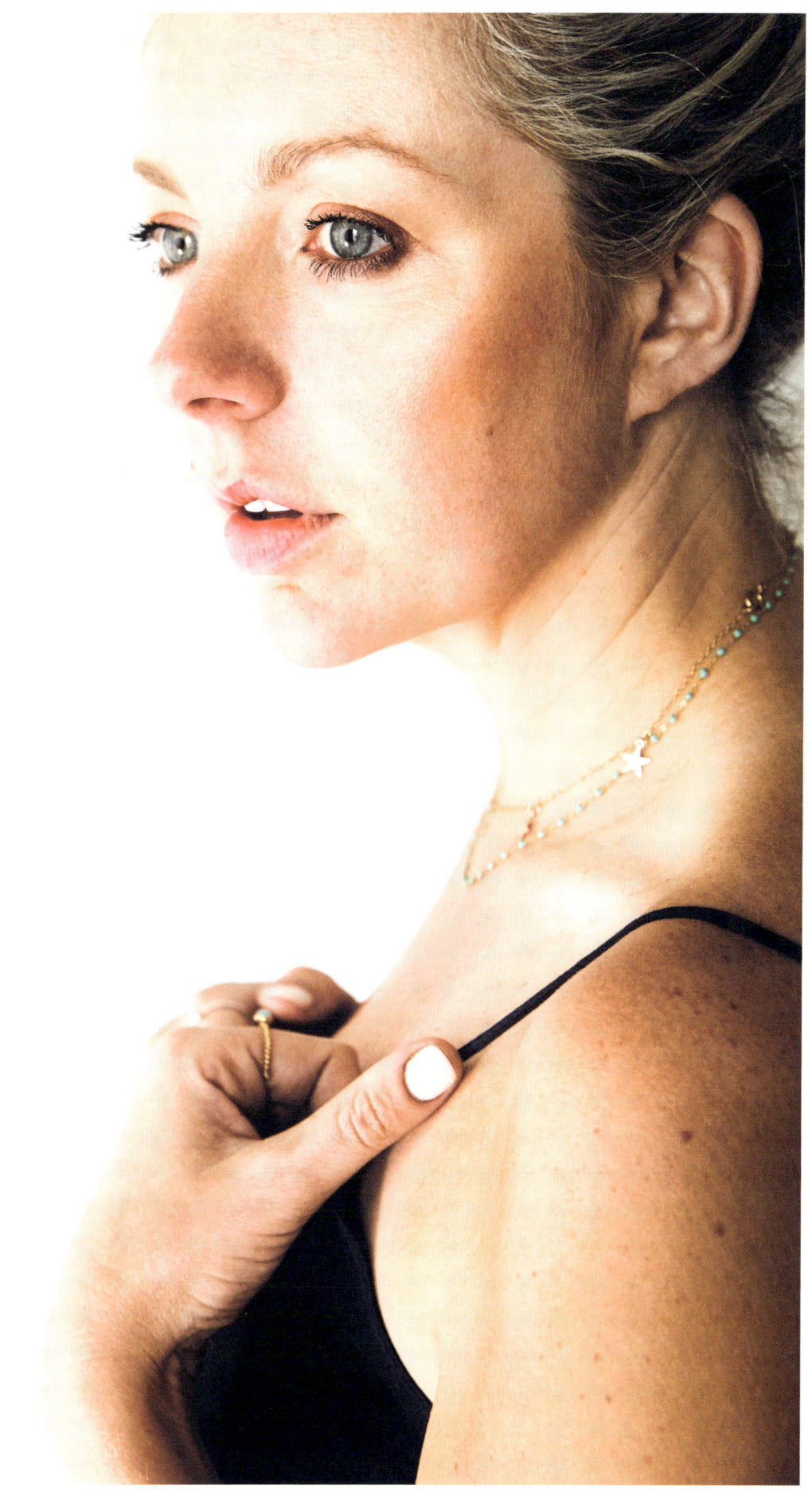

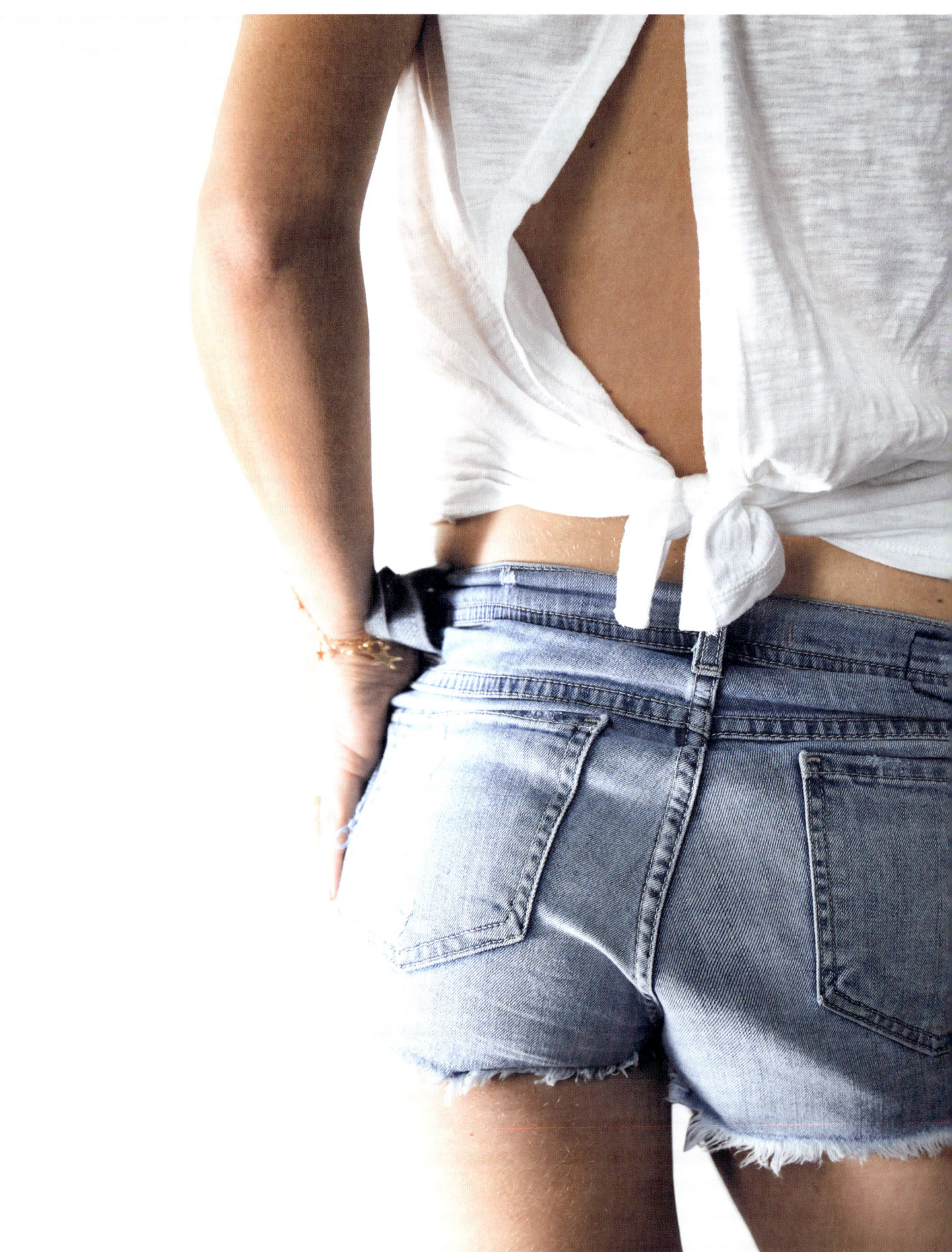

Be thankful for your life, spend time in nature, breathe deeply, let go of your worries, forgive yourself and others, and build your life around what you love.

We all want to be fit, healthy and happy. We all want to feel that we matter, that we have a purpose and that we belong. Yoga has given me all of this and so much more. Yoga helps me to feel 'whole', like I am putting forward a kinder, happier, more heart-filled version of myself. It has helped me understand that contentment is less about how much I have acquired or how much I have accomplished and more about how well I have participated in my own life. It has taught me to be grateful for the ordinary moments – the mundane, the everyday stuff – just as much as the extraordinary moments – the surprises and the magic. And it has taught me to live in the present rather than feel resentful about the past or worried about the future.

Yoga can give all of this to you, too. All you need to do is turn up on your mat and do your best. As you focus on your breath, and on where your body is in space, you can't help but be in the moment. When you have finished your yoga session, you will take that feeling of wellbeing and lightness into the rest of your day (or night). And you're more likely to honour your body by choosing nutrient-dense ('clean') foods that are close to their most natural state – fresh vegetables, fruits, whole grains, nuts and seeds, beans and a little dairy, fish or meat, if you like.

For me, yoga is food for the soul, and when I teach yoga, it feels like I share that nourishment with others. I want you to think of this book as a private yoga retreat – everything you need to heal your body, mind and soul is right here. In Part 1, I explain the amazing benefits of this ancient practice. I also teach you some of the core poses and give you a range of sequences to use for different life challenges, including yoga to help you sleep and to improve fitness and muscle tone. In Part 2, I explain the principles of clean eating and include fifty delicious recipes that go hand in hand with yoga practice. This section also includes a seven-day vegan cleanse, with pared-down recipes, a prep guide and simple eating plan. And in Part 3, I explore some of the ethical and spiritual principles that underlie a yogic way of life, and how these can empower you to be the best you, right now. So unroll your mat, open your heart and let's go!

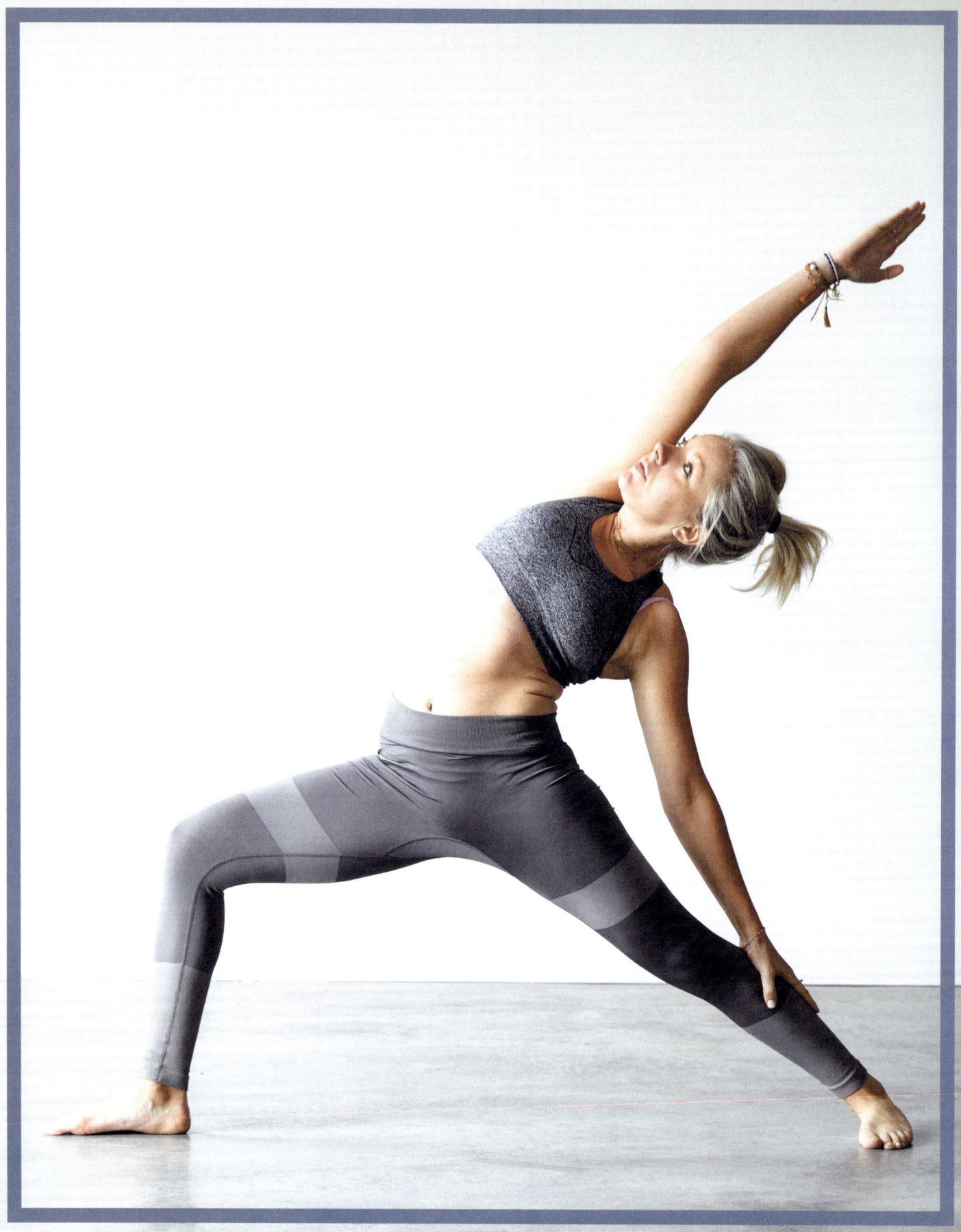

YOGA PRACTICE

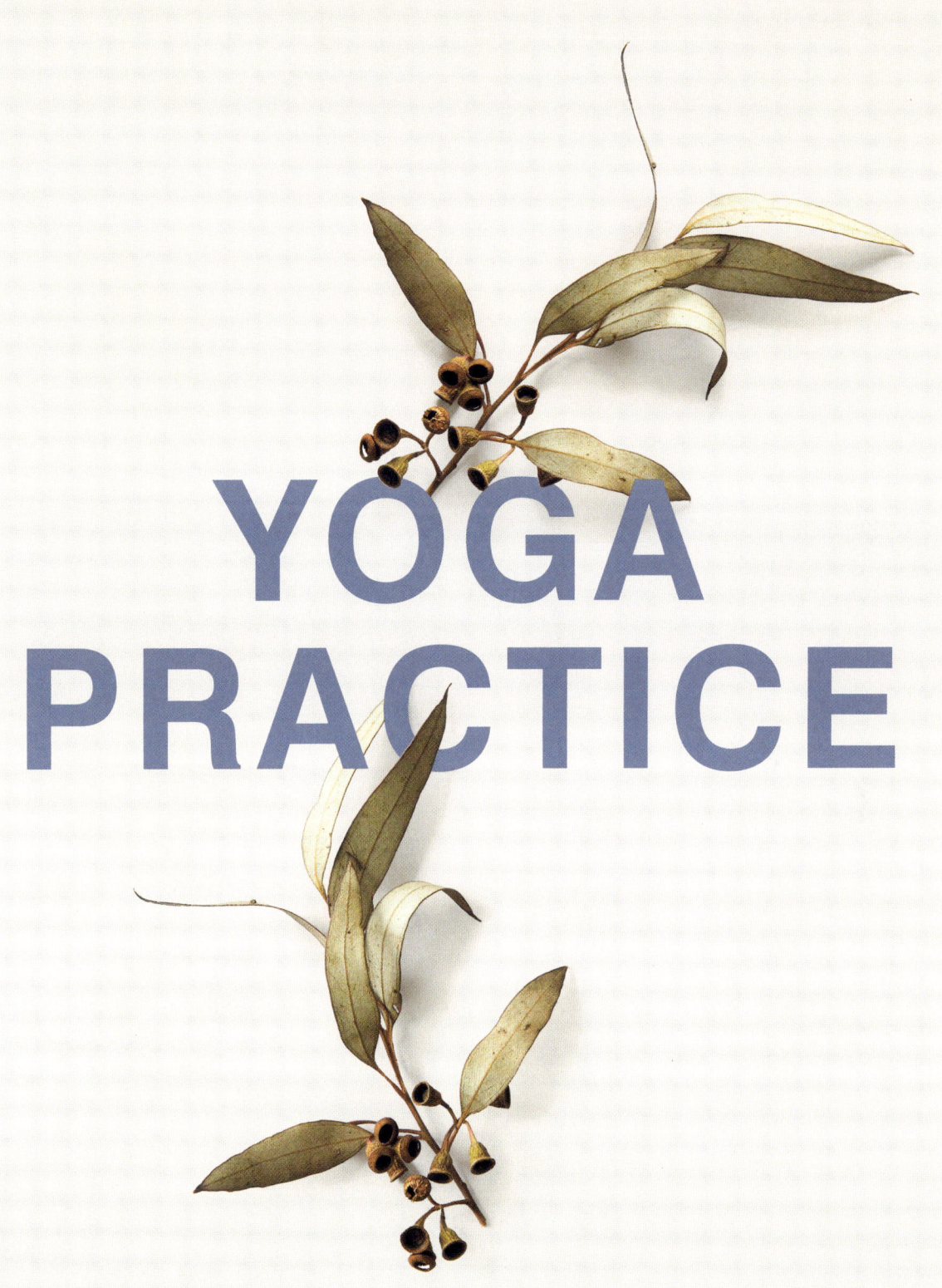

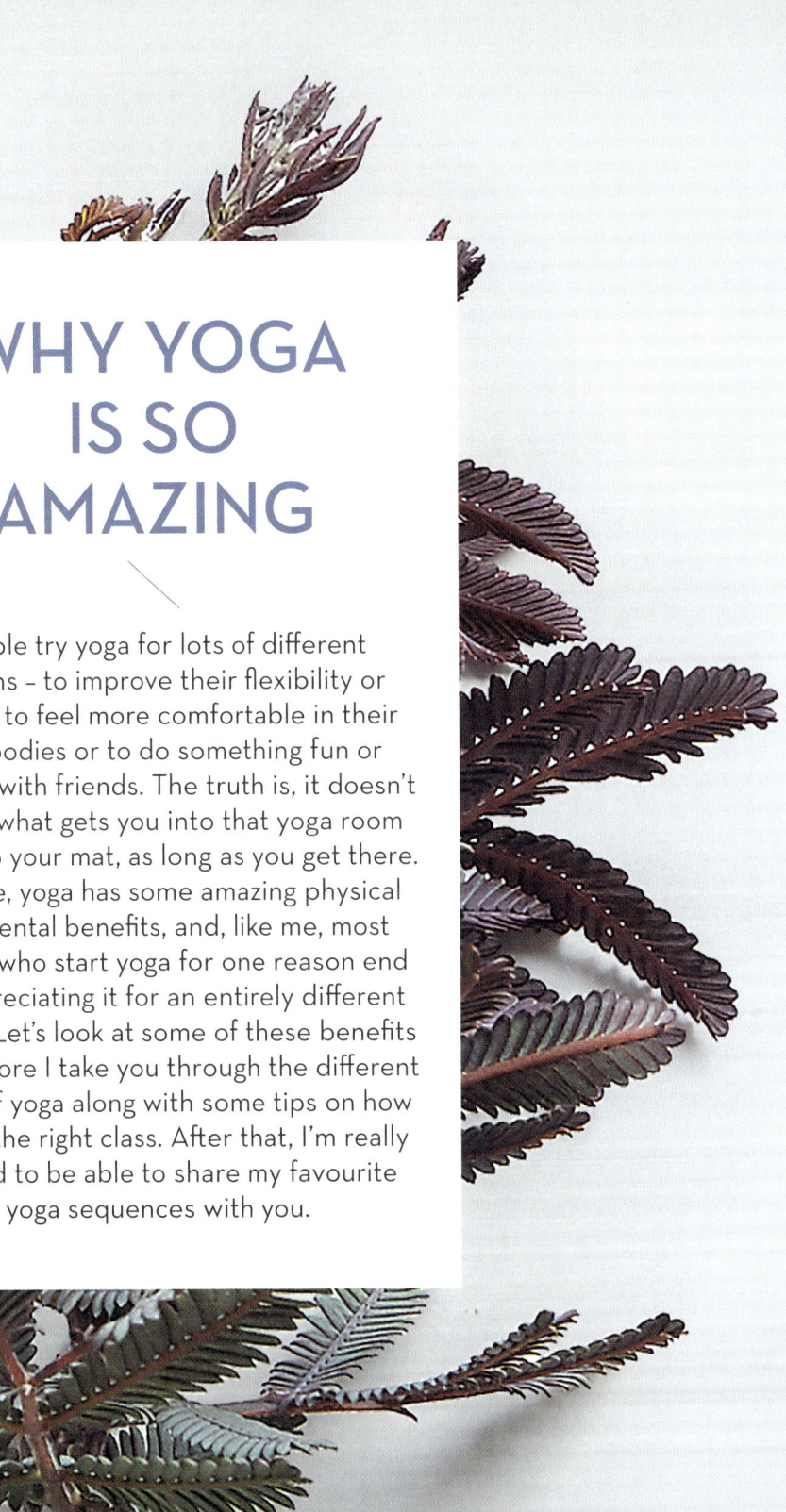

WHY YOGA IS SO AMAZING

People try yoga for lots of different reasons – to improve their flexibility or fitness, to feel more comfortable in their own bodies or to do something fun or relaxing with friends. The truth is, it doesn't matter what gets you into that yoga room and onto your mat, as long as you get there. You see, yoga has some amazing physical and mental benefits, and, like me, most people who start yoga for one reason end up appreciating it for an entirely different reason. Let's look at some of these benefits now, before I take you through the different styles of yoga along with some tips on how to find the right class. After that, I'm really excited to be able to share my favourite yoga sequences with you.

Yoga has been practised in India for at least 2000 years (scholarly types argue about the exact date), but it wasn't introduced to the West until the early twentieth century, and only really took off in the 1980s. Since then, there has been heaps of research into its positive effects on our physical, cognitive and emotional health.

Balance and coordination

Balance is a skill you develop in spades by practising yoga. Even a simple pose like warrior 1 (see page 41) requires balance, and every vinyasa class has a sequence of poses dedicated to balance.

Coordination is how smoothly your body parts work together to perform a particular action. It involves strength, balance and flexibility, as well as an understanding of where your body is in space (spatial awareness). Coordination is very important in vinyasa, as vinyasa requires the synchronisation of movement with breath. Studies have shown that yoga helps improve balance and coordination, especially among people over sixty.

Blood pressure

Many studies looking at the cardiovascular health benefits of yoga have concluded that it is particularly effective at helping to lower blood pressure (high blood pressure or hypertension is a significant risk factor for heart disease and stroke). Along with dietary modifications such as cutting out salty, fatty, sugary processed foods and increasing our intake of fresh, whole foods, exercise has long been known to reduce blood pressure, and since yoga is a form of exercise, scientists think that this may be part of the reason it works. Yet, stress is also associated with high blood pressure, so it makes sense that any activity that helps to reduce stress would help to lower blood pressure. And yoga most definitely activates the parasympathetic nervous system – the calming 'rest and digest' response, which is the opposite of the stressed-out 'fight or flight' response.

Bone density

Because yoga is a weight-bearing exercise, it's great for helping to build bone density. In fact, a 2016 study found that practising yoga for just 12 minutes a day reversed osteoporotic bone loss. This is great news for older people (especially women), whose bones can become brittle and porous due to ageing.

Brain function

Recent research has found that regularly practising yoga, along with breathing exercises (pranayama) and meditation (dhyana), not only helps to preserve brain function, but can also improve it. To put it simply, yoga prevents your brain shrinking as you age. In fact, pranayama has been shown to improve connectivity between the right and left hemispheres of the brain, which is great for problem solving.

> 'You've got to show up and suck before you can show up and shine.'
>
> **CHRIS WILSON, YOKE YOGA**

Flexibility

Flexibility is really about freedom of movement. Some people are naturally flexible in some joints but not in others, and their range of movement partly depends on the length of the muscles that extend across a particular joint (this is the stretchiness that improves in yoga). Some people are scared that they're not flexible enough to begin with, so they never take up yoga. But know this: you don't need to be flexible to *start* doing yoga, you just have to do it regularly enough and it will happen naturally.

Flexibility is brilliant at helping to prevent injury, which is why lots of sporty people use it to balance their strength and cardio training. There have also been studies on how yoga helps reduce the pain of osteoarthritis (the joint pain you get after a fracture or just wear and tear due to ageing).

Mental health

We've known for a while that exercise is an effective treatment for depression and anxiety. Since yoga is also a form of exercise, you'd kind of expect it to be good for mental health. The thing is, it's actually *way* better than other forms of exercise, especially for depression. In 2017, a comprehensive study of the use of yoga as a treatment for depression found that yoga was significantly better than relaxation practices and aerobic exercise. There is also emerging evidence that yoga may be an effective treatment for anxiety disorders. A 2016 study found, for example, that hatha yoga reduced anxiety for people with the most severe symptoms, and that symptom reduction increased the longer they'd practised yoga.

Now, most of us have experienced anxiety in one form or another: tightening of the chest, sweaty palms, constant worry, over-thinking and disconnecting from yourself. Here's where yoga comes in. Yoga is often referred to as nature's remedy for anxiety as it stimulates the production of GABA in the brain. GABA is the super-chilled neurotransmitter that calms over-excited neurons – sort of like a natural sedative. In a 2010 study, 12 weeks of weekly yoga practice for people who had never done yoga before resulted in a 13 per cent increase in GABA levels. In an earlier study, the same researchers found that experienced practitioners who did a one-hour yoga class increased GABA levels by 27 per cent.

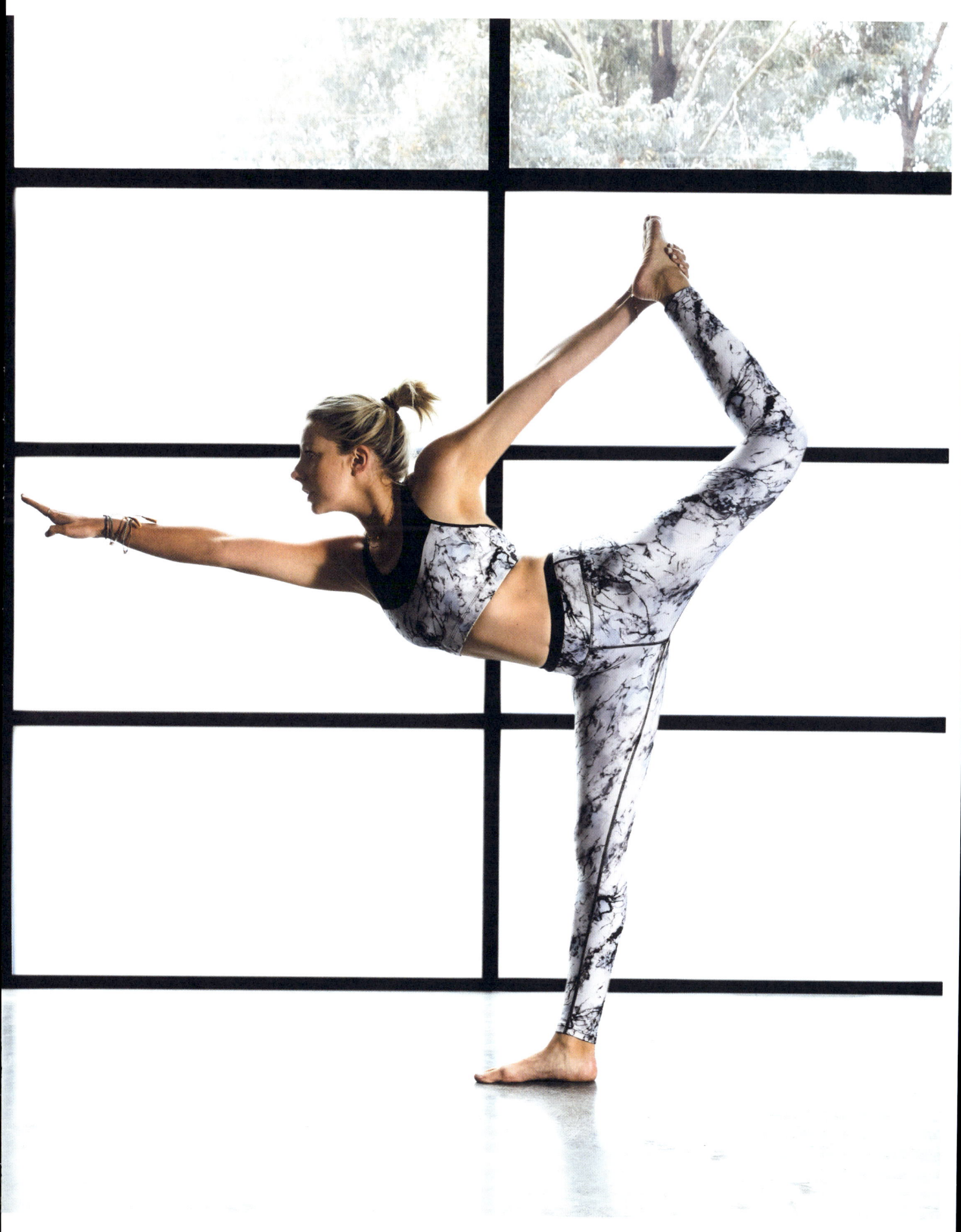

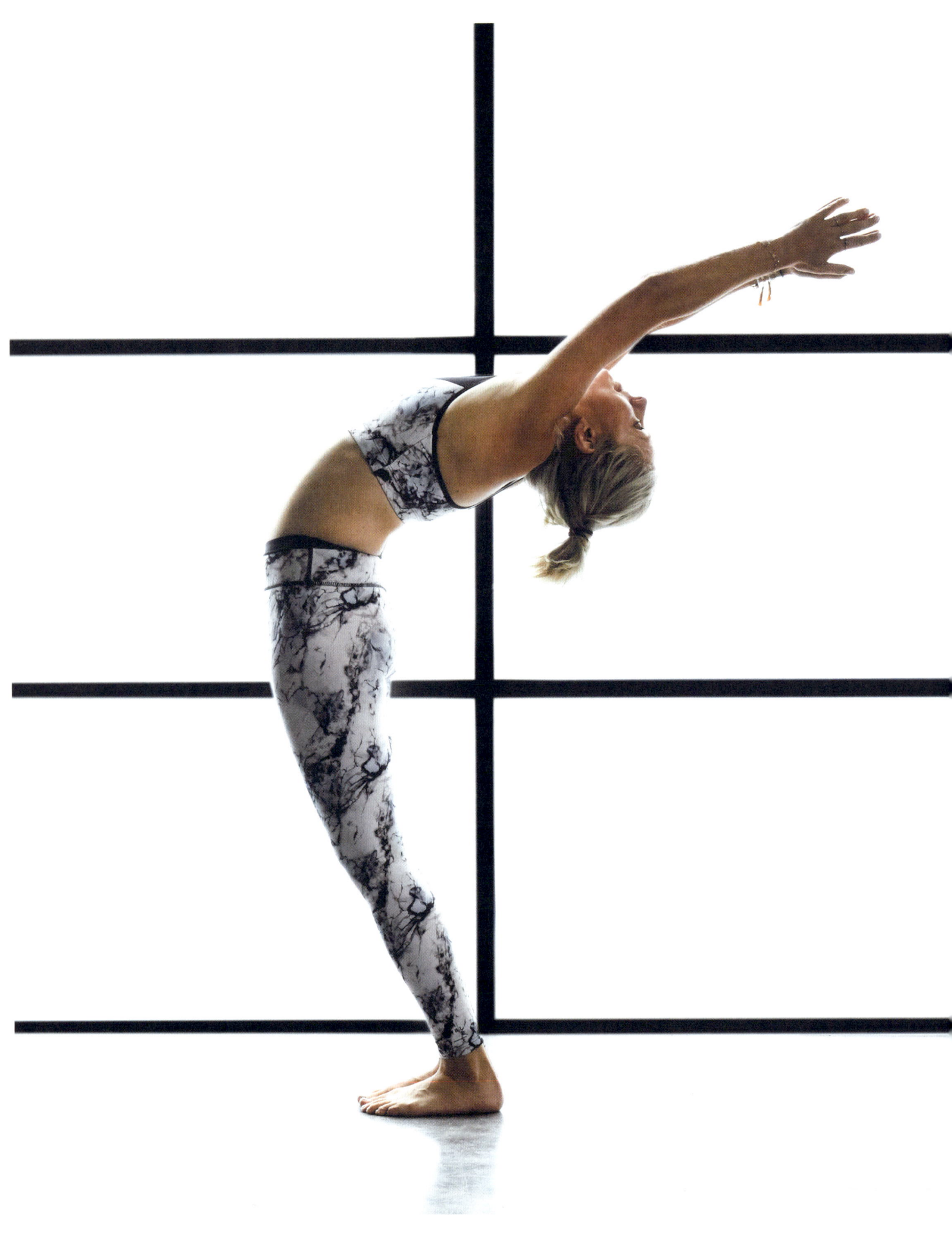

> I can walk into a yoga class stressed out or worried about something, and by the end of the class I have a clear head and am able to respond rather than react.

Strength and posture

Even though yoga is regarded as a gentler form of exercise, I can tell you that it *definitely* builds strength, especially when poses are held for longer periods of time. For example, if you hold chair pose (see page 40) for five or more breaths it will help to build strength in your leg and butt muscles, which in turn helps to protect against lower back pain and injury. Studies have also shown that it not only builds strength in the wrists and hands of people with rheumatoid arthritis, but that improvements in grip strength for women are double for those in men.

Yoga is also brilliant for posture. I've always tended to hunch over (especially over my phone and laptop!) and heaps of the poses I do have helped me to strengthen my back muscles and keep my shoulders back. In fact, any pose that can be described as a backbend is good for this (even upward facing dog pose is considered to be a backbend). I'm short, but I always feel longer, leaner and more open in the chest after yoga. It's a really nice feeling, and the more you practise, the better that feeling gets.

Stress

Stress is something I think we all experience at one time or another. To be honest, I reckon I get stressed out on some level at least once a week (it was way more than that before yoga became part of my life). When we're stressed out, things just don't flow – everything in life feels that little bit harder to do. A stressed mind is often linked to negative thoughts. We've all heard about the power of positive thoughts and that what we believe we manifest. Well, in yoga we use breath to relax our muscles and calm our thoughts. I know I can walk into a yoga class stressed out or worried about something, and by the end of the class I have a clear head and am able to respond rather than react.

One of the ways yoga helps with stress is by anchoring the mind in the present moment. By focusing on our breathing as we hold postures, we can't get caught up in negative thoughts about the past or anxious thoughts about the future. We're just trying not to fall over!

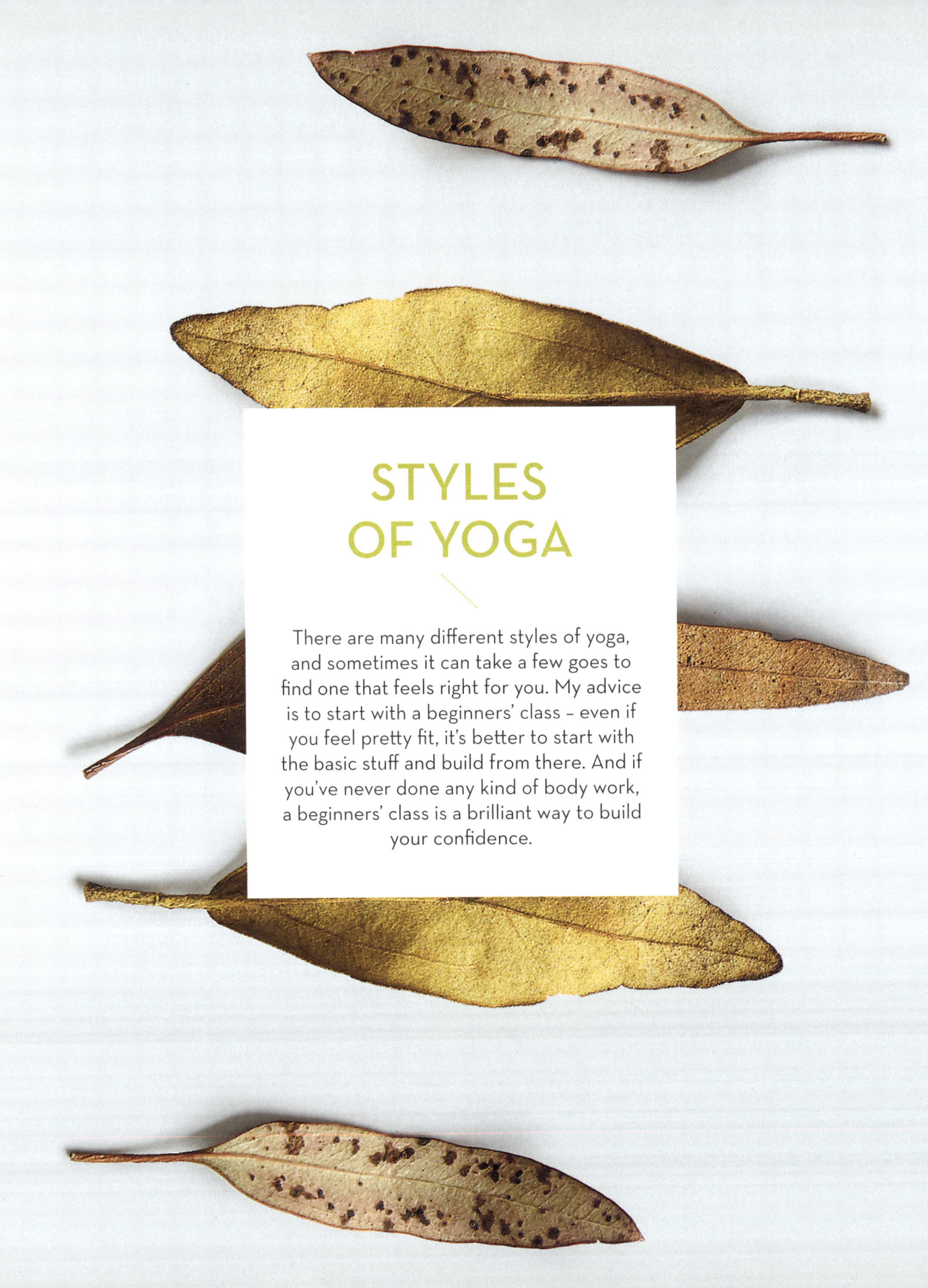

STYLES OF YOGA

There are many different styles of yoga, and sometimes it can take a few goes to find one that feels right for you. My advice is to start with a beginners' class – even if you feel pretty fit, it's better to start with the basic stuff and build from there. And if you've never done any kind of body work, a beginners' class is a brilliant way to build your confidence.

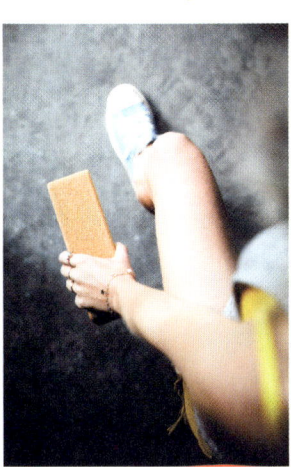

Which style of yoga to choose? To help you decide, here's a bit of a guide to the popular forms of yoga.

Acro

This is a blend of acrobatics and yoga, and is heaps of fun provided you have well-trained instructors and a buddy you can trust. Generally, one person is 'base' and the other 'flies'. It's actually quite safe (and easier than you might think), as long as you are taught correct alignment.

Anusara

Developed by American yogi John Friend in 1997, anusara is a relative newcomer to the yoga world. It has been described as a light-hearted version of Iyengar (see page 23). Classes feature various props (bolsters, blankets, straps and blocks) to assist physical alignment. Anusara is welcoming to beginners, and its classes are upbeat and accepting to people of all fitness levels.

Ashtanga

Ashtanga (literally 'eight limbs') is based on ancient yoga teachings and was brought to the West by K. Pattabhi Jois in the 1970s. It's a rigorous style of yoga that follows a specific sequence of postures, and is similar to vinyasa yoga, as both styles link every movement to a breath. The difference is that ashtanga always performs the exact same poses in the exact same order. This is a sweaty, physically demanding practice. I did my first-ever ashtanga class by accident in LA recently: I thought I was going into a vinyasa class, then I quickly figured out it was something else entirely. After we did a few simple stretches, we spent the whole class working on one particular arm balance. We focused so much on the correct alignment that it didn't feel I was doing much at all, but by gee I felt it the next day. I had been working muscles I didn't even know I had!

Bikram

This style of yoga was created by Indian yogi Bikram Choudhury in the early 1970s. Choudhury designed a sequence of twenty-six poses to be performed in a room heated to 40°C with high humidity – the aim being to help stretch and strengthen the muscles as well as detox the body. Every Bikram class, anywhere in the world, follows the same sequence of poses. It is a set 90-minute class and you start sweating the moment you set foot in the classroom.

YOGA PRACTICE

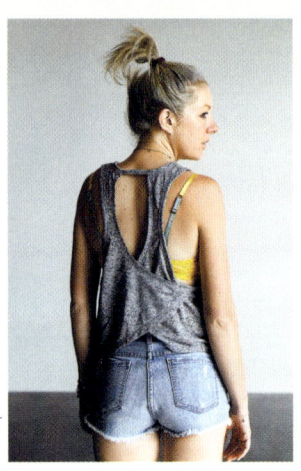

Broga

Yep. This is a form of yoga geared to men, where the focus is on strength and fitness as well as flexibility. It's been going for a few years in the USA, but has only just started in Australia.

Men generally have longer bones and larger, bulkier muscles than women, which is one reason they are often less flexible (the muscles have to stretch a long way to reach over joints). But this doesn't mean they can't do other forms of yoga. On the contrary, any kind of yoga is amazing for blokes, and more and more men of all ages are choosing to do it. Some do it for relaxation, others to lengthen and stretch muscles after weight training or running.

Hatha

Hatha technically refers to the physical practice of yoga (asanas as opposed to, say, chanting), so all of the popular styles of yoga in the West are actually hatha. However, studios who advertise hatha classes tend to focus on the asanas that are common to all. If you step into a hatha class, it will feel a tad slower than vinyasa, but you will learn the correct alignment for the basic yoga poses. You probably won't work up a sweat, but you should leave class feeling longer, looser and more relaxed.

Hip-hop

Don't worry, hip-hop yoga doesn't mean you have to bust out your breakdance moves, it just means you'll probably be doing down dog to Snoop Dogg! The idea is that synchronising poses to both breath *and* music will be even more effective at calming our chattering 'monkey minds'. (I did a whole class to Kendrick Lamar at Y7 in LA once. The room was candle-lit and heated with infra-red panels. It's one of my all-time favourite yoga experiences.)

Hot

If you see signs for hot yoga, it could mean Bikram, though it is more likely to deviate from the original sequence in some small way. This is because Choudhury trademarked his sequence and sued studios who called themselves Bikram but didn't teach the poses exactly the way he said they should. Hot yoga could also refer to vinyasa or hatha performed in a heated studio (usually between 26°C and 32°C). I did a hot yoga class in LA that used infra-red lamps rather than heaters, which is supposed to further enhance the detoxifying effects. Whatever style of hot yoga you choose, don't forget to bring a water bottle!

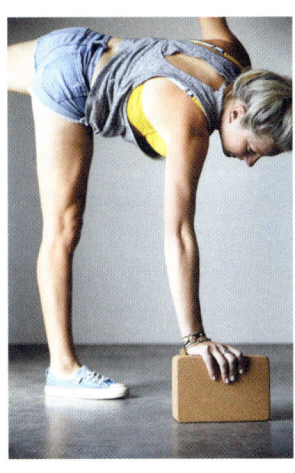

Iyengar

Iyengar yoga is a very meticulous style of yoga focused on correct alignment of the body. It was developed by B. K. S. Iyengar in the 1970s and uses a wide array of yoga props, including blocks, bolsters, blankets, straps, wall ropes and chairs. There isn't a lot of jumping around in Iyengar classes, so you won't get your heart rate up, but you'll be amazed to discover how physically and mentally challenging it is to maintain the poses. Iyengar teachers must undergo comprehensive training with certified Iyengar masters. If you have an injury or chronic condition, Iyengar is probably your best choice to ensure you get the knowledgeable instruction you need.

Jivamukti

Founded in 1984 by David Life and Sharon Gannon, jivamukti means 'liberation while living'. This is a vinyasa-style practice with themed classes, often including chanting, music and scripture readings. Jivamukti teachers encourage students to apply yogic philosophy to their daily lives.

Kundalini

Kundalini yoga has physical, spiritual and philosophical components. Classes include meditation, breathing techniques (such as alternate nostril breathing) and chanting, as well as yoga poses. I recently took a kundalini workshop, where I learned a lot about the chakras and awakening the kundalini energy through sound and movement. It's said that the kundalini energy is responsible for showing you what you are truly capable of – your true potential. It forces you to face your fears and connect to the faith in your heart.

Power

Like hot yoga, power yoga can mean different things. That said, the name does give you a hint that it's a strong practice and chances are you'll get a good sweat on. For me, power yoga is a strong heated vinyasa class (movement to breath). That said, I've also seen power yoga that uses an ashtanga style without heat and involves longer holds of five or more breaths. You'll see power yoga at some gyms, too, as a way to encourage gym-goers into yoga. My advice, as with all yoga, is to try it on and see what fits for you.

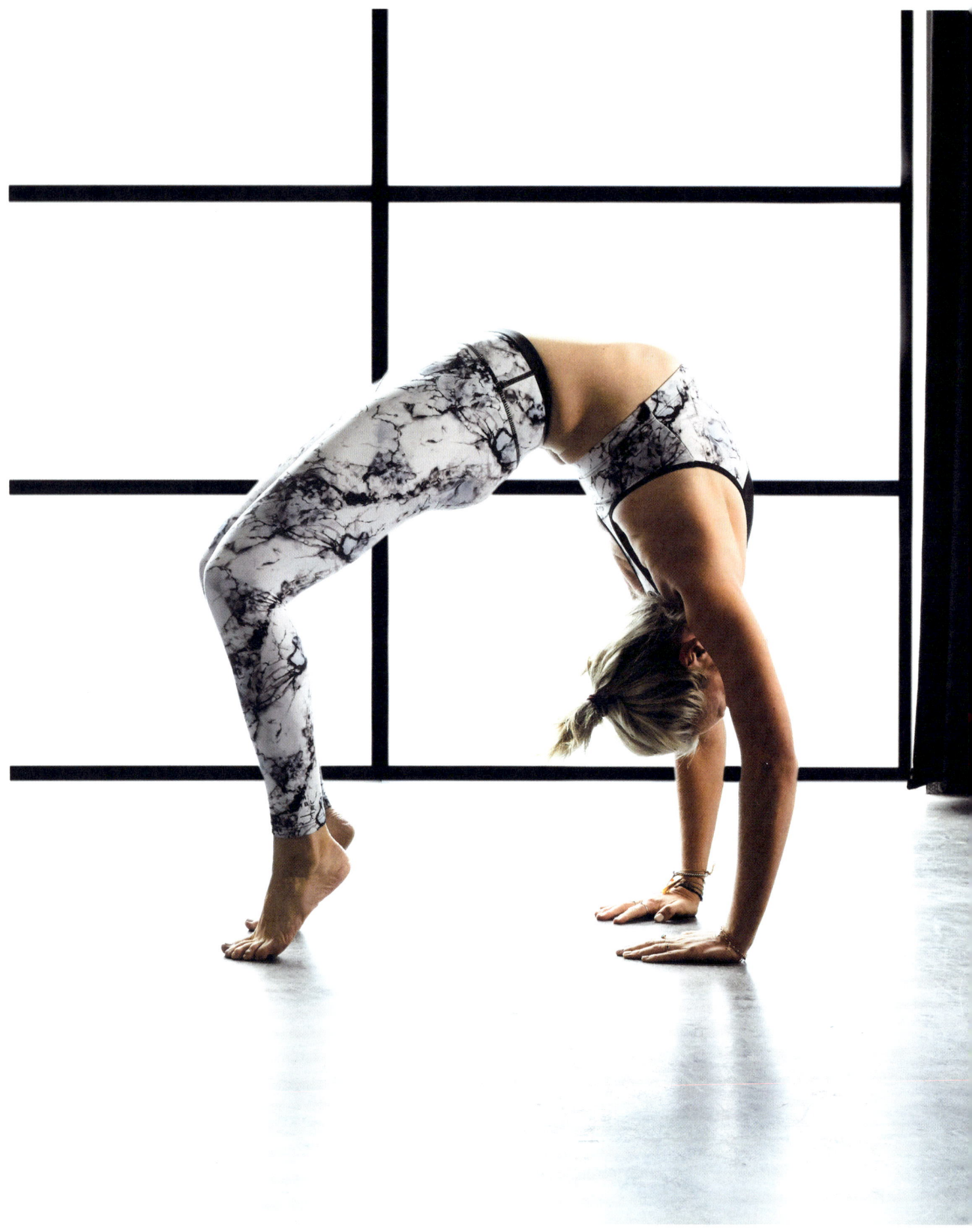

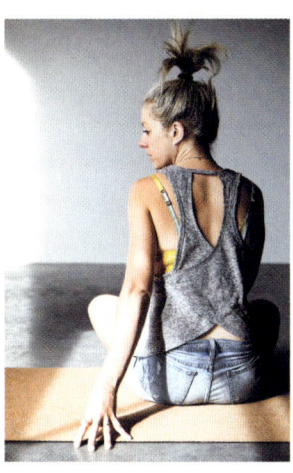

Restorative

This is similar to yin yoga (the two are often confused), but has less emphasis on flexibility and more on relaxation. Restorative yoga is all about healing the mind and body through simple poses, which are often held for as long as 20 minutes with the help of bolsters, pillows and straps. A good restorative class is more rejuvenating than a nap. It is a great class to do at night if you have anxiety issues or you just want to wind down – you'll sleep like a baby afterwards!

Vinyasa

Vinyasa is the kind of yoga I teach and practise the most. It's all about the connection of movement to breath, so poses are synchronised to your breathing. When you're in 'flow' you'll be doing one movement per breath for certain parts of the class, which not only gives you a good workout (building internal heat or 'tapas') but also helps to build mental discipline (I talk more about this on page 225). Like most forms of yoga, vinyasa is based around the sun salutation ('sun A' or surya namaskar – see page 36), but instead of stopping to talk about the finer points of each pose, I just maintain the flow.

It's no surprise, then, that some studios call it flow yoga, flow-style yoga, dynamic yoga or vinyasa flow. The intensity of the practice is similar to ashtanga, but the sequences vary from class to class. Also, some teachers like to use music in their classes (I do), as it helps people to relax and focus. If you're new to yoga, it is a good idea to take a few classes in a slower style of yoga, such as hatha or beginners' Iyengar, to get a feel for the poses first.

Yin

Yin is less about working muscles and more about improving strength and flexibility in tendons and ligaments. It focuses on passive, seated postures that target the connective tissues in the hips, pelvis and lower spine. It is much more of a meditative practice, as the poses are held for much longer – anywhere between 1 and 10 minutes. Yin yoga teachers use bolsters, blankets and blocks to prop students into passive poses, so the body can experience the benefits of a pose without having to exert any effort. The aim is to increase flexibility and encourage a feeling of release and letting go. Yin is also a wonderful way to learn the basics of meditation and stilling the mind, so is great for those who need to relax.

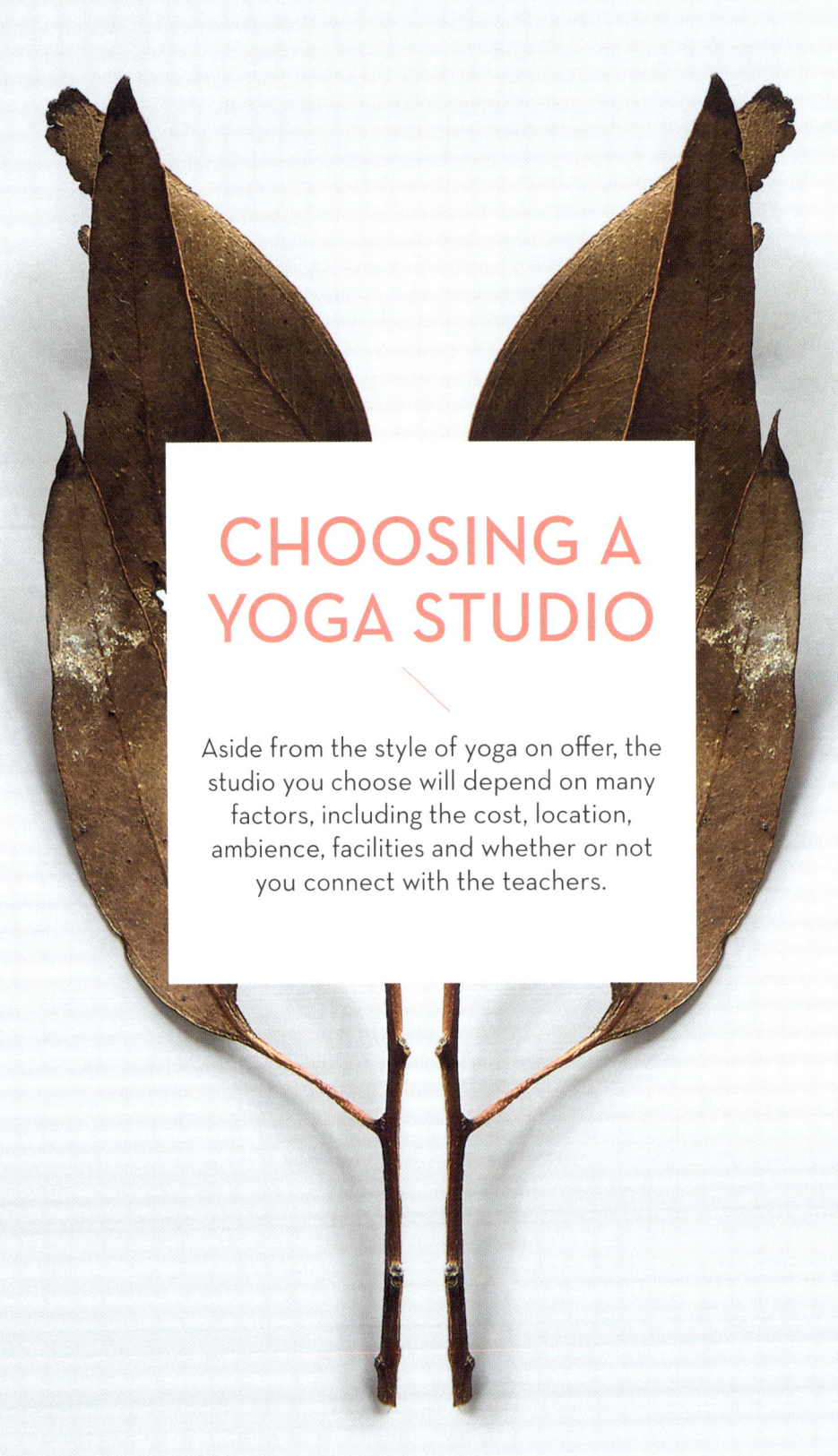

CHOOSING A YOGA STUDIO

Aside from the style of yoga on offer, the studio you choose will depend on many factors, including the cost, location, ambience, facilities and whether or not you connect with the teachers.

> Whatever style you choose, always look for studios that offer a beginners' class … It's better to start with the foundations and build upon them.

Ambience

Is the room spacious, bright and light? Can the lighting be dimmed for the relaxation part of the class? Do teachers burn incense or essential oils?

When I teach vinyasa, I like to use music to help people relax, especially in the slower parts of the class where thoughts can begin to creep in. Some people like to practise to music, others don't, so make sure you ask when you sign up if this is an issue for you.

Cost

Many studios offer rates for casual visits so you don't need to sign up for a whole block of classes. Others offer a free 'trial' lesson (or two) as part of a ten-week course. Sometimes this is all you will need to work out if the studio is the right fit for you.

Facilities

Is there a clean toilet and changing room in the studio (preferably more than one toilet if classes are larger than ten students)? Some studios will offer herbal tea before class – different schools will provide different things, so my advice is to take a few trial classes to see if everything feels right.

Location

This can be a big factor. Most people want to be able to go before work or school, or on their way home, without adding an extra hour of travel on top of the class time. Beginners' classes are usually 1 hour, and anything above that will be 90 minutes to 2 hours (or more), so you need to factor this in to your day.

Style

If you want to focus on fitness, strength and flexibility then hot yoga, ashtanga or any of the vinyasa styles may suit. If you are less interested in getting your heart rate up and more interested in improving your physical and mental flexibility then hatha, Iyengar or anusara could be good to try. If you really want to learn to relax and listen to your body, yin and restorative yoga are perfect. The spiritual stuff is a big part of kundalini and jivamukti, though it can also be a part of other classes depending on your teachers. See pages 20–25 for more about the different styles of yoga. Whatever style you choose, always look for studios that offer a beginners' class. If you walk straight into an inversion workshop, chances are you won't be back! It's better to start with the foundations and build upon them.

Teachers

Finally, a yoga studio is only ever as good as its teachers. Are they knowledgeable, friendly, helpful, approachable? More importantly, are they focused on their students? Depending on the style of yoga, a teacher should be floating about the room, helping to correct and adjust students' poses and giving alternatives to those who cannot do the full pose or have an injury.

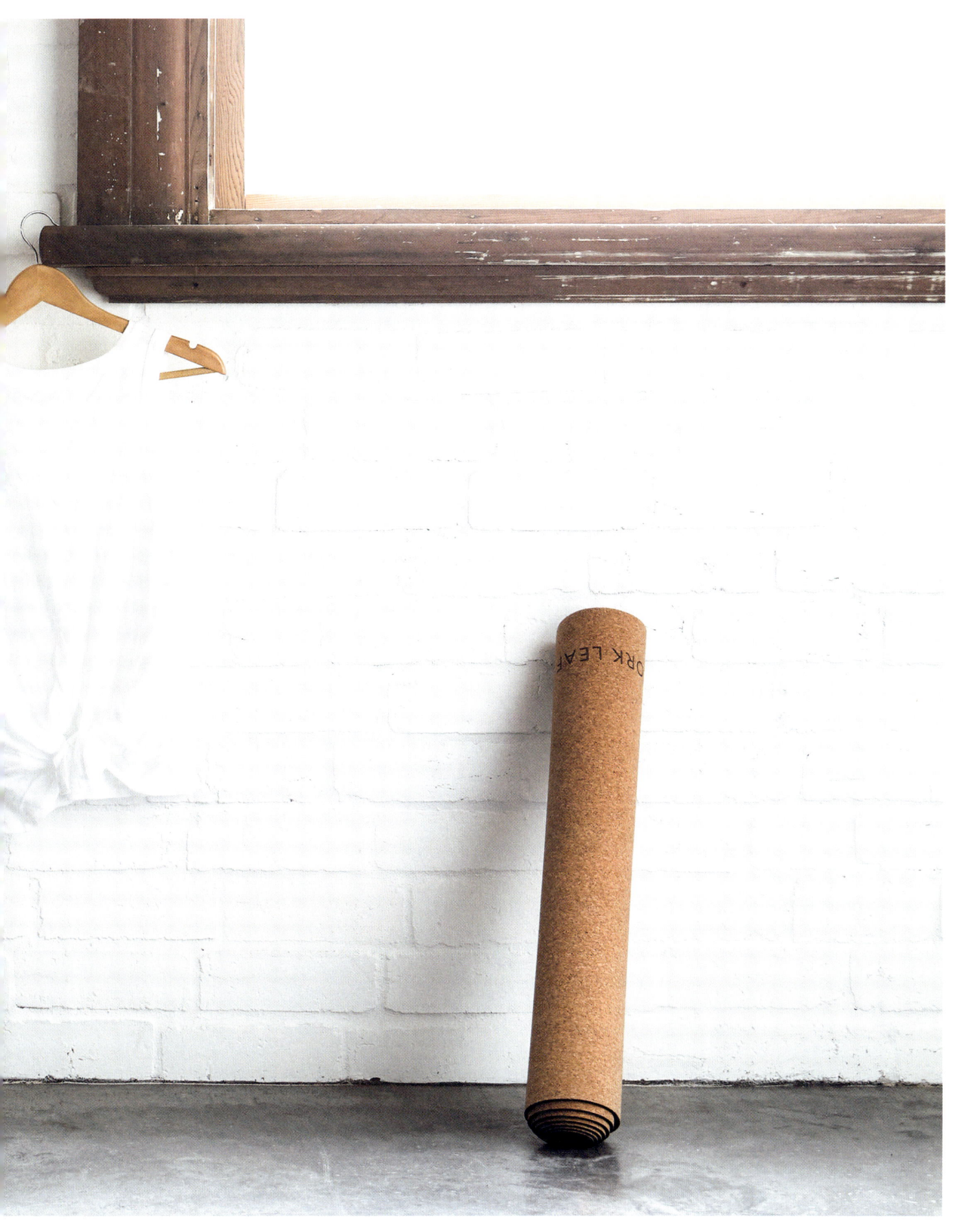

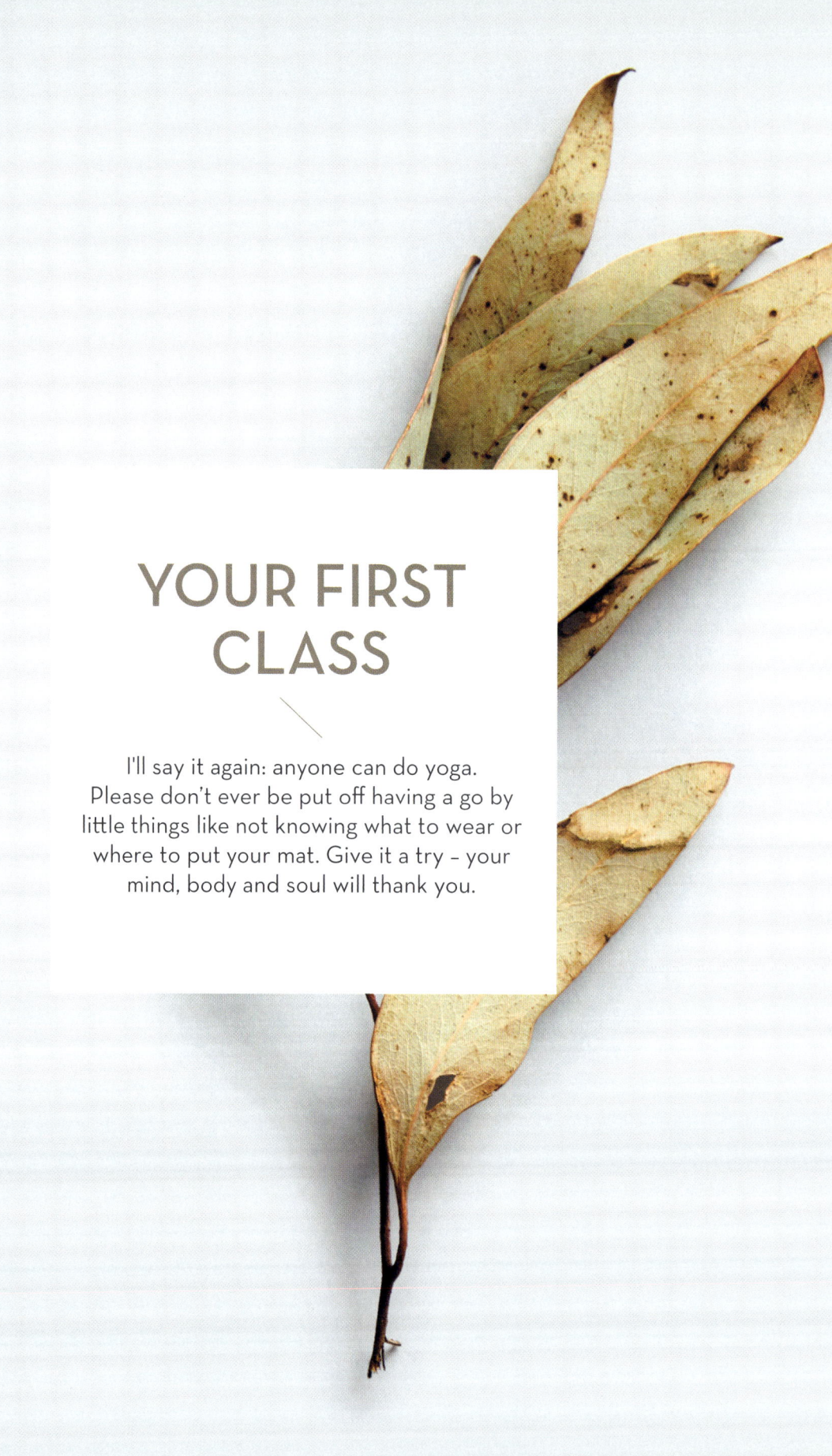

YOUR FIRST CLASS

I'll say it again: anyone can do yoga. Please don't ever be put off having a go by little things like not knowing what to wear or where to put your mat. Give it a try – your mind, body and soul will thank you.

It goes without saying that you need stretchy, comfy clothes to do yoga. You'll also be barefoot, so it's probably best to have footwear that's easy to get on and off. Many studios now have online registration and booking services, but if they don't, it's a good idea to get to your first class a bit earlier (by, say, 15 minutes) so that you can fill in any paperwork there. Here are some other things to consider.

Collecting props

Yoga studios will provide any props you need. In general, you will use a strap and two blocks for vinyasa or hatha classes; bolsters and blankets for yin and restorative yoga; and all of the above plus chairs and wall ropes for Iyengar. If you're not sure which props to collect and when to collect them, just ask.

Leaving early

If you go to a yoga class and decide that it's just not your jam, please don't walk out – it's considered very disrespectful to both your teacher and your classmates, plus it can throw people right off their practice.

If you know that you have to leave early for some reason, tell your teacher beforehand and keep your mat right near the exit so you don't disturb people.

What to bring

- **Bottle of water:** this is mainly for hot yoga or vinyasa flow, though you might still feel thirsty after an hour or two of the slower styles of yoga.
- **Towel:** you'll need one for hot yoga (or any style where they heat the room). You can also hire towels at the studio if you prefer.
- **Yoga mat:** some studios provide mats, others get you to bring your own or hire one (or buy a new one from them). Just make sure the mat has good grip – I find some rental mats can be a bit slippy (probably due to wear and tear) so I like to bring my own. I still use the one I bought when I was training to become a teacher.

Where to put your mat

For your first class, I recommend placing your mat in the middle and towards the back, so you have lots of people in front of you to follow. Some studios will have markers on the floor so that people know how much space to leave around their mats. If you're not sure, have a look at the people in the front row. In my experience, people who set up in the front row have been coming for yonks and know what they're doing.

Namaste literally means 'my soul sees and honours your soul' or 'I see the light within you, it's the same light that is within me'.

Yogic rituals

At the end of yoga class (and sometimes at the beginning), most yoga teachers will bring their palms together over their breastbone, bow their heads and say 'namaste'. It literally means 'my soul sees and honours your soul' or 'I see the light within you, it's the same light that is within me.' I think there's something very sacred and heartfelt about this exchange.

In some classes, the teacher might also call for an *aum* ('om') chant. This word is a sacred sound in Hinduism and refers to the source of the universe and everything in it. It might seem weird at first but just go with it – it's a lovely way to feel the connection with everyone in the room.

In my classes, after we say namaste, I shift my hands (still together in the prayer position) across to my heart and say 'to the highest love'. Then I bring them to my lips and say 'to the highest truth' and finally I touch them to my forehead and say 'to the highest consciousness – I give mine'. This is a grounding ritual you could use at the end of a meditation, or any time you decide to do some yoga at home.

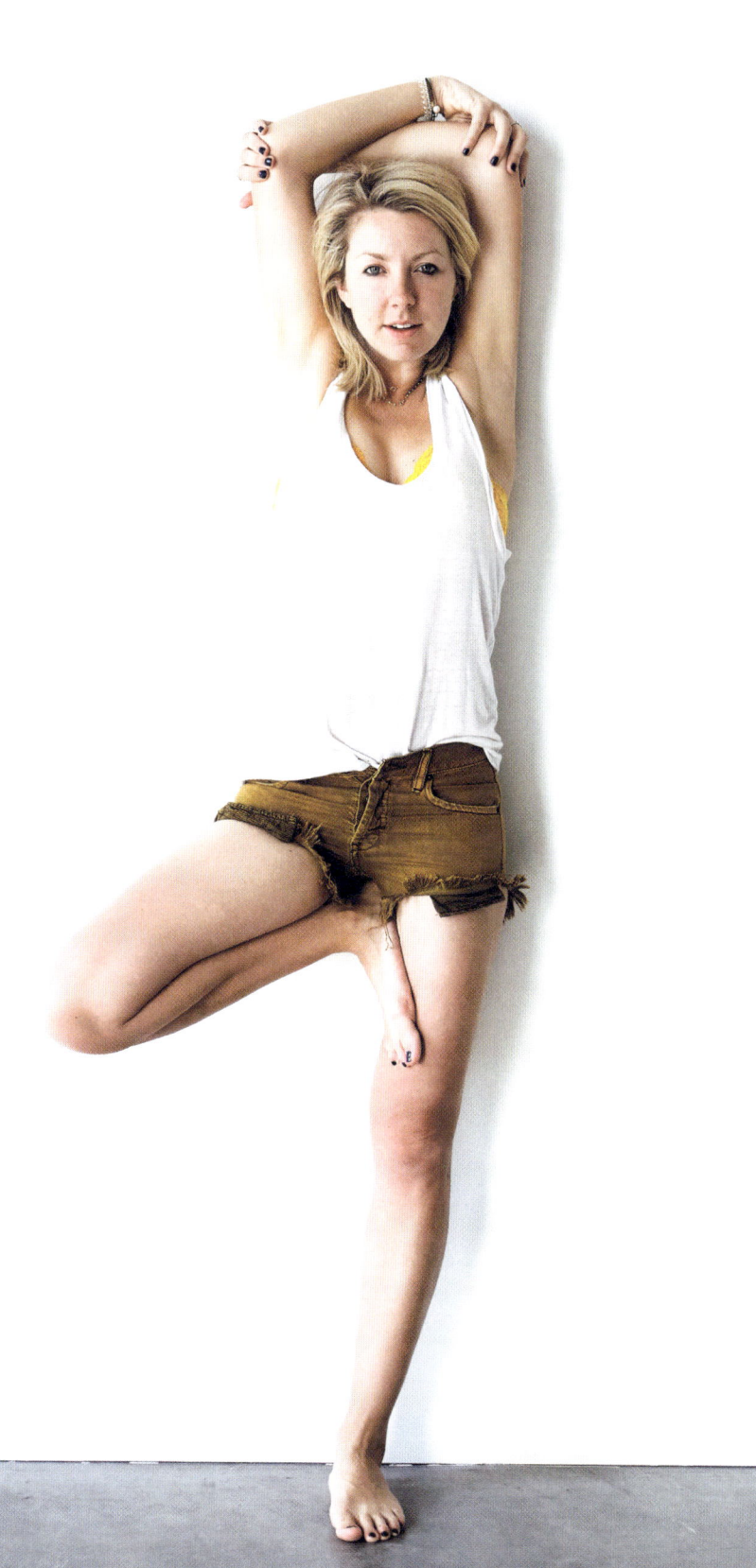

In this section, I will introduce you to some of the basic poses that are common to all styles of yoga. I've also put together some sequences that I love to use when I'm doing my own practice. These are sequences I use for warming up, for toning my tummy (and butt!), to help me sleep, deal with jetlag, or cope with sadness. I haven't included a specific sequence for stress because, to be perfectly honest, *any* yoga is wonderful for stress.

One of the reasons I adore yoga is that you can do it anywhere. Recently, I was staying in a tiny hotel in Singapore and there was no space in my room, so I ended up doing a sequence in the hallway of the hotel. It makes me smile to think about it! If you want to do yoga, you will always find a way. Oh, and if any of the poses look hard, don't worry – your body won't let you go too far.

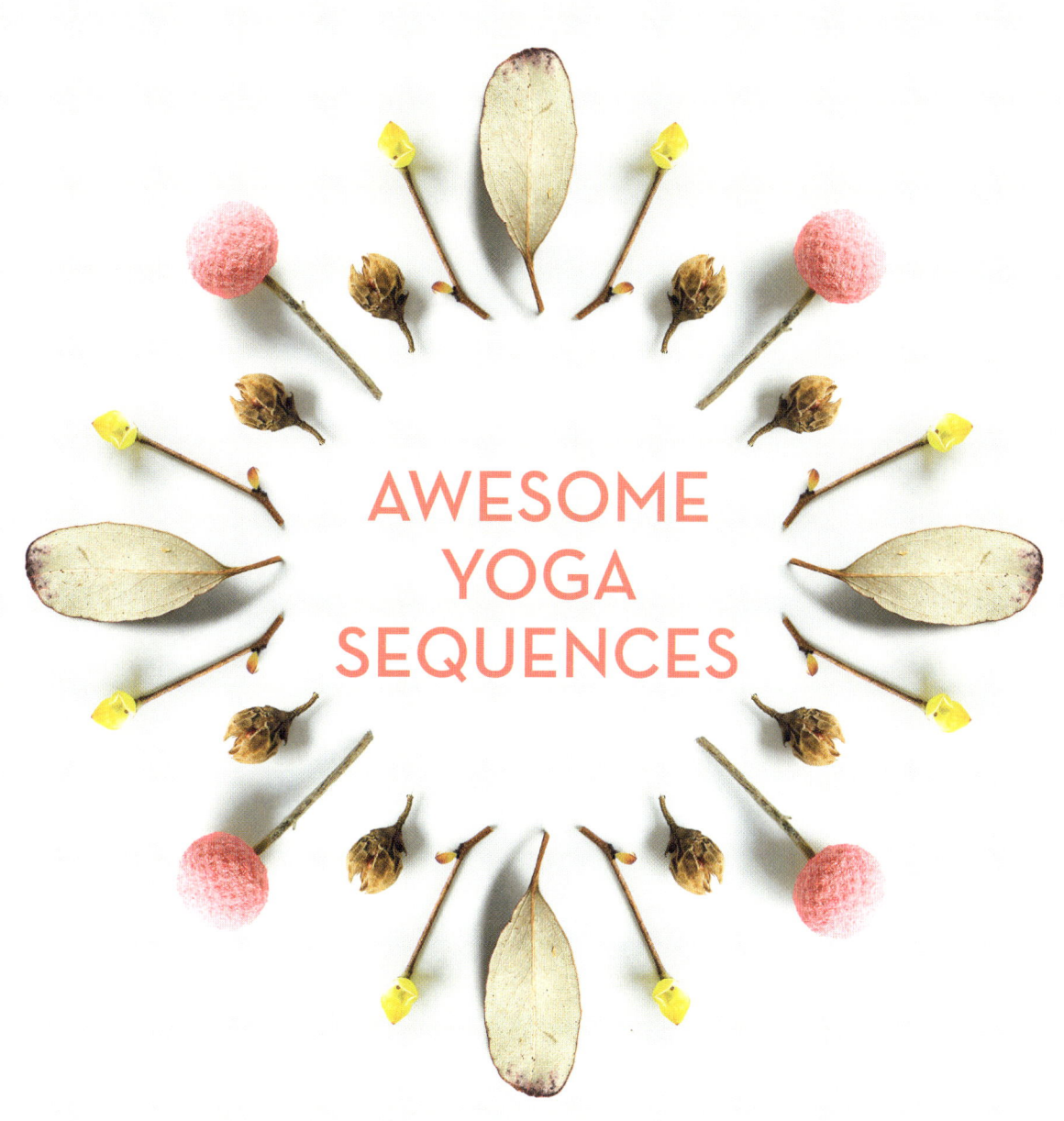

SUN A WARM-UP
(surya namaskar)

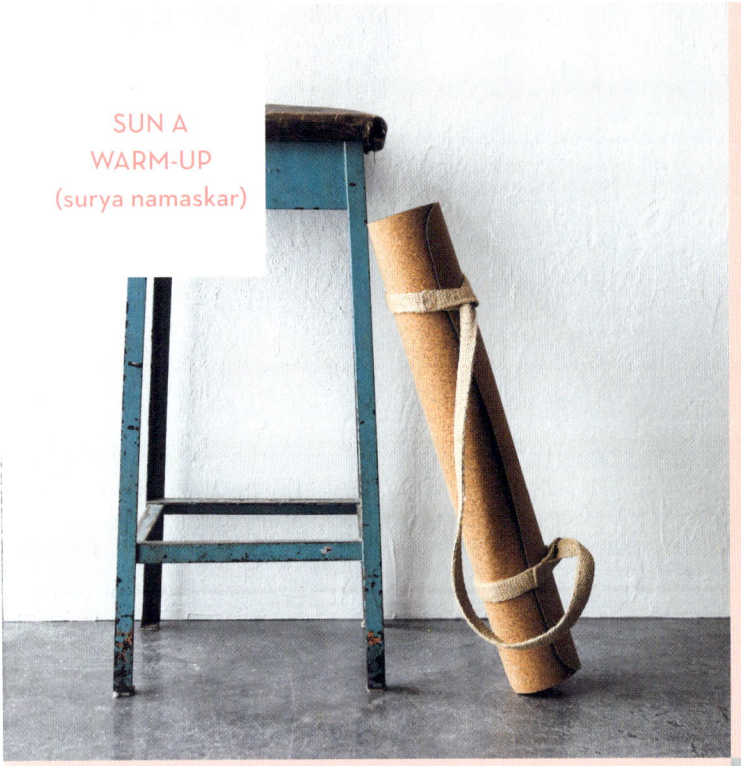

Sun A is a great way to get moving in the morning or to energise yourself if you've been sitting at a desk at work all day. You will find these poses in a lot of classes, as we always like to warm up the spine before we get into practice.

In Sanskrit, sun A is called surya namaskar (literally 'to bow to the sun' or 'to adore the sun'). When I perform this sequence, I always think about how lucky I am to be able to practise yoga.

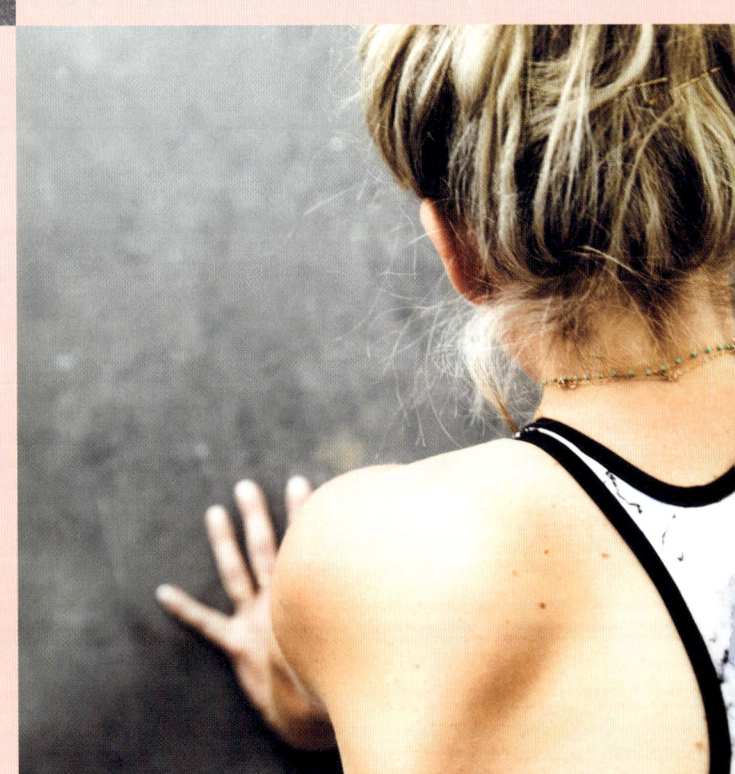

1 TADASANA (STANDING MOUNTAIN POSE)

Start with your feet together (or hip-width apart, whichever feels balanced and strong for you). Lift and spread your toes and then your heels, pressing them into the floor. Hold your arms by your sides, palms facing outward. Tighten your thigh muscles (this will lift your kneecaps) and turn your calf muscles outward. Suck your navel towards your spine, lift your shoulders up, then melt them down your back.

Tip: Some teachers will start in prayer pose, with the hands pressed together and both thumbs pressed gently over the centre of the chest.

2 URDHVA HASTASANA (UPWARD SALUTE)

Inhale, stretch your arms out to the sides and then lift them straight up, palms facing each other and fingers outstretched.

3 ARDHA UTTANASANA (HALFWAY LIFT)

Exhale, bend forward at the hips, looking ahead, and reach your hands towards your shins. Keep your spine long and flat (only grasp your shins if you can keep your spine and neck aligned). Now inhale.

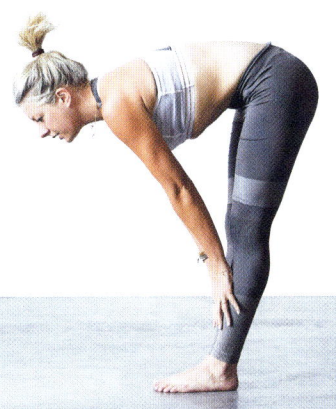

4 UTTANASANA (FORWARD FOLD)

Exhale, keeping your thigh muscles contracted (this helps to support your lower back), and drop your arms and let them hang loose. It should feel nice, and in the first set you can hang out down there for a few breaths; we call this rag doll. Place your palms flat on the floor (bending your knees if you need to).

Tip: Don't worry if you are nowhere near being able to touch your toes; your hands will get closer to the ground the more you practise.

5 *UTTIHITA CHATURANGA DANDASANA* (HIGH PLANK)
Inhale and step (or hop) your feet behind you, making sure your hands are flat on the floor and your arms are straight and shoulder-width apart. Take a full breath as you lengthen your spine.

Tip: It's really easy to have your butt too high in the air, or to slump your spine, so think about being really sturdy and strong in this pose, and stack your shoulders directly above your wrists.

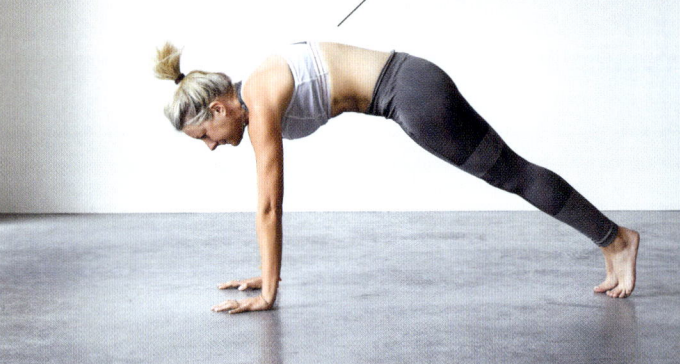

6 *CHATURANGA DANDASANA*
(LOW PLANK OR FOUR-LIMBED STAFF POSE)
Exhale, shift your weight forward slightly and bend your elbows as you lower your body, keeping your spine nice and straight. This is a very strong pose, so drop to your knees at first if you need to. (This one *really* builds your core muscles!)

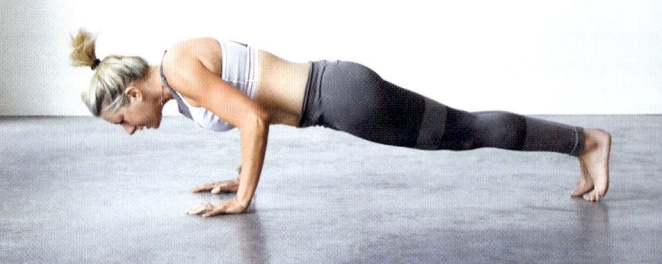

7 *URDHVA MUKHA SVANASANA*
(UPWARD FACING DOG OR UP DOG)
Inhale, roll forward on your toes so the tops of your feet are supporting your weight, and straighten your arms, keeping your thighs and legs off the mat. This is a really strong backbend so make sure you keep your thigh muscles switched on to protect your lower back. I like to keep my gaze forward, but you can look skyward.

Tip: If you're new to yoga, I recommend doing cobra pose here instead (see 8). I did cobra pose for the first three months until I had the strength to do up dog.

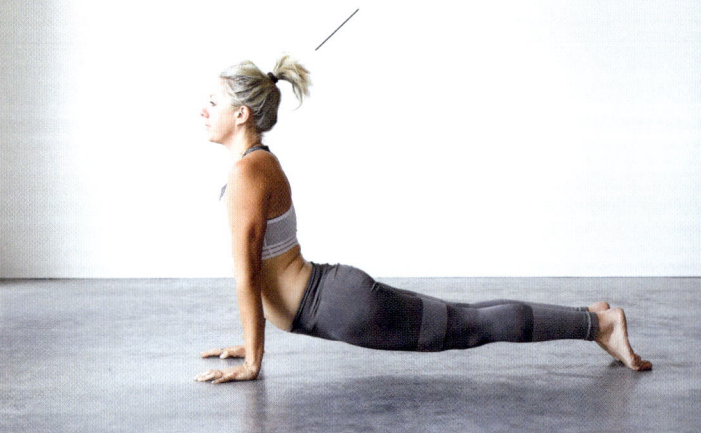

38 ____ YOGA PRACTICE

8 BHUJANGASANA (COBRA)

This is a good alternative to up dog for beginners. In this image, I'm showing you the first part of the pose before you peel back.

Roll forward on your toes to lower your torso onto the mat, keeping your hands flat and your legs straight. Inhale and lift your chest off the floor, straightening your arms as far as is comfortable. (I call this 'peeling my heart off the floor'). Try one set using your hands then another floating your hands off the mat, which will help build your core and lumbar strength.

Tip: Hug your elbows in and down, while keeping your gaze forward in front of your mat.

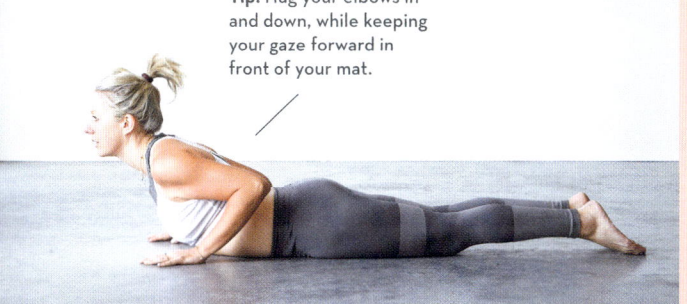

9 ADHO MUKHA SVANASANA (DOWNWARD FACING DOG OR DOWN DOG)

Exhale, roll the toes back, straighten your arms and lift your hips into down dog. Stay here for a few breaths. When you start out it's fine to have a bend in your knees. Press into the mat with your hands (imagine there's a suction pad in your palms), pushing down through your thumb and forefinger. Lengthen your spine (I think of this as melting my shoulders) and focus on pressing your heels down (this is a wonderful stretch, but will take practise).

Now inhale, bend your knees, look up and step (or hop) your feet between your hands so that you're back in uttanasana (forward fold). From there you jump up to urdhva hastasana (upward salute) and then drop your hands by your sides into tadasana (or prayer pose if you prefer), before starting the sequence again.

Once you learn the poses in sun A, and how to flow smoothly between them, you can do them as many times as you like. When you first start, as few as ten rounds can get your heart rate going and stimulate the flow of prana (energy). I know this sounds weird, but after I've done three to five rounds of sun A, I can feel the difference in my spine and I actually feel taller!

Tip: When a teacher says 'walk your dog out' they mean to gently push your heels down one at a time as if you are 'moon walking'.

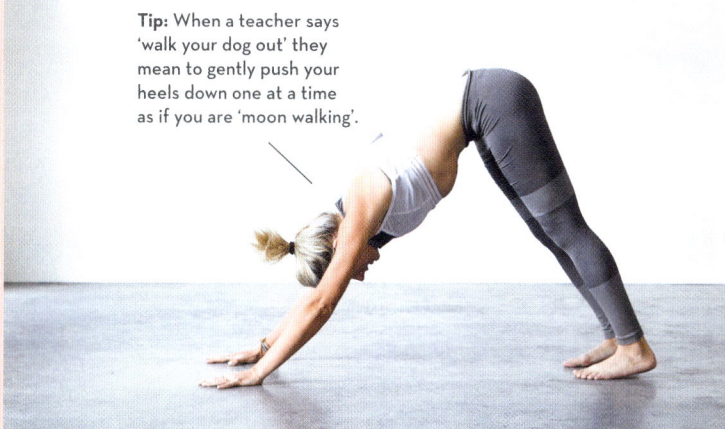

YOGA PRACTICE

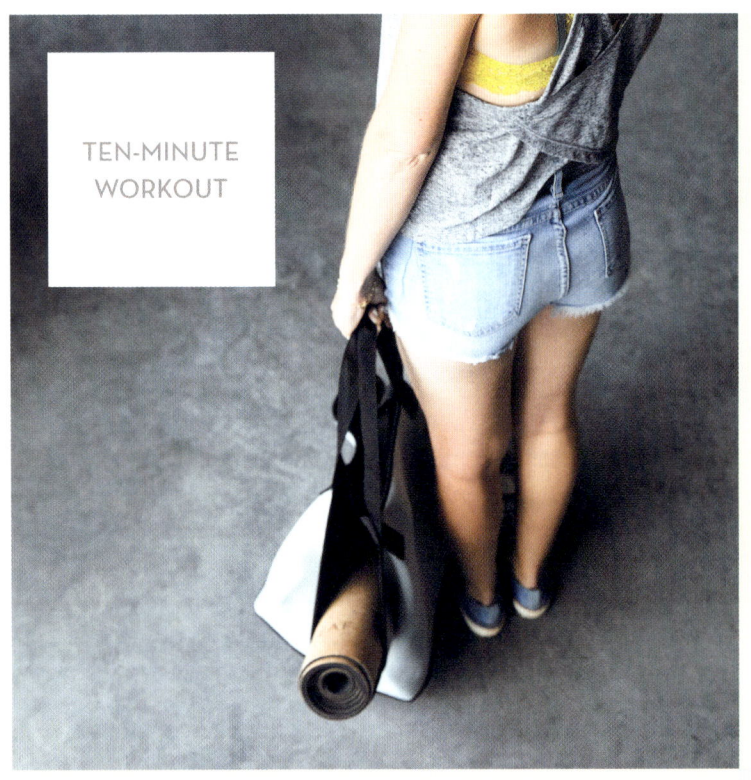

TEN-MINUTE WORKOUT

I love this little sequence, and like all yoga, you can make it as difficult or easy as you like. If you want to make it harder, sit deeper in the poses and hold for five full breaths. (I once did a class where a teacher got us to hold the chair pose for fifteen breaths!) Try not to lift up your body in your transitions, as the lower you stay the harder your muscles work.

1 UTKATASANA (CHAIR POSE)

- Start in tadasana (see page 37) with your feet together (or hip-width apart – whatever feels most stable for you). I like to have my feet together, big toes touching, with a slight gap between my heels so that my feet are perfectly parallel. Inhale, stretch your arms out to the sides and then lift them straight up, palms facing each other and fingers outstretched.
- Keeping your thigh muscles switched on, your chest open, your arms reaching upward and your fingers active, sit back in your seat and be comfortable with the uncomfortable.

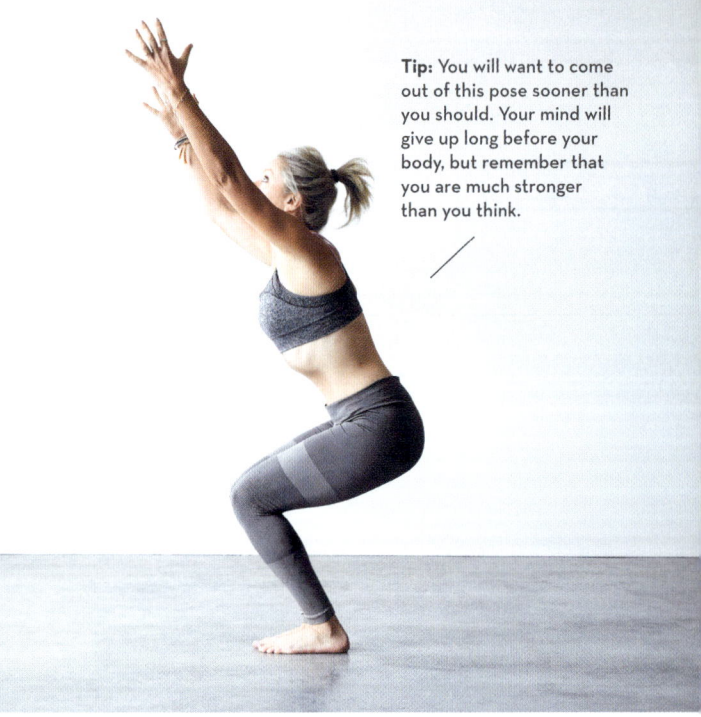

Tip: You will want to come out of this pose sooner than you should. Your mind will give up long before your body, but remember that you are much stronger than you think.

2 VIRABHADRASANA 1 (WARRIOR 1)

Start in down dog (see page 39).

- Look forward, lift your right leg off the floor and step it between your hands.
- Place your left (back) foot at 45 degrees and widen your stance so your hips are facing forward (they will want to be on the diagonal but try to keep them square).
- Reach for the sky, spreading your fingers and keeping a strong upward stretch.
- Deepen the front leg bend as far as is comfortable.

3 VIRABHADRASANA 2 (WARRIOR 2)

- From warrior 1 (see above), lower your arms, stretching them outward at the same time as you rotate your torso 45 degrees.
- Keep your eye line over your middle finger. Some people like the heel of their front foot to be aligned with the heel of their back foot, but I prefer a heel-to-arch alignment. Try them both to see what works for your body.

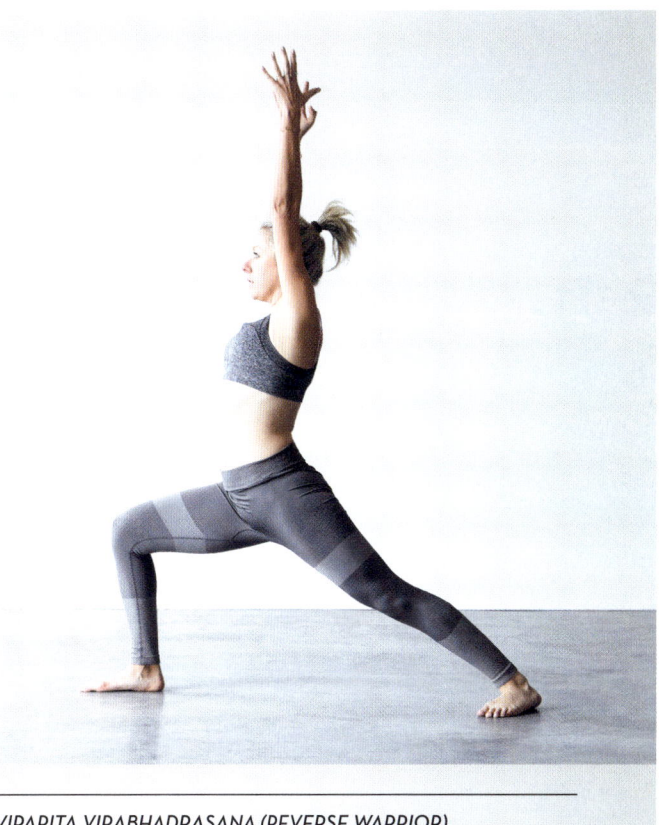

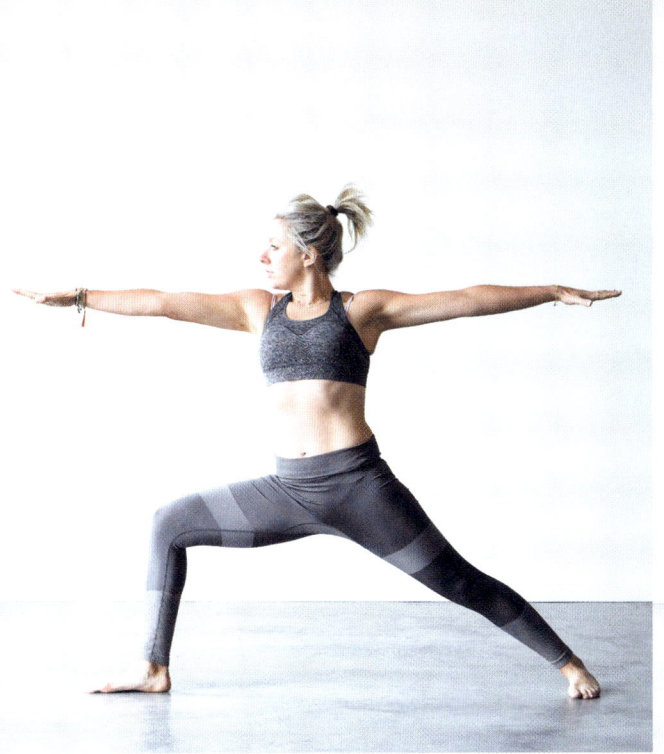

4 VIPARITA VIRABHADRASANA (REVERSE WARRIOR)

From warrior 2 (see left), lift your right arm skyward and arch your back, with the aim of resting your left arm on the calf of your left leg. It should feel like a nice stretch down both sides of the body.

Tip: Try to stay as low in the pose as you can to get the maximum benefits and build leg strength (it's easy to focus on the backbend in the upper body and cheat on the legs).

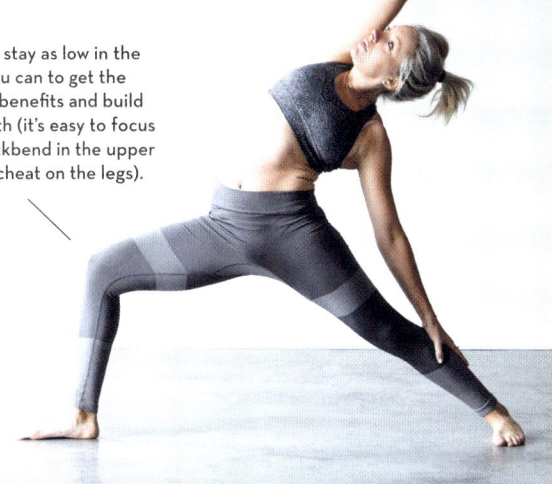

YOGA PRACTICE

BUTT TONER

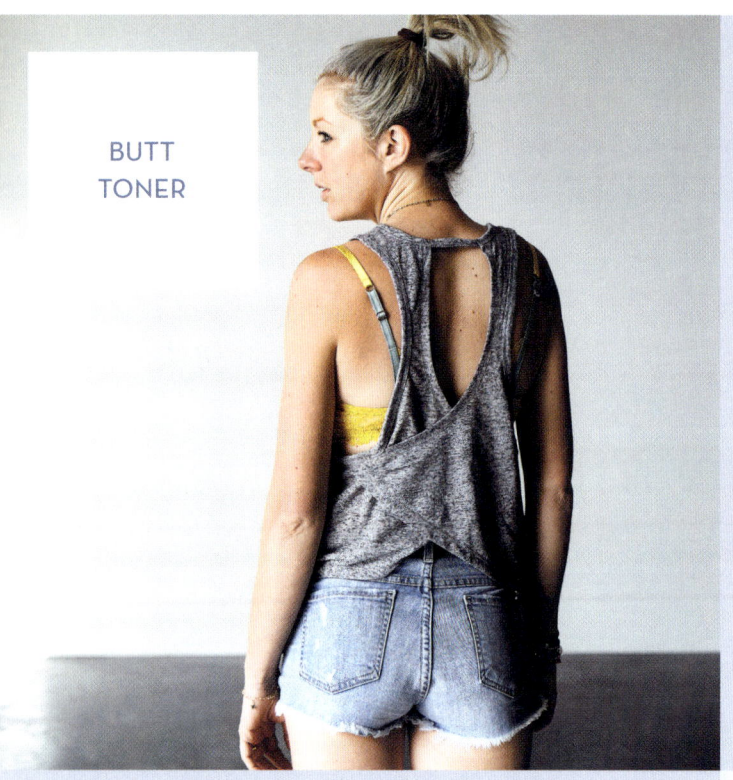

This combination of standing splits into half moon is a killer for the butt. It works a treat, and you will feel it the next day for sure when you're walking up stairs.

1 *URDHVA PRASARITA EKA PADASANA (STANDING SPLITS)*
This is quite literally a standing version of the splits, known as hanumanasana (monkey pose).

- Start in a forward fold (see page 37) with your hands on the ground (use blocks for support if necessary), then try to wrap one hand around your ankle followed by the other if you can. Your hips will want to flare open and stack here, but really focus on keeping them square facing towards the ground.
- Charge your core and thigh muscles, and keep your hips square as you lift your chosen leg. (You will naturally want to open the hips to get your floating leg up higher, but try to keep your hips closed at this point as you want to work your butt muscles.)
- Try wrapping one hand around your calf, then maybe the other hand.
- At this point you would usually return to a forward fold before repeating with the other leg, but instead you will transition to half moon (see 2).

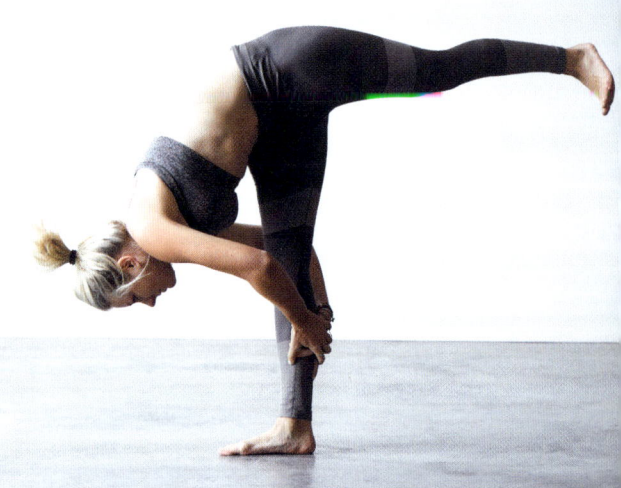

2 *ARDHA CHANDRASANA (HALF MOON POSE)*

There are many ways to enter this pose (see page 49 for another), but I'm pairing it here with the standing splits to give your butt muscles a real workout!

- From a standing split (see 1), rotate the hip of the floating leg outward (so your hips are stacked) and bring the matching arm up to rest on your hip (or stretch it skyward if you can). Hold it for three to five breaths then return to the standing split.
- Now return to a forward fold (see page 37) before repeating with the other leg.

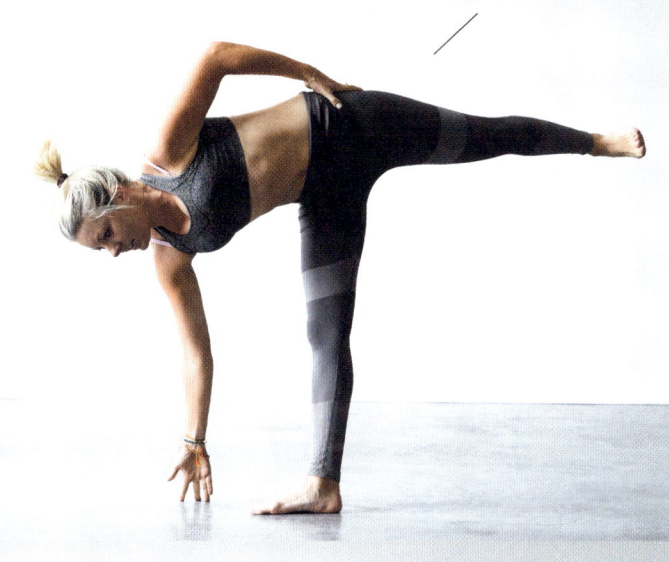

Tip: Switching between these two poses sounds fine in theory, but it's a bit of a challenge and you will feel the burn after a couple of rounds! Just remember that your hips are square in the splits, and then rotated and stacked in half moon.

3 *UTKATASANA (CHAIR POSE) WITH EAGLE ARMS*

Follow the directions for chair pose on page 40.

- Now slowly straighten your back and open your shoulders, raising your arms up while keeping your elbows slightly bent.
- Exhale as you fold forward to exit the pose.

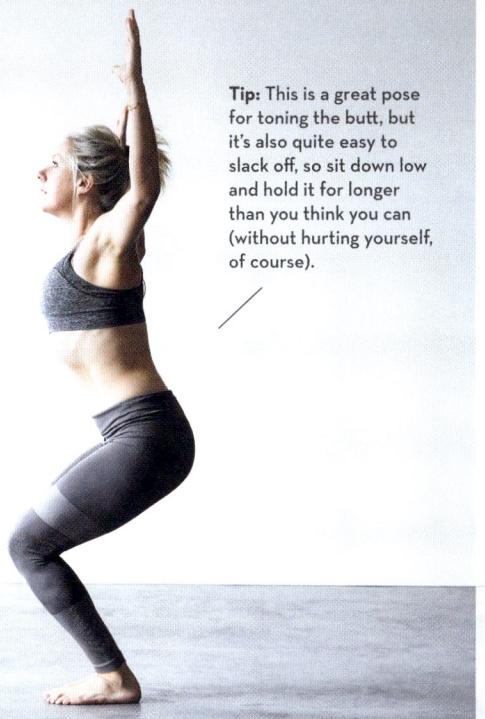

Tip: This is a great pose for toning the butt, but it's also quite easy to slack off, so sit down low and hold it for longer than you think you can (without hurting yourself, of course).

4 *SHOELACE POSE*

Like many poses, this one has a left and right version, so always do both to keep your body in balance.

- Start by kneeling on all fours.
- Lift one knee and tuck it in behind the other, then slowly sit back between your heels.
- If this feels too strong on the knee that's underneath, straighten that leg, or sit on a block or blanket.
- Hold for ten breaths, keeping your neck soft and letting your head hang.
- Repeat on the other leg.

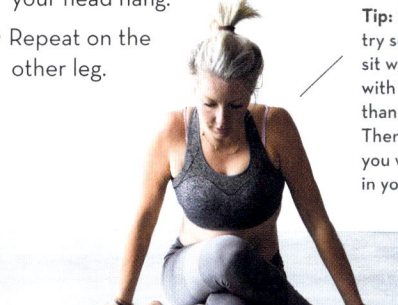

Tip: If this pose is too strong, try square pose, where you sit with your knees wide (as in with your shins aligned rather than crossed at the ankles). Then simply fold forward – you will definitely feel this in your glutes.

TUMMY TONER

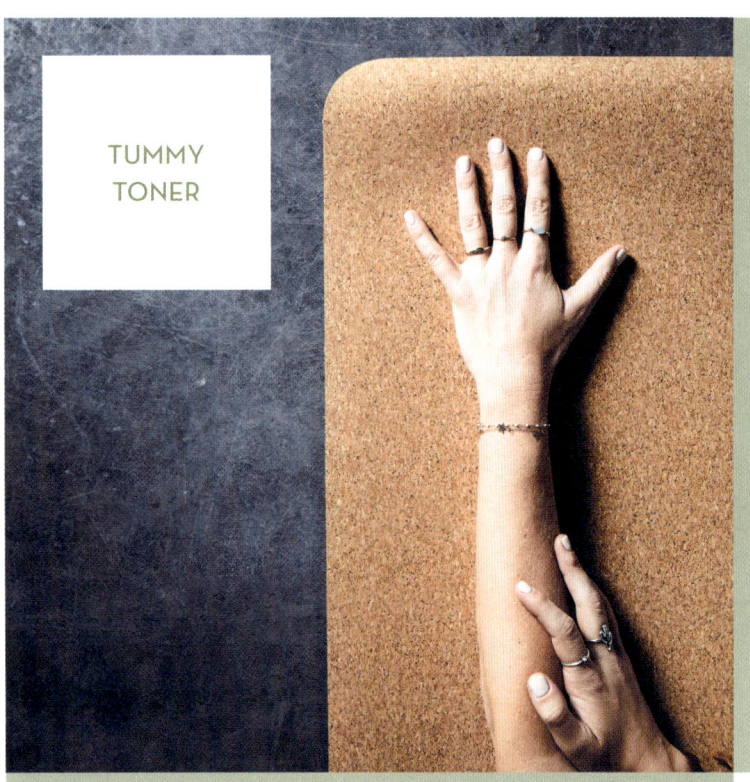

Core work is important in yoga as it helps to protect the spine when doing backbends and inversions. Most of the poses I describe in this book really work your core muscles, so if you do enough yoga you'll definitely have the best abs in town!

In kundalini yoga (see page 23), ab work creates heat and unlocks the base of the spine, which is said to be the source of kundalini energy – where your true potential lies untapped.

1 *NAVASANA (BOAT POSE)*

Boat pose is a core hold that can be varied to make it as easy or as hard as you like.

- Start by sitting on your butt with your knees bent and your hands flat on the floor beside your hips.
- Now inhale as you lift both feet in the air, keeping your knees together and your shins parallel to the floor, rocking back to maintain your balance.
- To make it a tad easier, keep your hands on the floor.
- To make it harder (or if you have a little more gas in the tank), straighten your legs out. Holding them higher is easier – keeping them lower will help you feel the burn!
- Hold the pose for as many breaths as you can while still feeling comfortable.

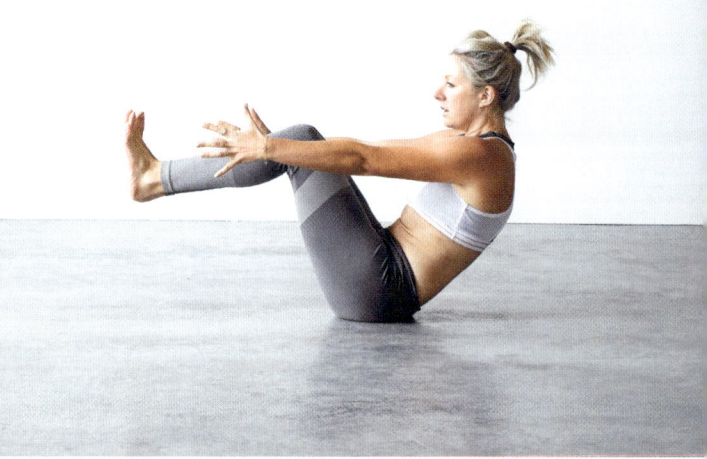

2 ARDHA NAVASANA (LOW BOAT OR CANOE POSE)

This is a version of boat pose that really fires up your abs, as well as your lower back and glutes.

- From navasana (see 1), simply straighten and lower your legs, keeping your leg and core muscles charged.

Tip: I will often hold boat pose (see 1) for ten breaths, then alternate between boat and low boat (see 2) for ten breaths, inhaling on boat and exhaling on low boat, then finish with low boat for ten breaths. It's a really quick and effective way to fire up your core!

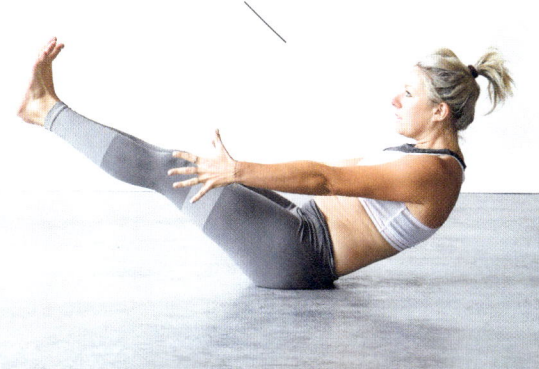

3 PHALAKASANA VARIATION KNEE TO NOSE (TIGER CURLS)

Tip: Teachers will say 'knee to nose', the idea being that you will be able to kiss your knee one day!

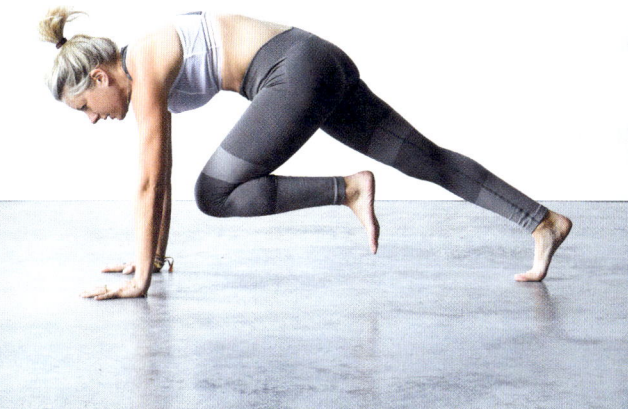

These are fun to do, but very challenging – a brilliant core workout. If you really want to step things up, do a few rounds of tiger curls. You will feel the burn, but it's worth it!

- Start in down dog (see page 39).
- Lift your left leg, kick it back, then bring it towards your left tricep (aim for the armpit, the higher the better).
- Hold it for one breath (or two if you can), then kick back, straightening the leg and lifting it up to the sky.
- Now bring it across to your right elbow, kick back up and swap to the other leg.

Tip: This works your core even harder, so is not something you should try until you are easily doing the sun A sequence.

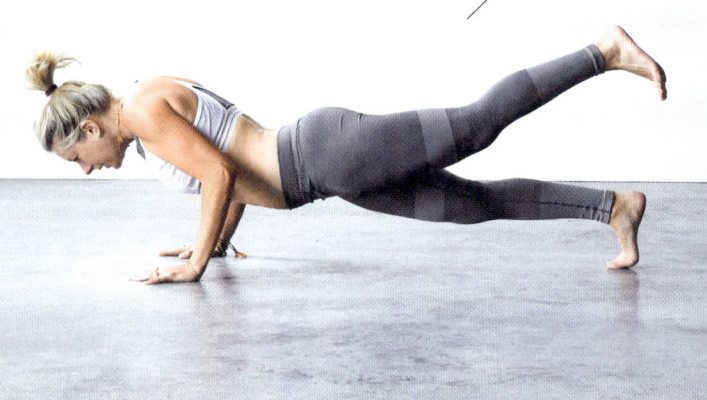

4 *EKA PADA CHATURANGA (ONE-LEGGED PLANK)*
Simply follow the sequence for sun A (see page 36), doing the high plank on one leg, then dropping to the low plank while still on one leg. Note that this is an advanced transitional pose and totally optional. It took me about three years to get it right!

5 *PARIVRTTA ANJANEYASANA (CRESCENT LUNGE TWIST)*
- Start this pose in crescent lunge (see page 56).
- Bring your hands into prayer pose, then lean forward over your right leg and twist to the right, activating your core muscles to help protect your spine.
- If this feels okay, open your wings here and fly. (If it feels too hard, stay in prayer pose, as the twist is already lovely and deep.)

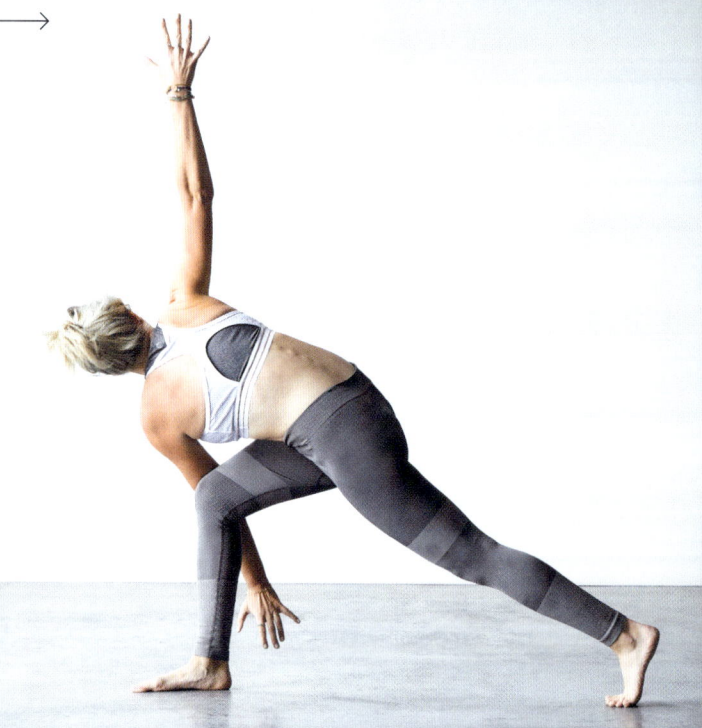

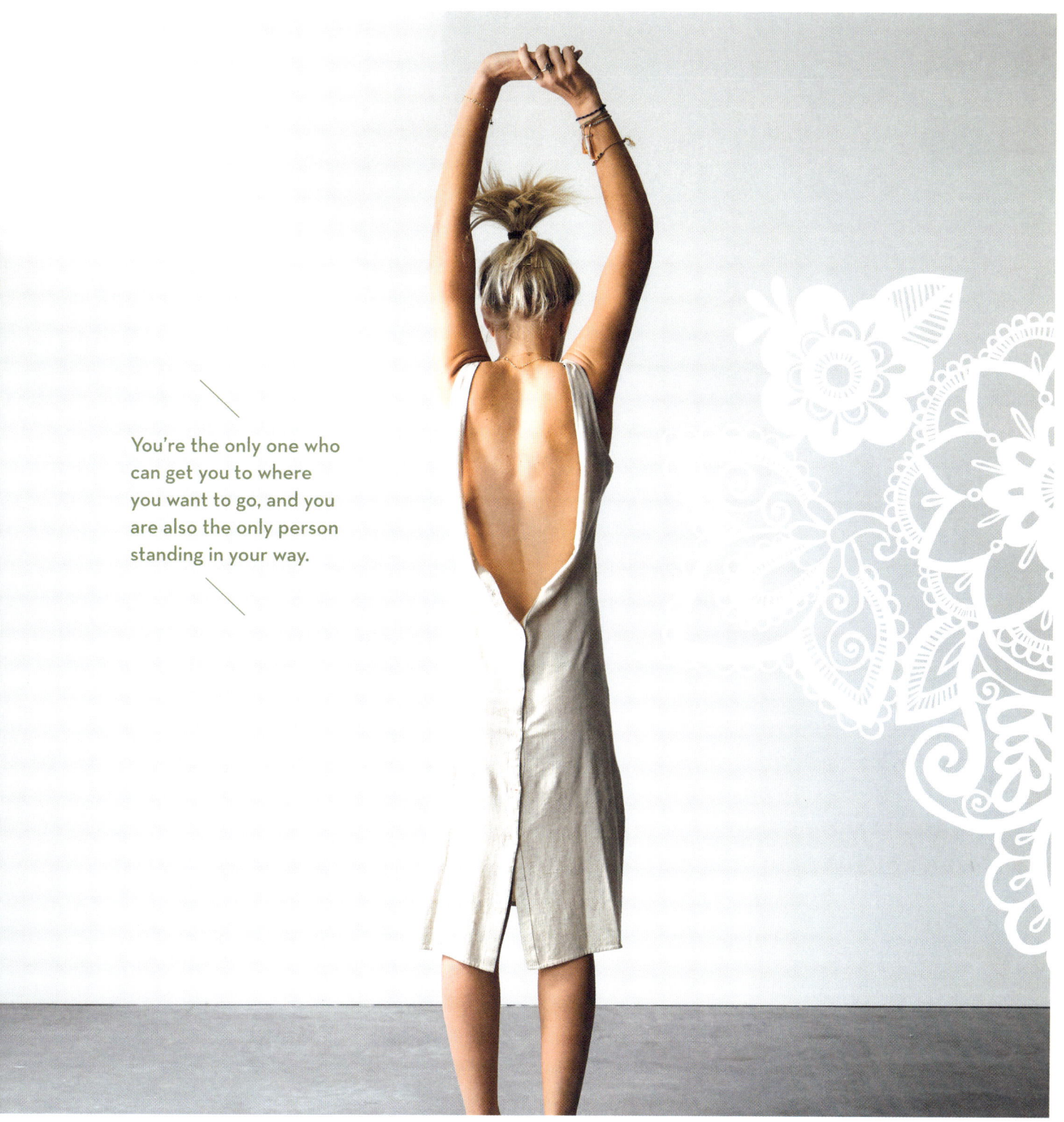

> You're the only one who can get you to where you want to go, and you are also the only person standing in your way.

TRAVELLER

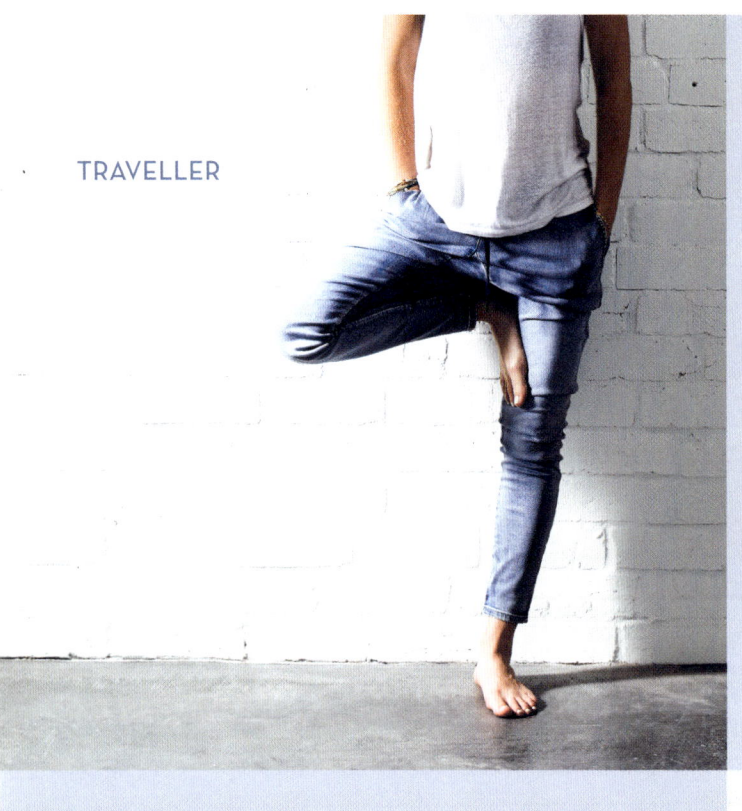

I do this sequence before I fly, during a flight (where possible) and when I arrive, and it really helps me to cope with that feral jetlag feeling. Camel pose is brilliant for long-haul flights as it helps to open your heart and chest. This is important, because unless you're lucky enough to be in first class, you'll usually spend most of the flight curled up in a ball trying to get some sleep without annoying the passenger next to you, which is not great for the spine!

On the plane, I walk to the toilet area and do forward folds while I'm waiting, and if there's space I'll even bust out a dancer's pose – it's a great conversation starter!

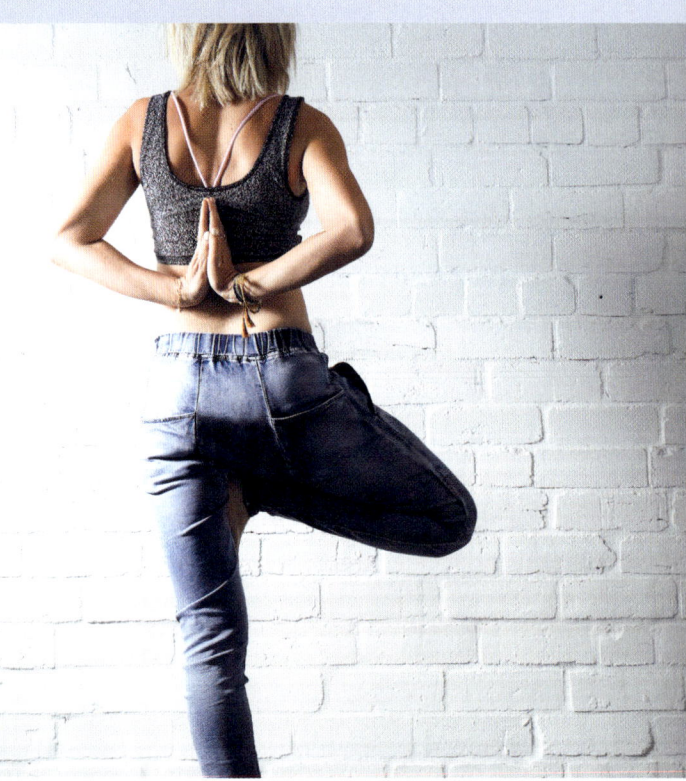

1 USTRASANA (CAMEL POSE)

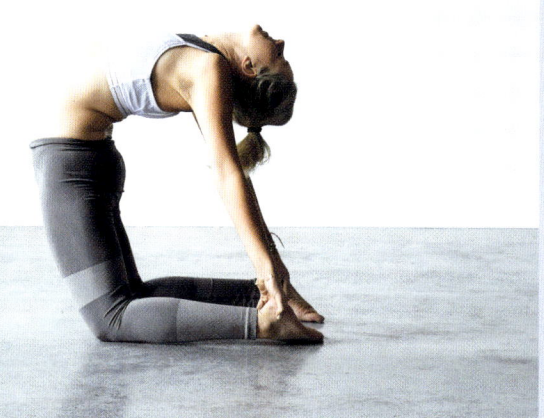

This is one of my favourite backbends. As with any yoga pose, you're in charge of how deep you go.

- Start in a kneeling position with your toes either curled to grip the floor or the tops of your feet resting on the floor.
- Now place your hands as if you're putting them in the back pockets of your jeans and slowly peel backwards, stopping when you feel your limit. (Only grab your heels if you feel no strain in your lower back.)
- Hold for five or so breaths and then very slowly straighten up, being careful not to slingshot yourself out of the pose.
- Now rest in a kneeling position, with your palms facing upward, and close your eyes.
- Repeat twice.
- After the third round settle into child's pose (see page 59).

2 ARDHA CHANDRASANA (HALF MOON POSE)

- Start in warrior 2 (see page 41).
- If necessary, place a block in front of your right foot, about a foot's length away (not pictured).
- Reach over to rest your hand on the block (if using) or floor, lifting your left leg high and opening your hips.
- Keep your right leg strong, pressing your toes into the ground and really activating your thigh muscles. (In yoga we say 'tight is light'.)
- At the same time, reach skyward with your left arm, keeping it straight and strong.

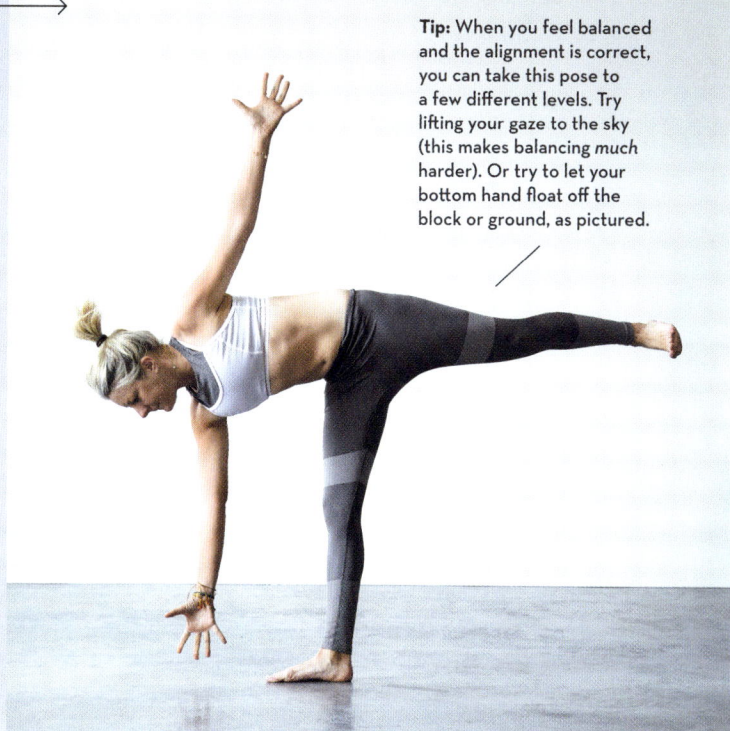

Tip: When you feel balanced and the alignment is correct, you can take this pose to a few different levels. Try lifting your gaze to the sky (this makes balancing *much* harder). Or try to let your bottom hand float off the block or ground, as pictured.

YOGA PRACTICE

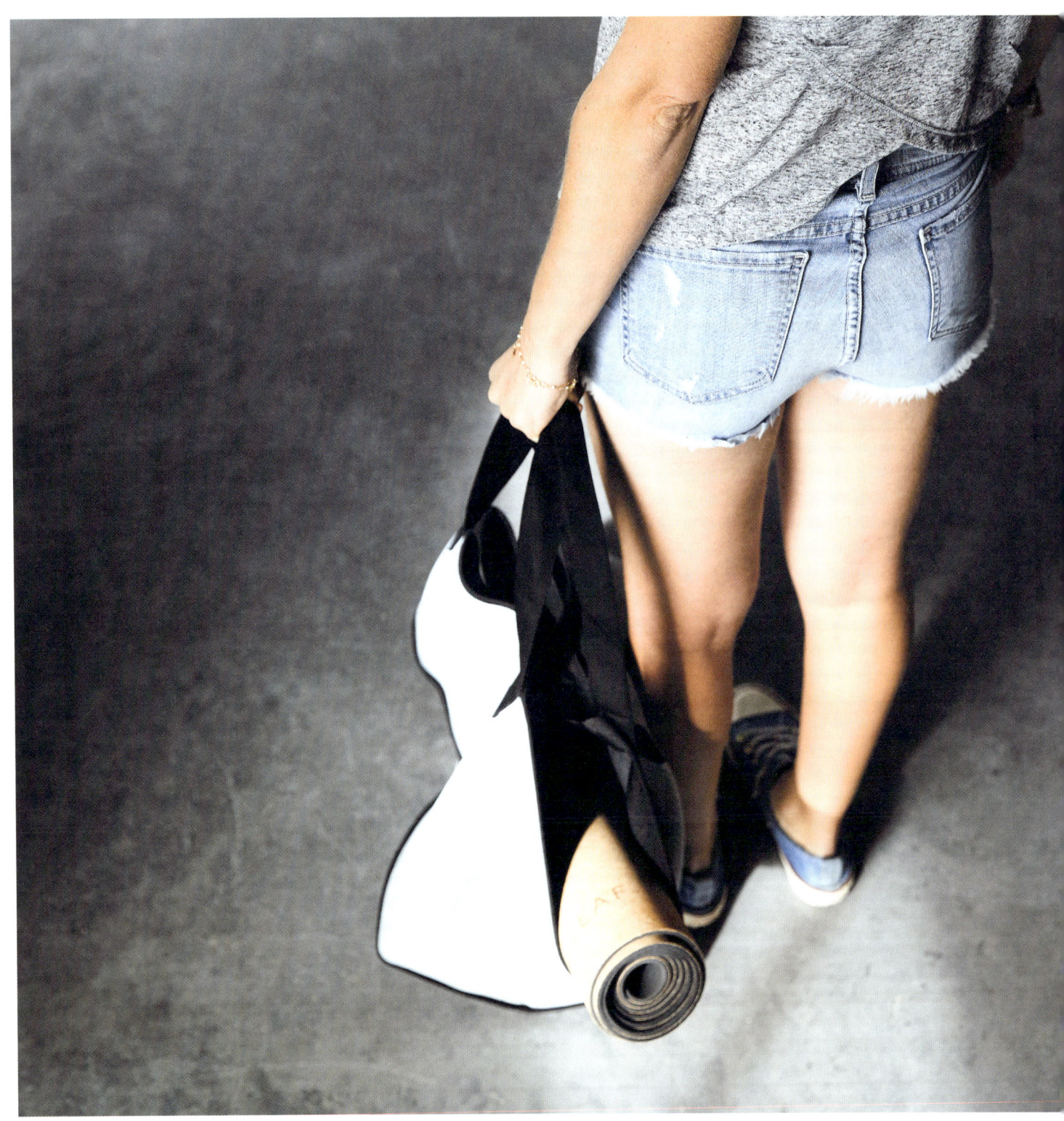

3 UTTANASANA (FORWARD FOLD)

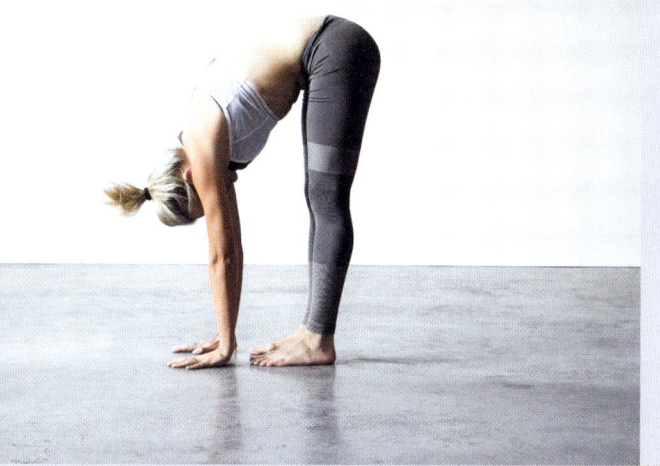

This pose is part of the sun A sequence (see page 36), but I include it here as a way to balance the strong backbend of camel pose.

- From tadasana (see page 37), exhale, keeping your thigh muscles contracted (this helps to support your lower back), and slowly bend forward from the hips, not the waist. In the version here, I don't bend my knees, but feel free to bend yours.

4 NATARAJASANA (DANCER'S POSE)

This pose is both a backbend and a balancing pose that looks wonderful and feels even better!

- Start in tadasana (see page 37).
- Inhale, bring your left hand out to the side, with the palm facing up, and reach forward with your right arm.
- Bend your left leg at the knee and reach down with your left hand to grasp your left foot around the top of the ankle.
- Turn your tummy muscles on and kick your left leg back, pressing your foot and hand against each other at the same time as tilting forward. If you fall out of the pose, just get back in.
- Now try it on the other side.

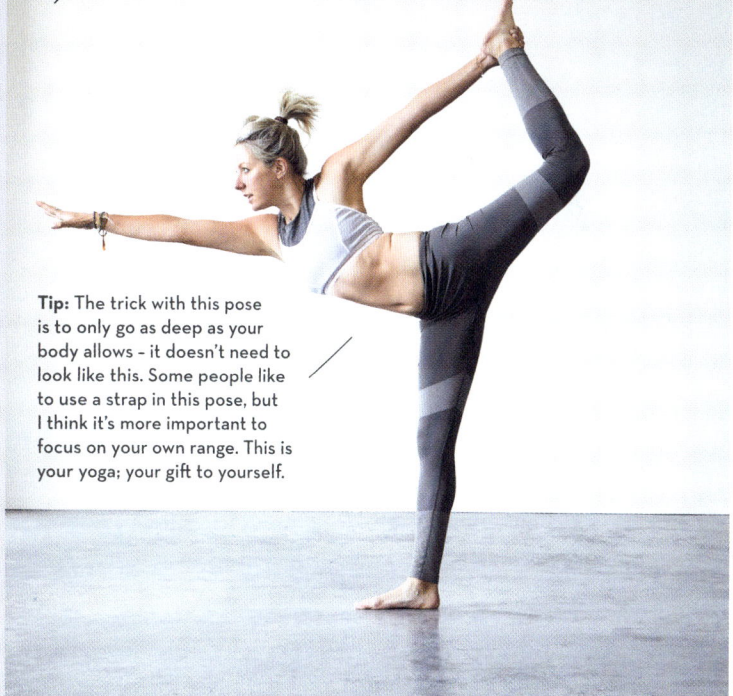

Tip: The trick with this pose is to only go as deep as your body allows – it doesn't need to look like this. Some people like to use a strap in this pose, but I think it's more important to focus on your own range. This is your yoga; your gift to yourself.

PRE-DATE

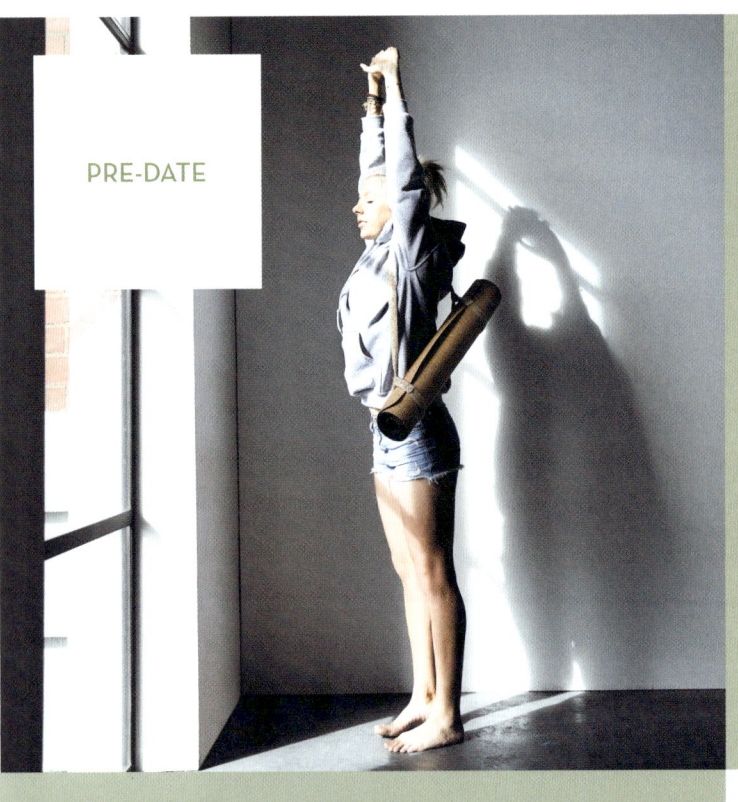

When we spend so much of our day in front of a computer screen or hunched over the steering wheel in a car, our bodies are closed in. This sequence is all about opening up your chest and cracking open your heart space. Try these poses before you meet up with someone on a date – I guarantee it will bring you some lucky love vibes.

1 *SETU BANDHA SARVANGASANA (BRIDGE POSE)*

- Start by lying on your back.
- Bend your knees and plant your feet hip-width apart (you need to be able to brush your heels with your middle finger).
- Press down through your feet and lift your hips off the mat, aiming to keep the tops of your legs as straight as you can and thinking about lifting your heart up and away from your feet.
- If you like, shimmy your shoulders towards your feet one at a time and interlace your fingers, keeping the palms touching (they'll always try to splay apart).
- Hold for five breaths if you can, then *slowly* lower your hips.

Tip: I like to do three rounds of this pose, and in between each round I 'windscreen wipe' my knees from side to side to release the muscles in my lower back.

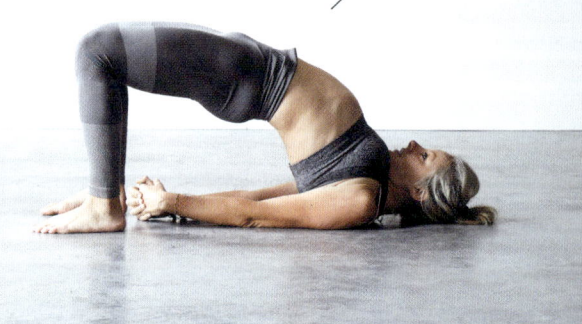

2 ARDHA ANUVITTASANA (STANDING BACKBEND)

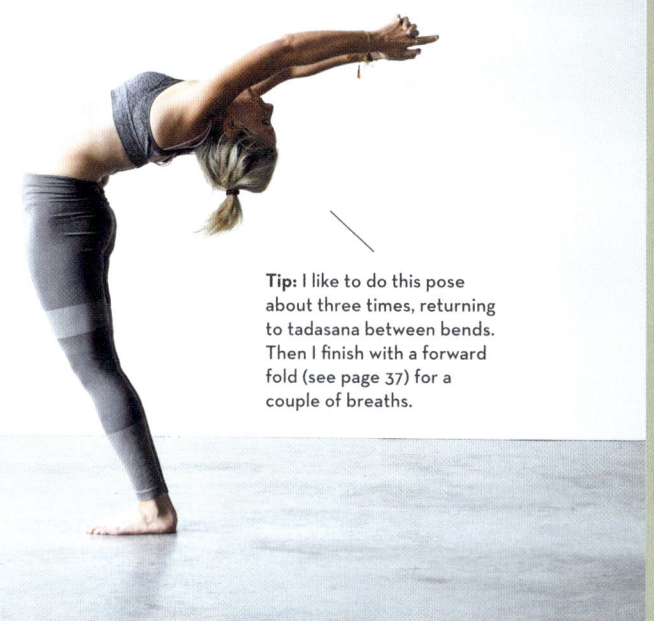

This is another heart-opening backbend.

- Start in tadasana (see page 37), then inhale and raise your hands above your head. I like to interlace all my fingers except the pointers (aka a pistol grip), but you can simply hold your palms together as in prayer pose.
- Now begin to peel back slowly. (Don't push yourself too far here; I've done it and ended up seeing stars. Just know that each time you do a round you'll find a little more depth.)

Tip: I like to do this pose about three times, returning to tadasana between bends. Then I finish with a forward fold (see page 37) for a couple of breaths.

3 URDHVA DHANURASANA (WHEEL POSE OR UPWARD BOW)

This pose is the next progression from bridge pose, and is quite advanced in the sense that you need openness in the shoulders and chest, length in the thigh muscles, and suppleness in the lower back. I would only try this in a class with the help of a teacher, but I've included it here to show you what is possible.

- Set up just as you would for bridge pose (see 1).
- Now lift your arms up and reach behind your head, placing your palms flat with your fingertips pointing towards your shoulders and hugging your elbows in close to your body.
- Exhale and press firmly into your feet and hands (activating your thigh and shoulder muscles) until you can rest the crown of your head on the mat.
- If you can, continue pressing upward until your head is clear of the mat. Try to hold this pose for five to eight breaths.
- Relax your muscles and lower your body gently, bringing your chin to your chest.

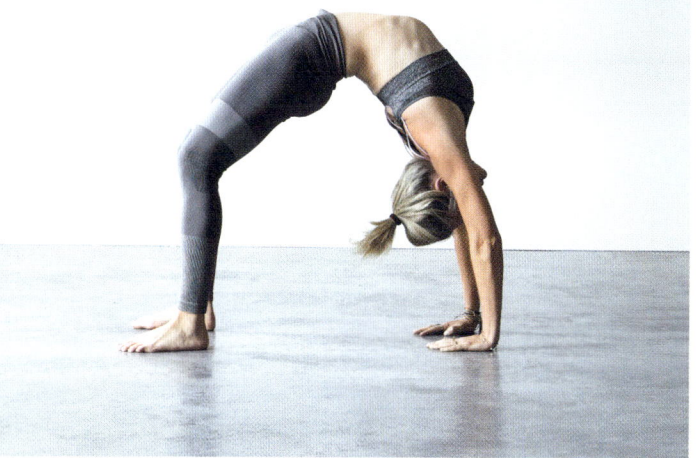

SADNESS

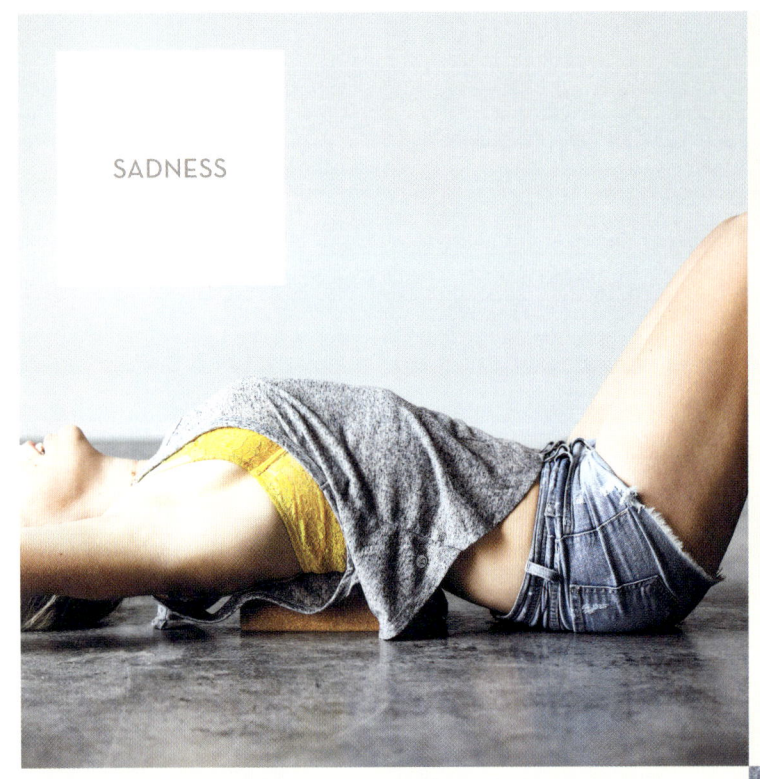

There are some beautiful yoga poses that are perfect for helping to let go of sadness, so that you can move on with your life.

Yoga is a very safe space to cry or let go of anything that's no longer serving you. Know that you'll be okay with whatever comes up, and that you will be open to new experiences.

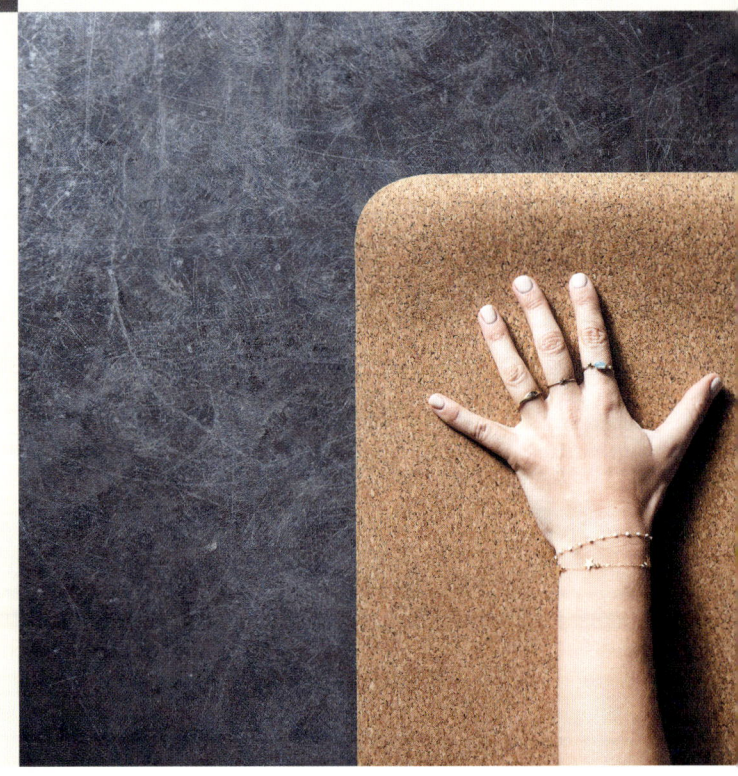

1 *USTRASANA (CAMEL POSE)*

I've already included camel pose on page 49, so I won't repeat the instructions here. But I do want to add that because this is a heart-opening pose, it can bring up emotions. When I was going through a break-up I found that this pose would make me a bit teary, so be ready for that.

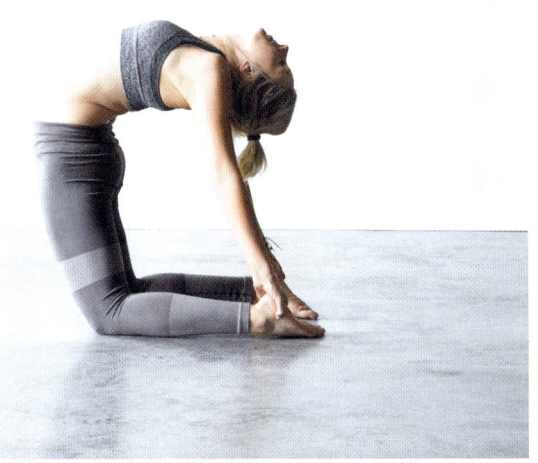

2 *SAVASANA (CORPSE POSE)*

This is the final pose of pretty much any yoga class, and although it's the least active, it's believed that this is where the magic happens. The idea is not to fall asleep but to 'relax with attention'. Many teachers will do breathing exercises or a guided meditation during this part of the class.

- Start in a seated position with your knees up and your feet flat.
- Gently uncurl your spine as you lower your back onto the floor.
- Now stretch out each leg, one at a time, keeping them about hip-width apart.
- Place your arms by your sides (not touching your body) with your palms facing upward to receive new energy or downward to ground yourself.
- Close your eyes and imagine your whole body is sinking into the floor. Stay in this position for at least ten breaths, or longer if you like (you can cover yourself with a blanket if the room is a bit cold).

Tip: When you're coming out of savasana the teacher will say 'bend your knees and turn to your right side'. They do this to maintain the sense of calm. However, if you are doing a morning sequence, and you want a burst of energy, you can try rolling to the left (I often do).

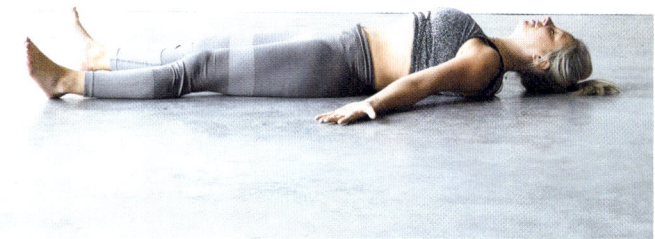

YOGA PRACTICE

3 ALANASANA (CRESCENT LUNGE)

This pose is a powerful step forward, moving away from the past and standing strong in the present.

- Start in down dog (see page 39).
- Now tilt your head up and look forward, then bend your right knee and step your right leg between your hands, aligning your knee over your heel. Your back (left) foot will still face the front but the heel will lift off the mat.
- Turn on the thigh muscles in your left leg (it should feel like you're 'zipping' your back leg up), inhale and raise your torso upright, sweeping your arms wide to the sides then raising them overhead, palms facing and fingers outstretched.
- To deepen the pose, settle into that front leg; the longer you hold it the tougher it will get. It really helps you to be in the here and now.
- When you are ready to come out, exhale, step your right foot back as you sweep your hands back to the floor and return to down dog.
- Hold for a few breaths and repeat with the left foot forward.

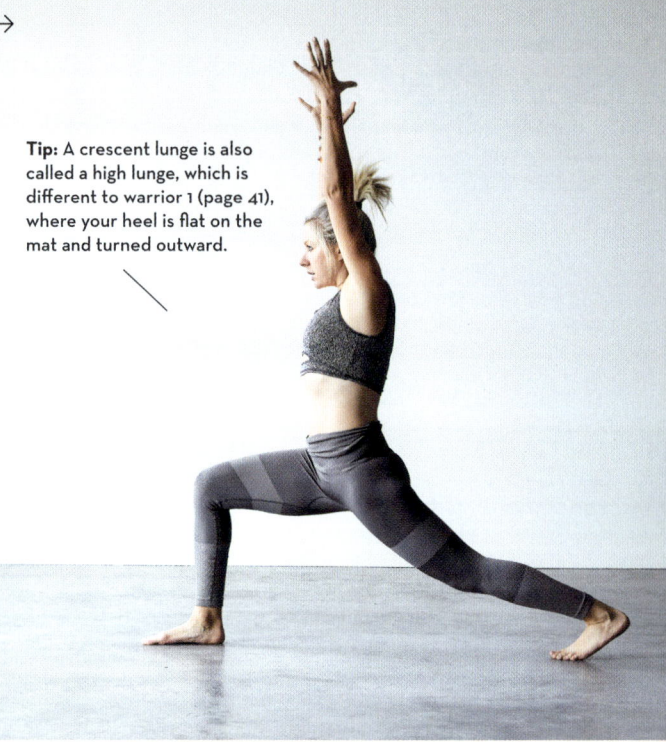

Tip: A crescent lunge is also called a high lunge, which is different to warrior 1 (page 41), where your heel is flat on the mat and turned outward.

4 VIRABHADRASANA 3 (WARRIOR 3)

Tip: If reaching forward like this too challenging, try holding your arms straight by your sides, or crossing your forearms over your heart.

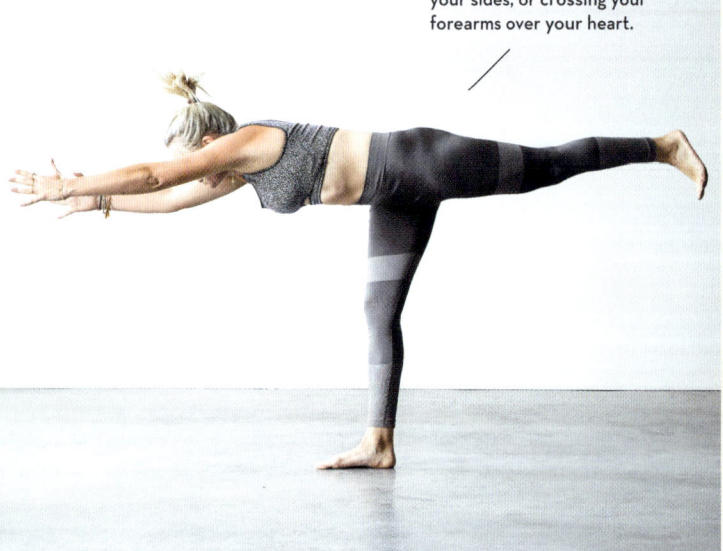

There are several ways to enter this pose, but I like to do it from a crescent lunge (see above).

- From crescent lunge, stretch your arms forward, parallel to the floor, palms facing.
- Press the heel of your forward (right) foot into the floor as you straighten your knee, while at the same time charging your left leg as you lift it off the floor. (Don't be tempted to lunge with your torso, as you'll lose your balance. Let your legs do the work.)

56   YOGA PRACTICE

5 UPAVISTHA KONASANA
(SITTING WIDE LEG FORWARD FOLD)

This pose is great for helping to calm the mind.

- Sit on the floor with your legs together and straight out in front of you. Place your arms by your sides with your palms on the floor beside your hips and your fingers pointing forward (this is dandasana, or staff pose). If this feels too tight in the hamstrings (backs of your thighs), sit on the edge of a folded blanket.
- From dandasana, lean back slightly on your hands so that you can slide your legs out wide.
- With your thighs charged and pressing into the floor, bend forward from the hips and slide your palms out in front of you.

Tip: Tight hips can be linked to current emotions. According to the teacher at a recent kundalini workshop I attended, financial freedom can also be stuck in the hips.

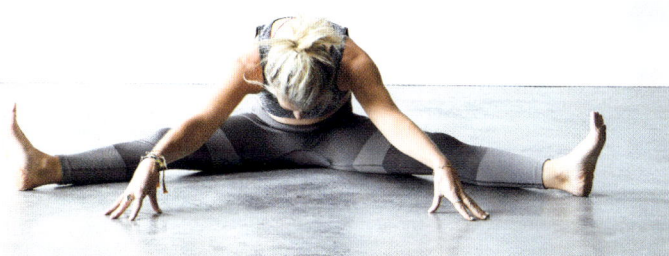

6 CHAPASANA (SUGAR CANE POSE)

- Start off in half moon pose (see page 49).
- Reach back with your floating arm and grab the ankle (outside or inside depending on how it feels in your spine and shoulders) then kick back (you'll look a bit like a bow and arrow). It becomes a bit more of a backbend, which helps to open your heart energy.

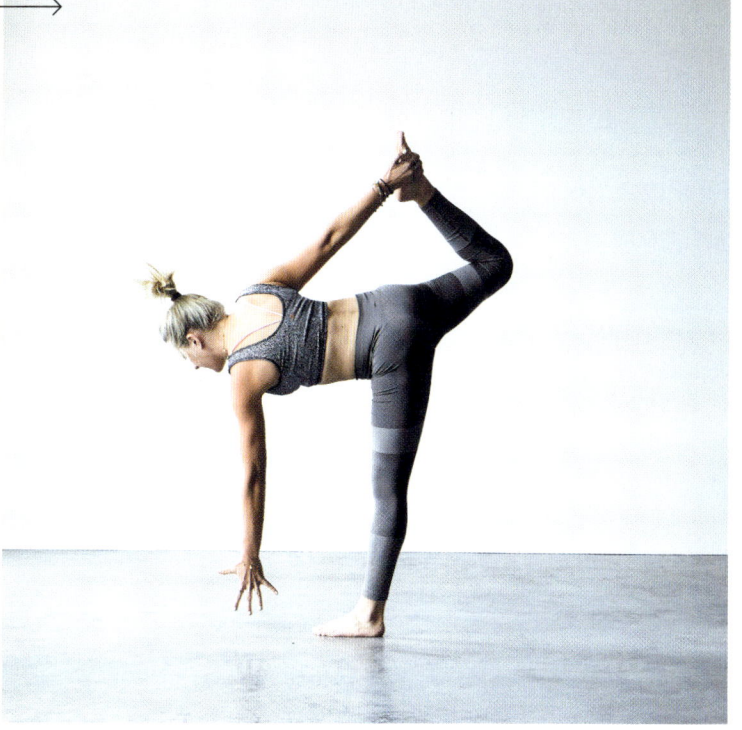

SLEEP

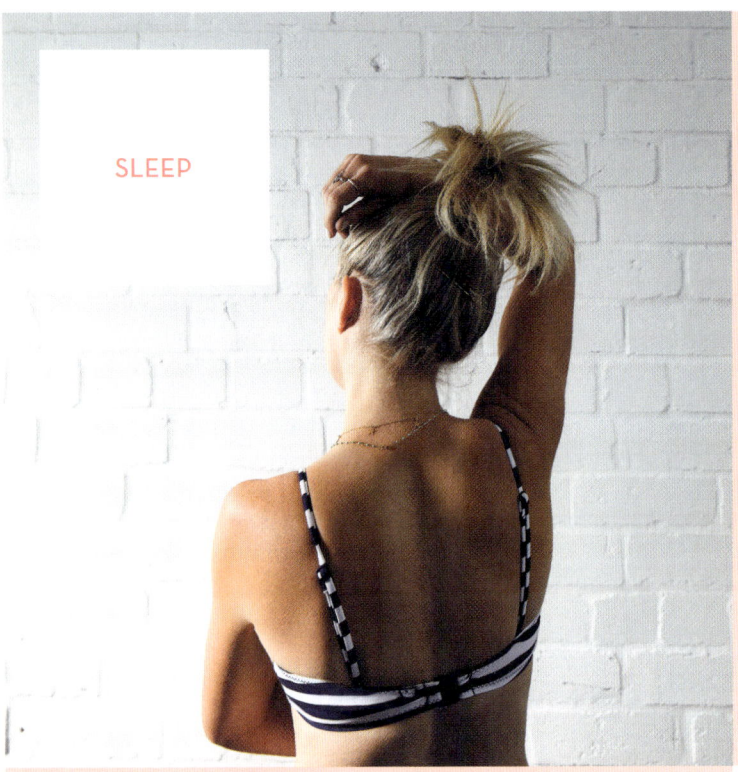

These poses are all about calming the nervous system and letting go of things that are preventing you from relaxing. This is also a great sequence to help cope with a stressful event.

In yin yoga, the spine is said to be a store for old emotions, so don't worry if old feelings arise in these poses. Observe them, love them and let them go.

1 *VIPARITA KARANI (WIDE LEGS UP THE WALL)*
This pose is unbelievably calming and relaxing.
- Start by sitting close to the wall with your legs together and stretched out to one side. (Some people like to place a folded blanket under the buttocks so the pose is even more relaxing, but it's up to you.)
- Shimmy your butt until it's really close to the wall, then bring your legs up until they are resting comfortably against the wall.
- Now let your legs fall into the splits (or you can just stay with your legs together if the splits are too strong).

Tip: Your butt needs to be really close to the wall or you won't get the full relaxing benefits of this pose.

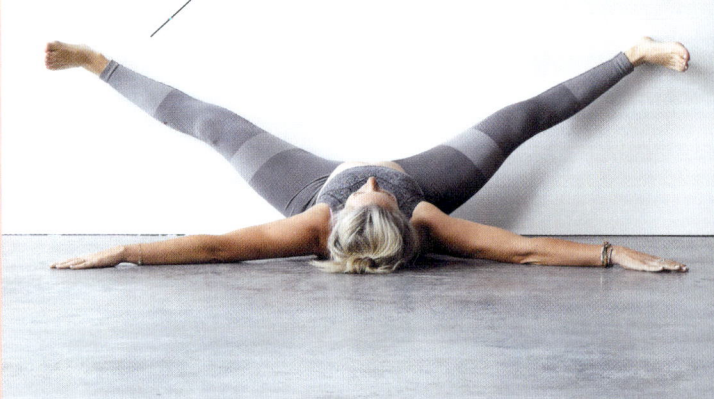

2 *UTTANASANA (FORWARD FOLD WITH SUPPORTED ELBOWS)*

This is the most relaxing version of this key pose.

- Stand with your feet hip-width apart (or closer if that is more comfortable for you) and grasp each elbow with the opposite hand.
- Charge your thigh muscles (your kneecaps will lift) to help support your lower back.
- Now fold forward at the hips, letting your head hang heavy.
- Stay in this pose for five to ten breaths.

Tip: You can take some 'elephant swings' here, too: just let your arms drop and sway from side to side.

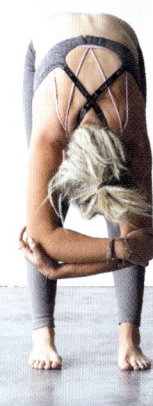

3 *BALASANA (CHILD'S POSE)*

This is a fantastic resting pose, and the wider your knees, the more restful it feels. Feel free to use this any time you feel exhausted or overwhelmed in a yoga class – your teacher will understand, as it's super calming for both the mind and body.

- Start in a kneeling position, then splay your knees really wide.
- Now slide your palms forward and let your forehead rest on the mat. Feel your body melt into the floor.

Tip: You can also bring your hands behind you beside your feet, though this doesn't open your shoulders.

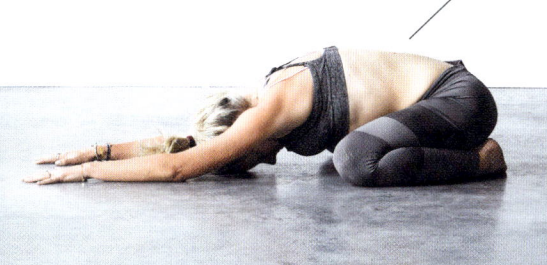

4 *TWISTED ROOTS*

This is a brilliant yin yoga pose to do after a stressful day at work. It can be done as a standalone pose, and will definitely help you sleep!

- Start by lying on your back with your legs together and outstretched.
- Now coil your left leg over your right leg (this is part of garudasana or eagle pose) and move both legs over to your right. (You may need to shimmy your hips a tad to find a comfy position.)
- Now spread your arms out wide into a T shape, turn your gaze to your left hand, shut your eyes and melt into the pose. Hold for about 5 minutes.
- Bring your hips back to the centre, uncoil your legs and repeat with the other leg.

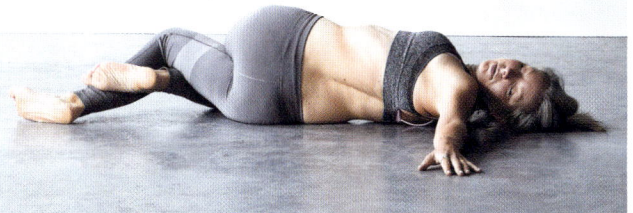

YOGA PRACTICE

CLEANSING

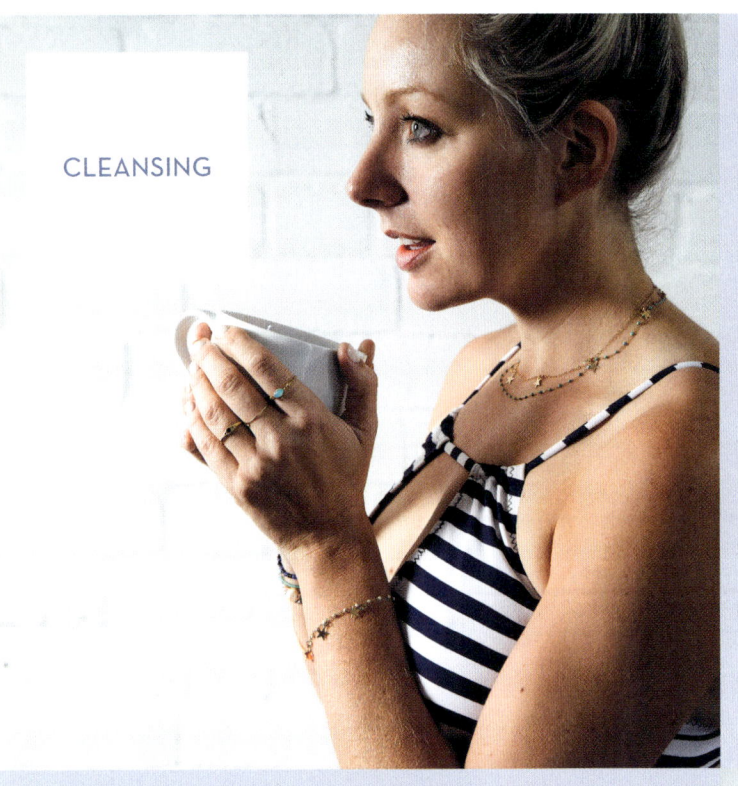

When it comes to cleansing, it's all about rinsing and twisting postures. These types of poses help to stimulate your organs of elimination, thus promoting detoxification in the body.

1 *TRIKONASANA (TRIANGLE POSE)*
  We usually come into trikonasana from a warrior 2 pose or reverse warrior (see page 41).
- From warrior 2, keeping your arms outstretched, bring your back foot in by about 30 cm (walk or hop).
- Straighten the front leg, reach forward and then windmill the arms open and peel your heart open to the sky, spreading your fingers and lifting your gaze to your thumb.

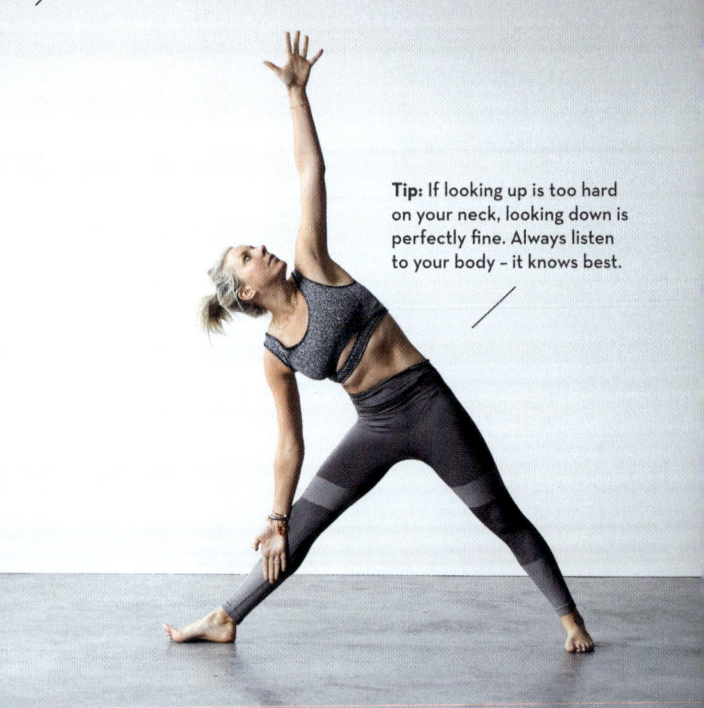

Tip: If looking up is too hard on your neck, looking down is perfectly fine. Always listen to your body – it knows best.

2 PARIVRTTA UTKATASANA (CHAIR TWIST)

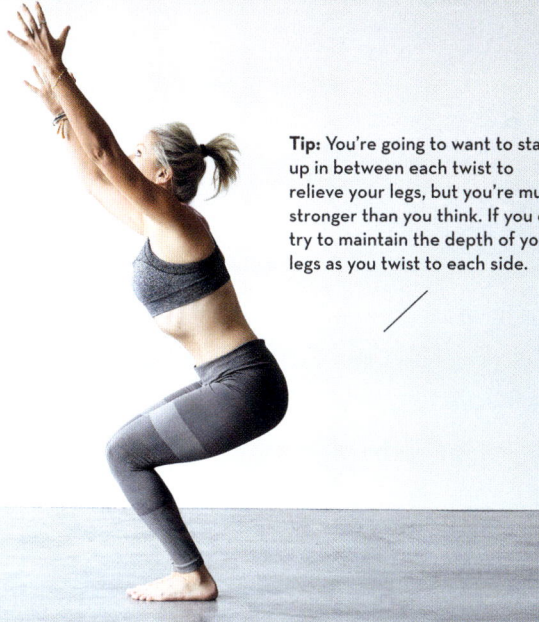

Tip: You're going to want to stand up in between each twist to relieve your legs, but you're much stronger than you think. If you can, try to maintain the depth of your legs as you twist to each side.

- Start in chair pose (pictured here, see page 40 for instructions).
- Cross your hands over your heart and twist to the right, keeping your knees aligned (one will want to jolt forward). Hold for three to five breaths.
- Come back to chair pose, then twist to the left.

3 APANASANA (KNEES TO CHEST POSE)

This pose is literally like giving yourself a hug. It also massages the digestive system, which is why it's great to add into your daily yoga during a cleanse. Some yoga teachers refer to this pose as 'egg of the universe', which is pretty cute.

- To get into the pose, start from a seated position (dandasana) and squeeze your knees into your chest.

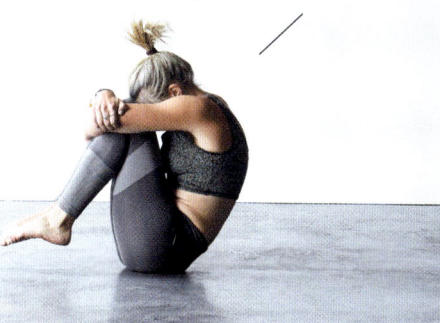

Tip: This is a lovely pose to do before savasana (see page 55). I inhale, say 'thank you' to myself, and as I exhale, I lower myself into savasana. Blissful!

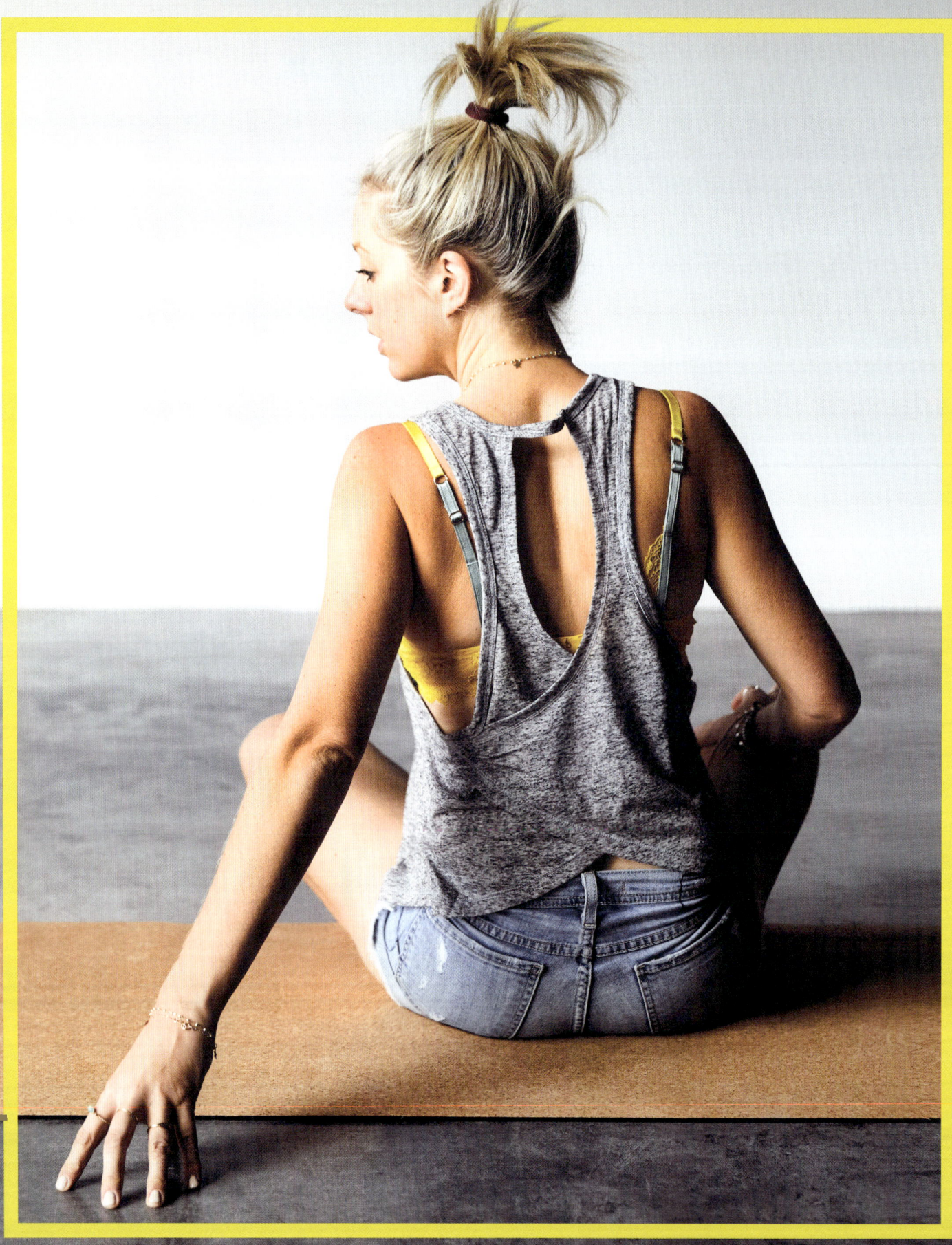

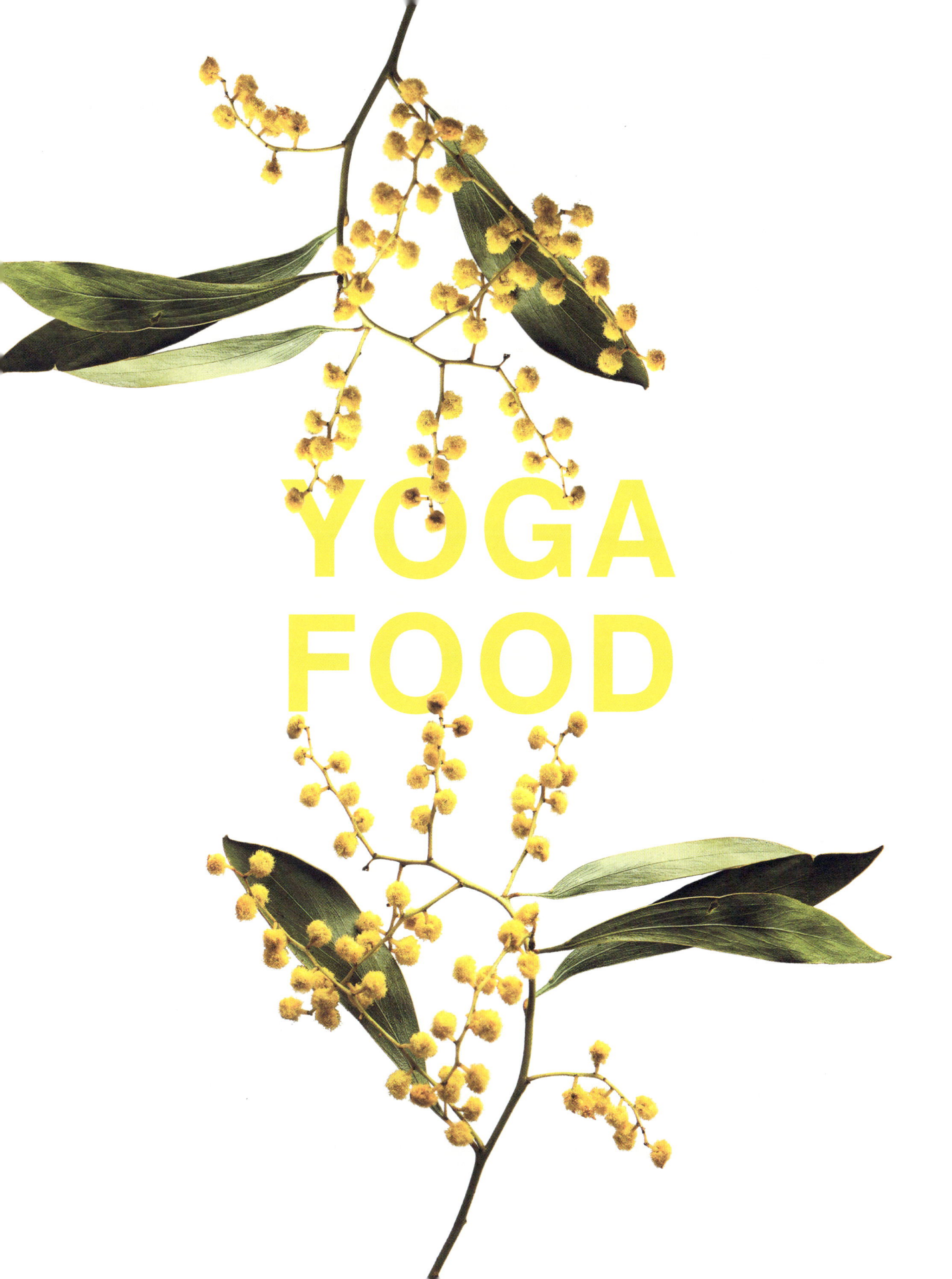

YOGA FOOD

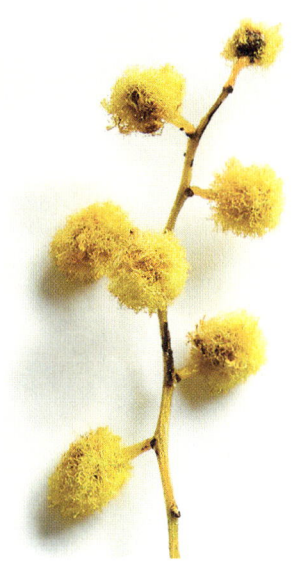

TIPS FOR CLEAN EATING

Nourishing your body with whole foods is a beautiful way to support it to be the best it can be. The tips in this section are ones that I follow every day to feel super confident in my mind and body.

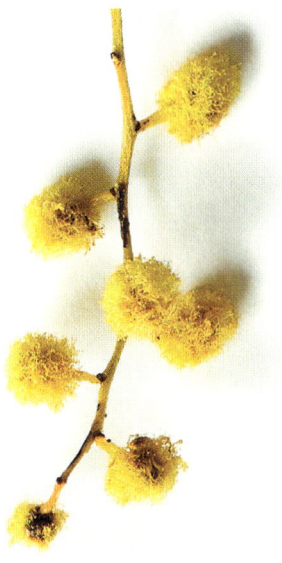

Eat like you love yourself.
Move like you love yourself.
Speak like you love yourself.
Act like you love yourself.

If you really want to make the most of your yoga practice, you need to start from the inside. We've all heard the old saying 'you are what you eat' and there is a lot of truth in that. If you fuel your body with nutrient-dense food as close to its natural state as possible, then you will feel vital and energetic all day long. I call this clean eating. If you eat sugar-laden refined carbs for a 'quick fix', yes you will get an initial surge of energy, but it will always be followed by a slump and you'll feel tired and moody, and crave those same carbs again. This not only undoes all of your hard work on the yoga mat, but also sets up the vicious cycle that, over the long term, can lead to weight gain and other health issues.

DITCH HIGHLY PROCESSED FOODS

When I say 'highly' processed, I really mean foods that are a long way from their natural state. You see, not all processed foods are bad. Ingredients such as butter, coconut oil, rolled oats, nut flours, brown rice and wholegrain flours are all 'processed' to a certain extent, but their nutrients are still intact. Pretty much all takeaway foods, bakery goods and packaged meals (pizza, pies, sausage rolls, tinned soups, sauces for pasta and noodles etc.) are made with refined wheat or corn flour, unhealthy oils and lots of extra salt and sugar to increase shelf life (and food manufacturers' profits). Basically, if you pick up a packet, can or jar and the ingredients list reads like a chemistry class, put it back. If you are serious about taking care of your body, then you've got to minimise these foods (or better still, ditch them completely). The alternative? Cooking from scratch. For some people, this is the daunting bit – having the right ingredients on hand and the time to chop your fruit and veg and do some cooking. But here's the good news – it's *heaps* easier than you think, and once you get into the swing of it, it will just become second nature.

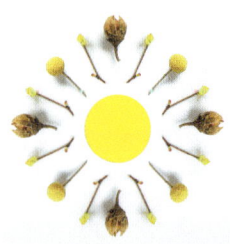

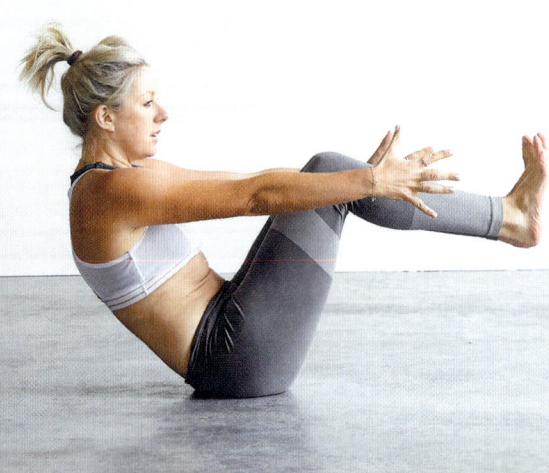

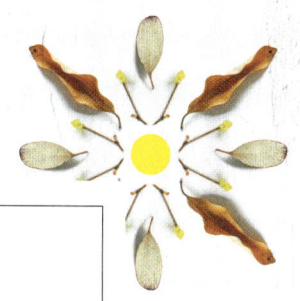
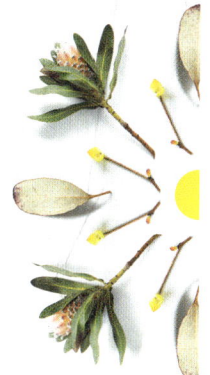

Processed carbs

Some people think carbohydrates are only found in pasta, cakes, bikkies and bread, but they are actually found in every food we eat except meat (even milk has carbs, along with all veggies, fruits, grains, nuts and seeds). Some carbs are called sugars, and others are starches. The sugars include the monosaccharides glucose and fructose and the disaccharides sucrose, dextrose and lactose (sucrose, aka table sugar, is actually made up of equal molecules of glucose and fructose). As I mentioned, sugar gives us an instant energy hit, but while glucose can be used by every cell in the body (our brain cells can ONLY use glucose), fructose (fruit sugar) can only be broken down in the liver, which can take a while. Meanwhile, the extra fructose is instantly converted to triglycerides (fat). This is because when our ancestors were hunting and gathering, they rarely found berries and other fruits, so they needed to be able to gorge themselves when they did to store the energy as fat. That's why we don't have a switch to tell us we've had enough fructose. This doesn't necessarily mean that fruit is bad, it just means that you should enjoy it in its whole form rather than via the concentrated sugars found in fruit juice or excessive amounts of dried fruit.

The other main type of carbohydrate is starch (and cellulose), which is found in fruits and veggies, nuts, seeds, legumes, wholegrain cereal (oats and brown rice) and wholegrain flour. Note that I said *whole*grain. Refined or highly processed grains (e.g. the white flour in bread, cakes, bikkies, pasta and noodles) have had the outer husk and germ removed, which means the starches are more rapidly converted to glucose in the body. In other words, they have the same effect as sugar. If you're going to eat bread or pasta, make it wholegrain, or better still, replace it with paleo bread, cauliflower rice or zucchini pasta.

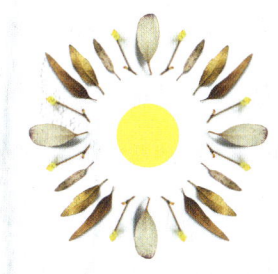

EAT *LOADS* OF VEGETABLES AND FRUIT

Yoga is about purity and clarity, so go for foods in their natural state. Veggies and fruit are the obvious choices here, as you can pretty much eat whatever you dig out of the ground or pick off a tree. The more serves of vegetables you can squeeze into your day, the better you will feel. The dark leafy greens (spinach, watercress, silverbeet, mustard greens, kale, Asian greens) always win first prize for nutrient content, but it's also important to get your rainbow happening. Red-, orange- and yellow-coloured veggies have loads of vitamins, as well as the carotenoids lycopene and beta-carotene, which are important sources of antioxidants (our bodies need antioxidants to reduce oxidative damage – aka ageing – and to fight inflammation).

To ramp up your veggie intake, try making my broccoli bites (see page 166); or use cauliflower rice instead of rice; or try making some zucchini pasta. I've even included a recipe for choc-chip cookies made from chickpea flour (see page 204), which means you're not only sneaking in more plant foods, but also more protein – plus they're gluten free.

I like to think of all veggies and fruit as super foods, but mushrooms are an especially great vegetarian source of protein and iron. I love how they have an almost 'meaty' texture, which is why they make delicious vegan burgers!

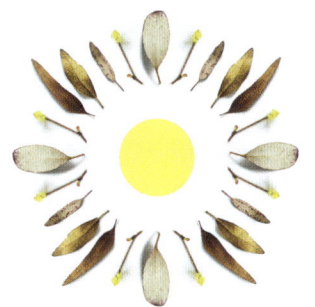
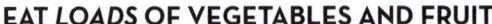
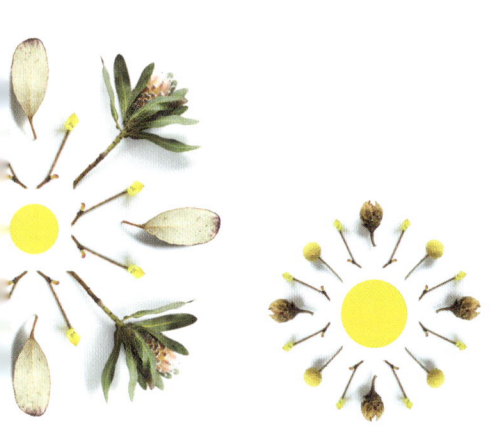

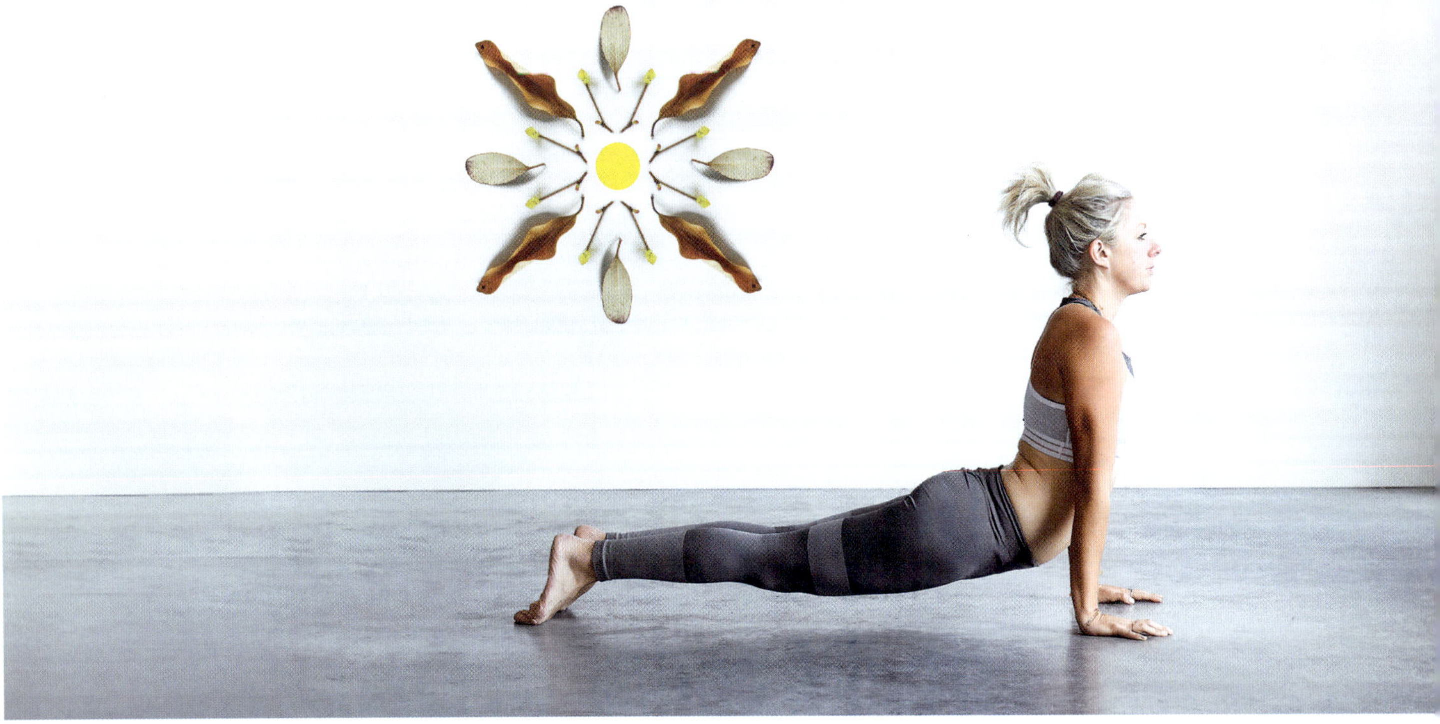

Yoga and vegetarianism

Many people who regularly practise yoga also choose to be vegan or vegetarian. Personally, I eat meat, though I do understand the reasons people follow a strictly plant-based diet. But when I'm training and doing yoga every day I feel that I get much more out of my body when I consume meat. So listen to your body – what foods make you feel vital and strong in both mind and body? What foods leave you feeling bloated or tired? The truth is, your dietary needs will change at different times of your life, so if you're open to change then it becomes a pretty lovely journey. And whatever your eating plan, you can always make it healthy.

In Hindu philosophy, food is the creator of prana (life force) and the types of foods we eat reflect our vitality and health. Food is also our first interaction with the world around us, and unless we eat with a sense of love, connection and peace then we will suffer. This is the concept of Sattva, which is one of the three Gunas or primary qualities of Nature. The others are Rajas (passion, activity, egotism) and Tamas (disorder, ignorance, apathy). Each of us possesses these qualities in various amounts, which can change depending on our life situation. A Sattvic diet is an Ayurvedic form of eating believed to promote a calm and compassionate mind by:

- avoiding all foods that involve the killing or harming of animals
- eating foods grown harmoniously with nature that are cultivated and ripened naturally
- preparing food with love and positive intention.

> If you're eating an abundance of veggies, fresh fruit, raw nuts and seeds and ethically sourced protein, you won't need to count calories. Think real food and real nourishment and watch the body respond – it wants to thrive.

EAT PLENTY OF PROTEIN

Protein gives you sustained energy because it keeps you feeling fuller for longer. I love fish (especially white fish) and eggs (they're like little nutrient bombs), and while I enjoy lean red meat and chicken, I don't have them every week.

If you're vegetarian, dairy food is a great source of calcium and protein, provided you can digest it. You may find that cheeses made from sheep or goat's milk are much easier to digest than those made from cow's milk. People who are sensitive to dairy often find that they have no problems with sheep's milk yoghurt.

Ricotta is something I love as it's a tad easier to digest than other cheeses and it's very high in protein. And who says you have to have all of your protein with your main meal? One of my favourite treats is a bowl of mixed berries mixed with two heaped tablespoons of ricotta, a couple of drops of stevia and a sprinkle of cinnamon.

Legumes are an important protein source for vegans and vegetarians. Sprouted mung beans add a nutritious crunch to salads, sandwiches and wraps, and I love a big handful on top of hot dishes. Try chickpeas or red kidney, cannellini or black beans in soups and stews, and lentils make amazing curries.

Protein combining

If you're vegan, it's important to understand protein combining. Proteins are made up of chains of amino acids. There are twenty amino acids, nine of which we have to get from our diet because our bodies can't 'make' them. These nine essential amino acids are phenylalanine, valine, threonine, tryptophan, methionine, leucine, isoleucine, lysine and histidine. A protein source is considered 'complete' if it contains enough of each of the essential amino acids for us to stay healthy.

Generally, all of the proteins from animal foods (meat, fish, poultry, milk, eggs) are complete. But the proteins in plant foods (nuts, beans, seeds, grains and vegetables) are usually not complete, because there's either not enough of each essential amino acid for optimum health or they're missing one or more of the essential amino acids. This is why it's important to combine legumes (beans, peas, lentils) with grains/seeds (rice, quinoa, millet, amaranth, spelt, barley) or grains/seeds with vegetables to create meals that are high in all of the essential amino acids. And if you think about it, this combo features in vegetarian dishes from heaps of different cultures, such as Indian chickpeas or dhal (lentils) and rice, Mexican beans and corn, and Japanese soybeans and rice.

Food	Amino acids in low supply	Complementary food (to help boost amino acids in low supply)	Sample meal ideas
Legumes (beans, chickpeas, lentils, peanuts, peas)	Methionine Tryptophan	Grains Nuts and seeds	- Lentil dhal with rice or quinoa - Broadbean stir-fry sprinkled with sesame seeds - Chickpea and tahini dip - Chickpea, quinoa and almond salad
Grains (barley, corn, kamut, oats, rice, rye, spelt, wheat) (amaranth, buckwheat, millet and quinoa are seeds/ancient grains that can be used in place of regular grains)	Isoleucine Lysine Threonine	Dairy (my recipes are reasonably low in dairy, but do often contain goat's cheese, ricotta and yoghurt) Legumes	- Tortillas with chilli beans and rice - Oats with a dash of plain yoghurt - Rye bread with avocado and goat's cheese
Nuts and seeds (almonds, brazil nuts, cashews, macadamia nuts, millet, pecans, pistachios, pumpkin seeds quinoa, sesame seeds, sunflower seeds, walnuts)	Isoleucine Lysine	Legumes	- Lentil salad with almonds - Beetroot hummus with walnuts - Macadamia and pea pesto - Navy bean salad with your favourite nut

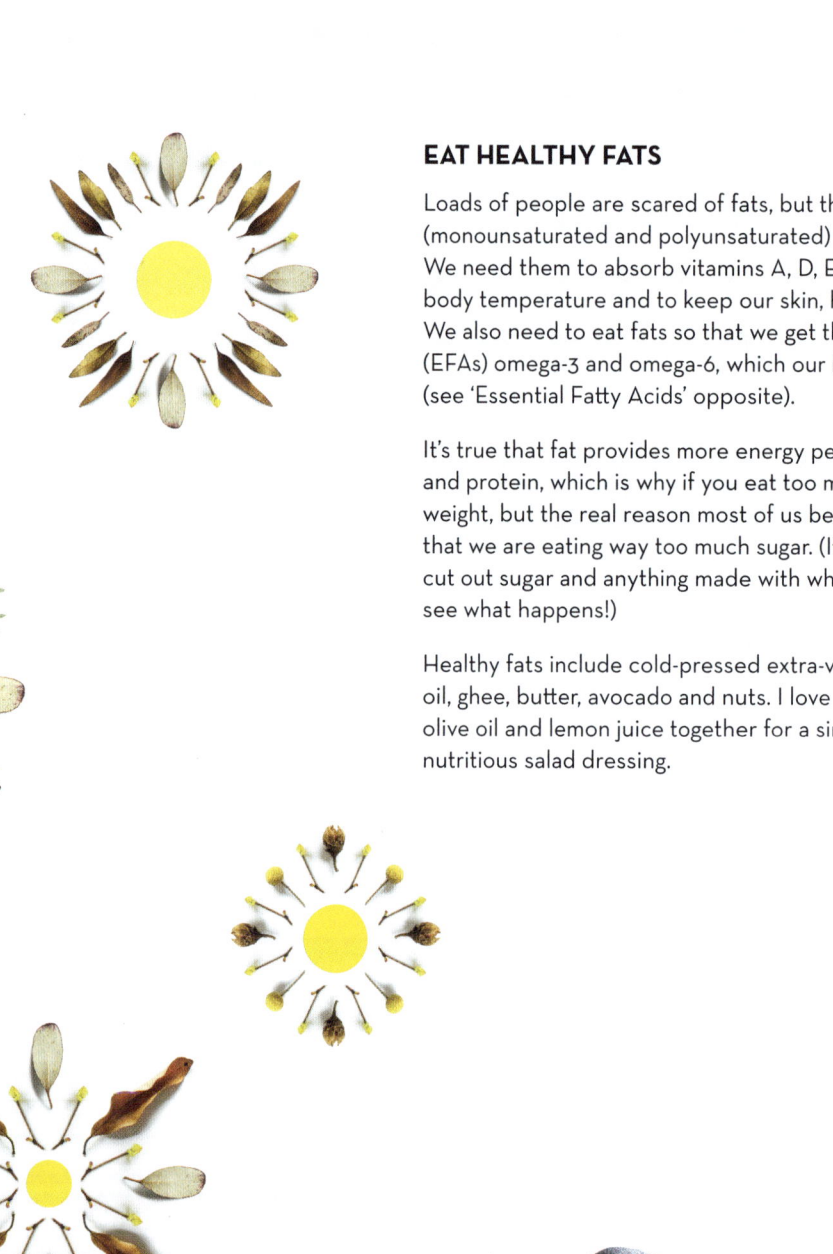

EAT HEALTHY FATS

Loads of people are scared of fats, but the healthy fats (monounsaturated and polyunsaturated) are super important. We need them to absorb vitamins A, D, E and K, to maintain body temperature and to keep our skin, hair and nails healthy. We also need to eat fats so that we get the essential fatty acids (EFAs) omega-3 and omega-6, which our bodies can't make (see 'Essential Fatty Acids' opposite).

It's true that fat provides more energy per gram than carbs and protein, which is why if you eat too much of it you will gain weight, but the real reason most of us become overweight is that we are eating way too much sugar. (If you don't believe me, cut out sugar and anything made with white flour for a week and see what happens!)

Healthy fats include cold-pressed extra-virgin olive oil, coconut oil, ghee, butter, avocado and nuts. I love mixing almond butter, olive oil and lemon juice together for a simple, delicious and nutritious salad dressing.

Essential fatty acids

There are several different types of omega-3 polyunsaturated fatty acids, but the long-chain omega-3s have been shown to have the most health benefits, particularly docosahexaenoic acid (DHA) and eicosapentaenoic acid (EPA), which are found in cold-water fish such as salmon, tuna, mackerel, sardines and herring.

Alpha-linolenic acid (ALA) is a short-chain omega-3 that's found in linseeds (flaxseeds), chia seeds, pumpkin seeds, canola, tofu and walnuts. However, ALA must be converted by the body to DHA and EPA, and because this synthesis is pretty inefficient we have to eat a lot more to get the same benefits as DHA and EPA.

When it comes to essential fatty acids, the balance is crucial. If we get lots more omega-6 than omega-3 (and in Australia, some researchers estimate that we're getting eight times more omega-6 than omega-3), it will interfere with the absorption of omega-3, an imbalance that some believe to be a contributing factor in the rise of cardiovascular disease, autoimmune diseases like arthritis, inflammatory disease and even cancer.

The best way to ensure you are getting enough omega-3 is to reduce your intake of omega-6. This means avoiding polyunsaturated oils that are high in omega-6, such as sunflower oil, safflower oil, grapeseed oil, rice bran oil and anything labelled 'vegetable oil'. Canola oil, walnut oil and soybean oil contain some short-chain omega-3s (ALA), but they've still got a lot more omega-6, which probably cancels out any benefit you'd get from the ALA – you're better off with a sprinkle of pumpkin seeds or chia seeds so you get the extra nutrients and fibre.

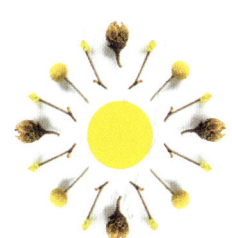

Always choose minimally processed ingredients that are as close to their natural state as possible.

EAT WHOLE GRAINS

If you're okay with gluten, please make sure you're eating foods made with whole grains, otherwise you may as well be eating sugar (see Processed Carbs on page 67). Personally, I feel bloated, gassy and uncomfortable whenever I eat gluten, so I prefer to get my slow-release carbs from quinoa, buckwheat and millet, which also happen to be high in protein, vitamins and fibre. (Despite the name, buckwheat doesn't contain wheat or gluten at all; in fact, it's more closely related to the rhubarb family.) Brown rice, wild rice, spelt, kamut and oats are also great options, though with all grain foods, make sure they don't take up too much of your plate. You want *at least* half of your plate to be veggies, about a quarter protein (this will be legumes and/or nuts if you're vegan and include some healthy fats) and about a quarter grain foods.

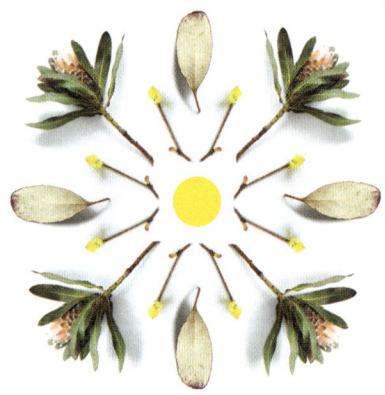
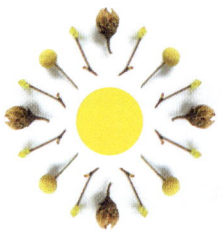
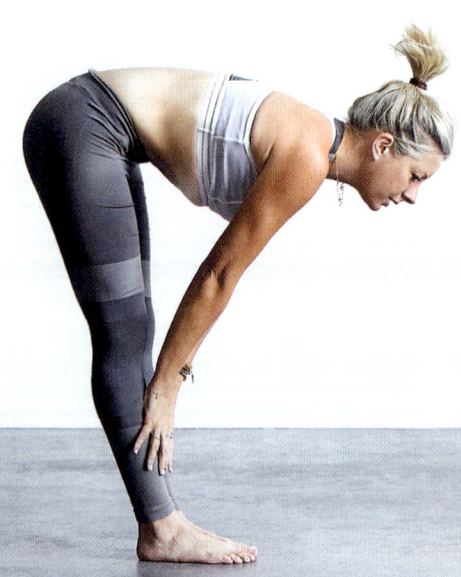

Gluten

Gluten is a protein found in wheat, rye and barley, and about one in one hundred Australians are allergic to it. This is called coeliac disease, where a sufferer's immune system reacts abnormally to gluten, attacking the lining of the gut. This reduces nutrient absorption and leads to serious symptoms, including chronic diarrhoea with foul, frothy or floating stools, anaemia, weight loss, muscle wasting and anxiety. Oats do not contain gluten, but they are often grown close to wheat, barley or rye crops, or processed on the same equipment, so most coeliac sufferers do not take the risk. They also contain a protein similar to gluten, which some people may react to.

Gluten intolerance, on the other hand, does not involve an immune response – people simply feel a bit gassy or bloated after they eat wheat-based foods, but are often okay eating ancient wheat varieties such as kamut and spelt. If you're not sure if you are gluten-intolerant, it's best to see a health professional rather than self-diagnose. And whatever you do, keep away from the highly processed 'gluten-free' foods in supermarkets – they are made with the same undesirable ingredients (sugar, salt, unhealthy fats and refined white flour). The only difference is that the flour has been even more chemically messed with to remove the gluten.

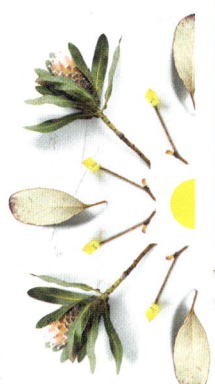
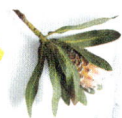
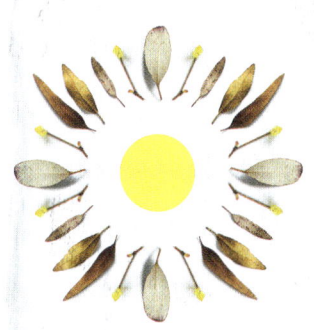
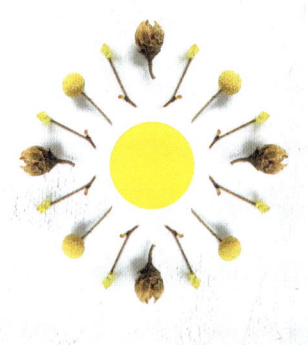

Fresh herbs and spices are the key to adding flavour to your food creations, not to mention the antioxidant hit you'll reap from them.

USE AYURVEDIC SPICES

Ayurveda is an ancient Indian form of healing that people still practise today. As with most traditional medicine, there are philosophical principles as well as the use of herbs and tinctures. Practitioners believe that each of us is made up of three different types of energy (doshas) – *vata*, *pitta* and *kapha* – and that the balance of these energies determines our health and wellbeing. Certain foods, herbs and spices can help increase or reduce doshas if they are out of balance.

Vata types	Pitta types	Kapha types
Light build	Strong, muscular build	Heavier build
Creative	Passionate	Stable
Soft-natured	Fiery-natured	Easygoing
Gentle	Productive	Methodical
Prefers warmth and humidity	Prefers cold climates	Prefers warm, dry climates
Dry skin	Fair skin	Oily skin

Asafoetida

In Ayurvedic medicine, garlic and onion are said to stimulate too much fire and passion, so this ground root is used instead as a flavour substitute. Even though it smells really strong, it has a calming effect on the body. People with fructose malabsorption may be familiar with asafoetida (also called hing), since it has a similar flavour to garlic and onion without the fructose.

Coriander

Coriander is another plant prized in Ayurvedic healing for its antioxidant and anti-inflammatory properties. Fresh coriander leaves are high in vitamin A and vitamin C, which means they're good for eyesight and skin health. The ground dried seeds are said to stimulate digestive secretions and to contain anti-fungal and even pain-relieving properties. Coriander is a key ingredient in making curries from scratch (I use the whole root – it's just as delicious as the leaves). I also love to toast the seeds and add them to salads, sprinkle them over roasted or barbecued meat or veggies – anything, really!

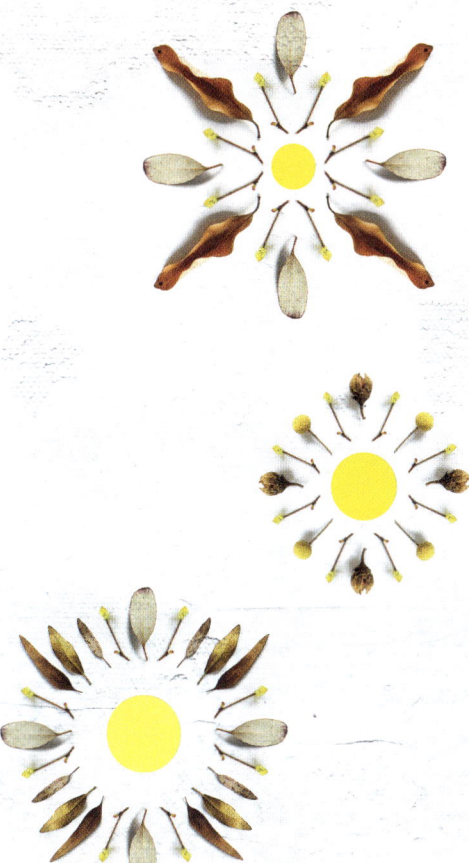

Cumin

Ground cumin seed is brilliant for digestion. It's said to stimulate bile secretion, so we're talking liver detoxification and the breaking down and digestion of fats. Cumin also provides the body with a nice whack of antioxidants, which help to prevent free-radical damage in the body. I like to add a pinch of cumin to avo mash (an ex-boyfriend taught me that trick).

Fennel

Fennel is actually a member of the carrot family, and the fresh bulb and fronds are an excellent source of vitamin C and potassium. (If you've never tried fennel before, my Fennel and Orange Salad on page 154 is a gorgeous introduction!) In Ayurvedic medicine, fennel seeds (whole or ground) are used as a digestive support, carminative (prevents flatulence) and vasodilator (helps reduce blood pressure). Due to their subtle, sweet liquorice flavour, fennel seeds are often confused with anise. They're used in chai tea blends and spice blends (especially five-spice powder), and are especially delicious with white fish, cucumber and soft cheeses like ricotta. If using the whole seeds to make tea or in cooking, make sure you crack them open with the flat side of a large knife to release the fragrant oil.

Ginger

Ginger, like most Ayurvedic spices, is known for its anti-inflammatory properties. It's great for digestion, and has long been used to combat nausea. It's also very warming so is good for circulation in the colder months. Use it freshly grated in your juice combos, salads and raw treats. Add a slice to boiled water to make fresh ginger tea. And if you don't have fresh ginger, ground dried ginger still has anti-inflammatory properties.

Turmeric

Turmeric is related to ginger, and, like ginger, its root (rhizome) is the main part used in cooking. (Its leaf is sometimes used in Indian cooking to wrap food.) Turmeric has been used in traditional medicine in India for over 2000 years to treat skin complaints such as eczema, certain allergies, and stomach and liver problems. Its active ingredient is curcumin, which has been shown to have potent antioxidant and anti-inflammatory properties. Population studies have even linked it to lower rates of diabetes and certain cancers, and research is now underway on its potential to help prevent Alzheimer's disease.

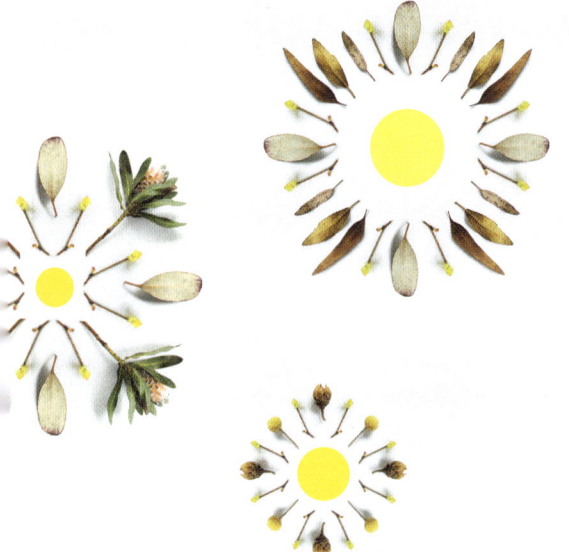

DRINK HERBAL TEAS

Herbal teas are a wonderful way to hydrate your body, and when you select the best herbs, you are also giving your body a lovely hit of antioxidants and other healing nutrients. Always go for teas in leaf form or use unbleached tea bags, so you're not introducing any unnecessary chemicals into your cuppa.

Chamomile

The tiny, delicate flowers of the chamomile plant are a well-known calmative, which means they help to calm your nervous system if you feel anxious or want help to fall asleep. Chamomile tea is also used to aid digestion and relieve flatulence.

Fennel

The seeds of this aromatic herb make a naturally sweet tea. I love drinking fennel tea after dinner to aid digestion. I buy organic fennel tea in unbleached teabags, but you could steep half a teaspoon of seeds in just-boiled water if you prefer.

Ginger

The roots of the ginger plant make a spicy tea that's great for digestion and circulation. (I love having it in the wintertime, as I get very cold fingers and toes.) Steep one or two thin slices of fresh ginger in a cup of boiled water for at least 5 minutes. It is very strong, so adjust with extra boiled water as you need. You can also buy organic ginger tea in unbleached teabags.

Liquorice

Liquorice root tea is naturally sweet and a great way to deal with sugar cravings when you are weaning yourself off sugary, processed foods. Although technically not an Ayurvedic herbal remedy, it is used in many traditional and alternative medicines for its potent anti-spasmodic, anti-inflammatory and anti-viral properties.

Tulsi

I've recently taken to drinking tulsi (holy basil) tea at night, as a great natural source of magnesium. In Ayurvedic medicine, it's said to stimulate digestive fire with its hot, sharp properties, and to be purifying and peaceful in nature. In India, this sacred plant is thought to bring blessings, so it is often found in people's homes or gardens.

Turmeric

Turmeric lattes are all the rage. I like them made with coconut milk and a touch of cinnamon and honey. They're caffeine free so totally fine to have at night time. See page 94 for a recipe.

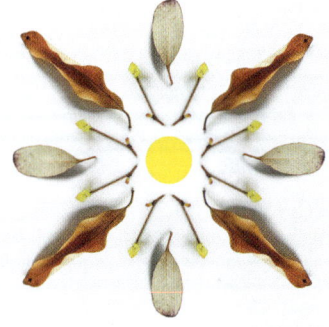

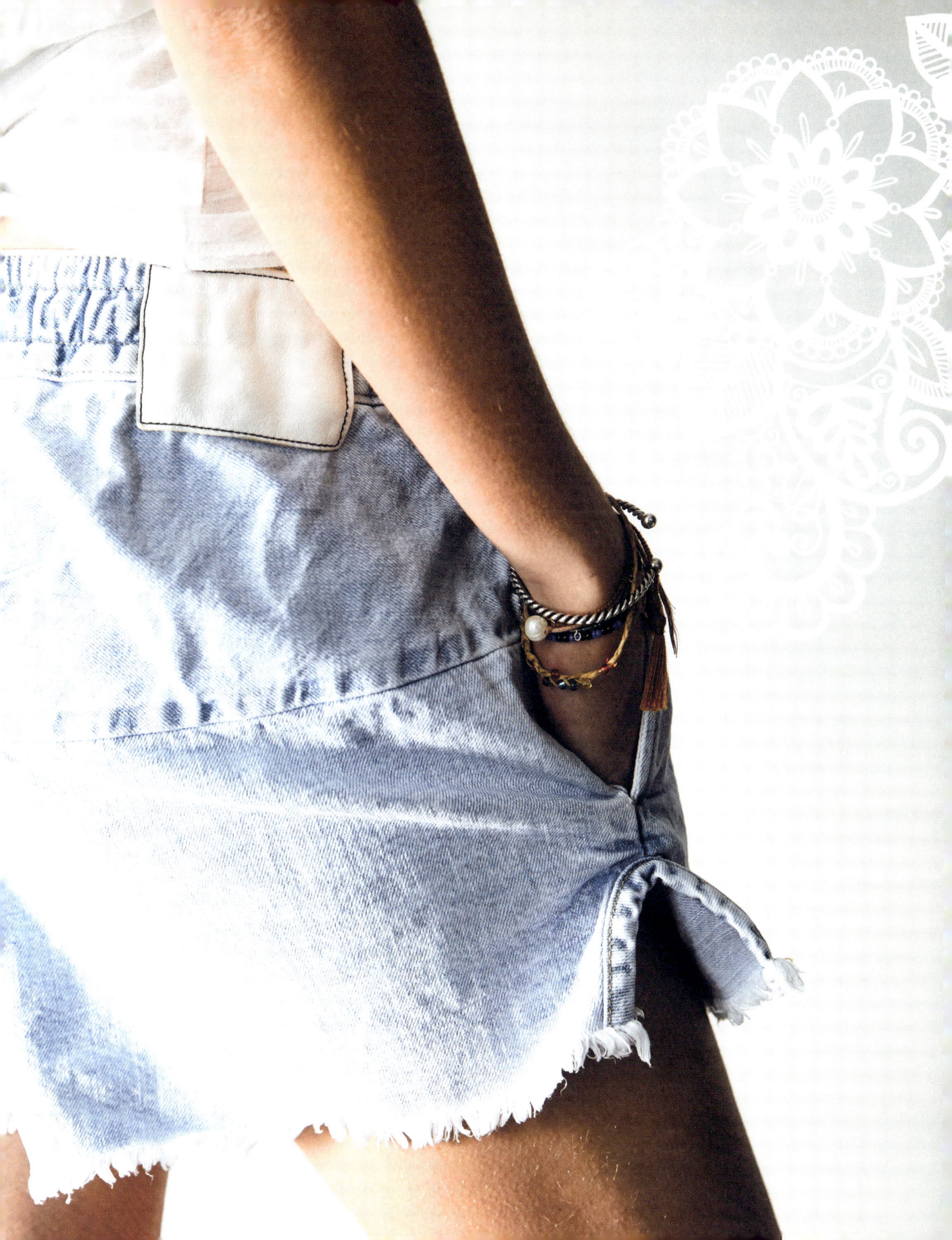

Eating is such a primal experience for us that we often do it on autopilot, shovelling in the food without really tasting it. Mindful eating is the practice of bringing your attention back to the present moment and noticing what you are doing, thinking and feeling.

STAY HEALTHY WHEN EATING OUT

This might sound like a challenge, especially when you are forced to eat out because you are travelling a lot. But, as my friend Karina once said to me, 'You can be healthy anywhere in the world and you can be unhealthy anywhere in the world.' I've never forgotten that comment, because it's so empowering. Yes, you're in charge.

When you're out for a meal, own it. Don't feel embarrassed. Check out the venue's menu online or phone ahead to see if they can accommodate your dietary requirements (they usually can). If not, just go somewhere else.

> **Here are some tips for clean eating when you're away from your own kitchen:**
>
> - Order grilled protein (no batter, no deep-frying)
> - Ask for any sauces and dressings to be served on the side so you can decide how much you want
> - Ask for extra veggies or salad instead of chips
> - Say no to the bread basket (or give it to someone else at the table who wants it)
> - Split a treat with a friend, or ask for it without cream or ice cream.

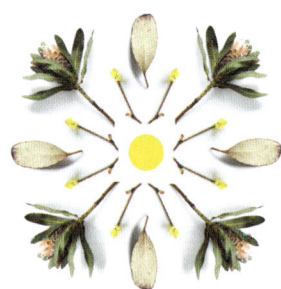

When I'm out, I always go for a protein that I rarely cook at home, or one that I haven't tried before. I also don't beat myself up if I have a treat (especially when I'm sharing a birthday cake with a friend!). If you choose to eat a treat, enjoy every morsel. Eating mindfully is a way to nourish your body, mind and soul.

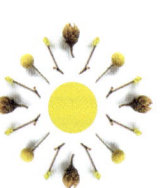
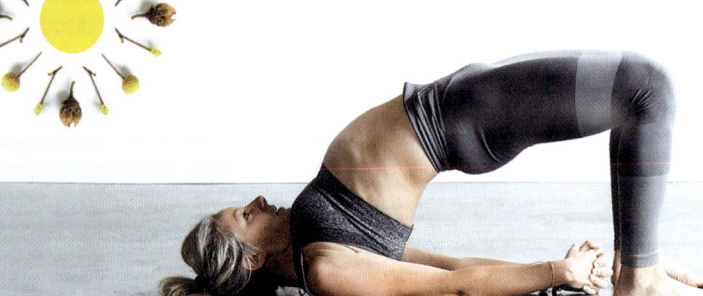

A typical day in my yoga life

I start the day with yoga – either a 60-minute vinyasa flow class, or if I'm doing my own practice, it's usually 20–30 minutes. I pop on some chilled music and start with a few rounds of sun A (see page 36), then I do a bit of a flowing sequence followed by a balance or backbend, and then I open the hips and chill in savasana (see page 55).

Breakfast for me is usually a green smoothie or, in winter, a quinoa porridge. Lunch is usually something like the Zenned-out Veggies on page 160 (kale, sweet spud, goat's feta, sunflower seeds and a couple of boiled eggs). For a midafternoon snack, I'll have raw nuts (or energy balls if I've done more training).

For dinner I always come back to a simple meal of protein (usually fish, chicken or eggs) with green veggies and some kind of healthy fat. One of my favourite green veggie combos is broccoli, spinach and avocado topped with extra-virgin olive oil and lemon zest. Sometimes I'll throw a few crushed brazil nuts or macadamia nuts on top for added texture and flavour.

If I'm having a treat I'll go for a small serve of berries or chopped pineapple with coconut yoghurt and a pinch of sugar-free granola. Or even better, a little slice of Paleo Chamomile and Lemon Loaf (see page 136) with a dollop of coconut yoghurt – it's super calming and really hits that sweet spot without any stimulating ingredients. (I avoid chocolate after dinner, as it's a natural source of caffeine and tends to keep me awake.)

I try not to eat in front of my laptop, phone or TV. If I do take a snap for Instagram I'll always pop my phone aside afterwards and really enjoy the meal that I've created. Just before I eat, I take a moment to feel grateful that I have such nourishing food, and I savour every mouthful.

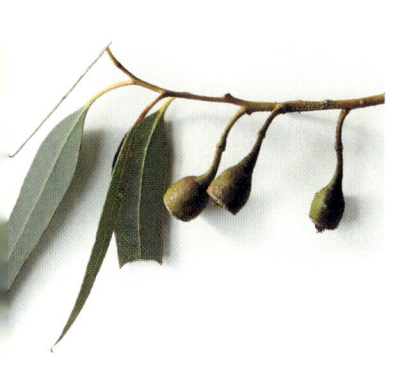 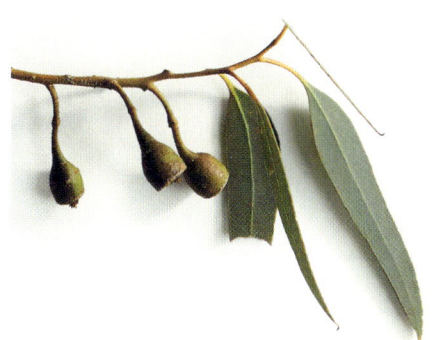

SEVEN-DAY VEGAN CLEANSE

Pressing 'reset' on your body, mind and soul with a simple seven-day cleanse is a great way to get into the yoga zone.

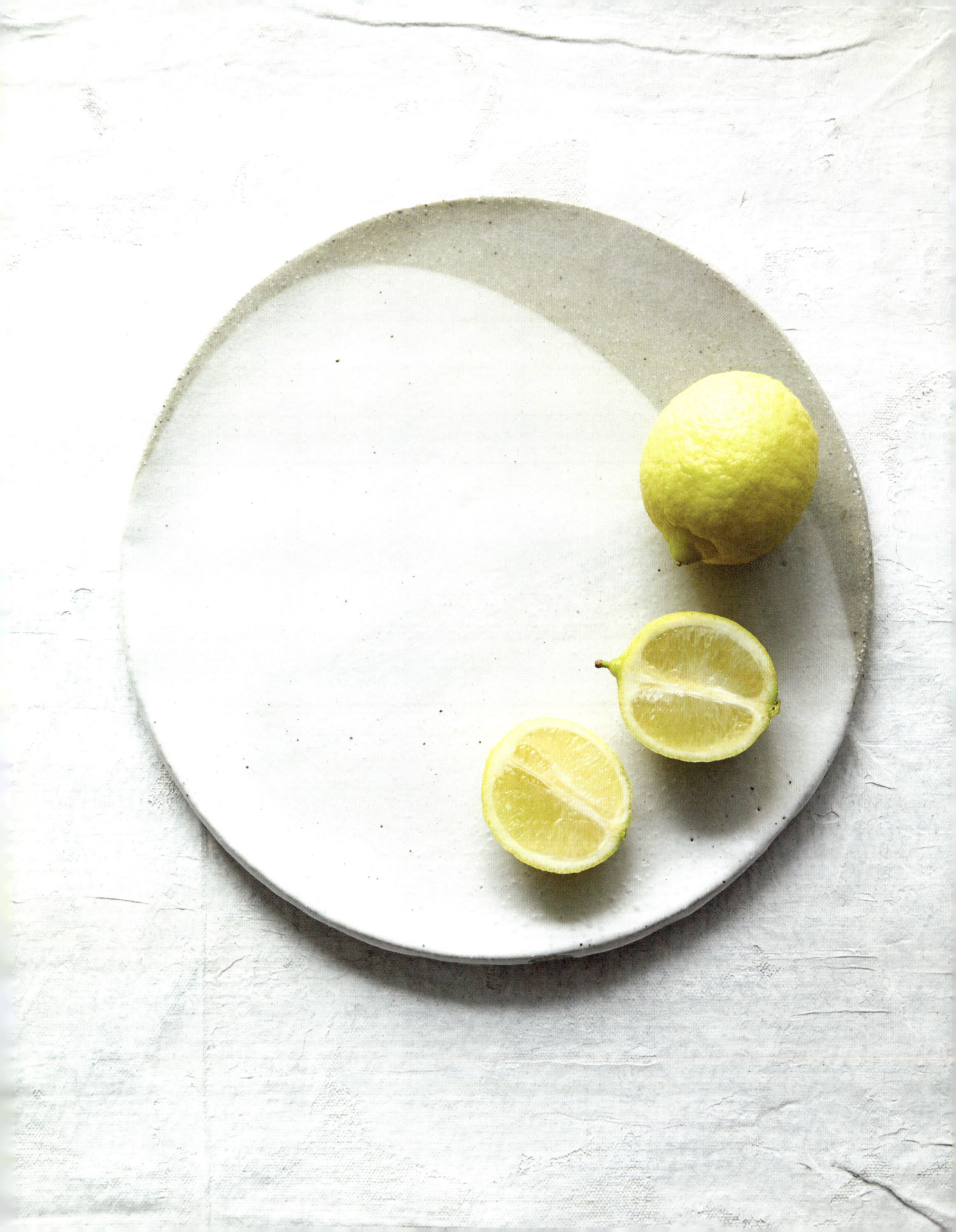

> 'Often the pain we feel is the breaking of the shell that encloses us.'
> **BARON BAPTISTE (POWER YOGA TEACHER)**

During my training to become a yoga teacher, I spent a week on a vegan retreat. It was a great experience, as it not only helped me to detox physically, but also emotionally. I kept a journal to write about old issues that came up for me, and afterwards I felt like I had pressed 'reset' on my body, mind and soul.

To help you experience that same clarity, I have created a seven-day vegan cleanse. The recipes contain no meat or dairy, though there is protein in the form of sprouts, nuts, seeds and quinoa. I've also left out wheat, onion, chilli and garlic, as wheat is known to cause digestive issues for some people, and onion, garlic and chilli stimulate too much pitta (fire) – we are going for a calming effect with this cleanse. This might sound scary if you are used to eating loads of these things – I'm a chilli head! – but don't worry, I use plenty of fresh herbs, salt flakes and freshly ground black pepper for flavour.

If you feel you need to up the protein at any point, simply add two boiled, poached or scrambled eggs to any of the meals (or add sesame seeds, dulse flakes, yeast flakes or chia seeds if you're vegan). I'm not a fan of soy-based products, as most soy grown is genetically modified, but feel free to include some tofu or tempeh if you like. Tempeh is preferable as it is fermented and therefore easier for the body to digest.

To be clear, this is a short-term eating plan to use for one week only – it is not an eating regime to follow long term. There are no cheat meals, or healthy-but-still-sweet treats. It is designed to give your digestive system, liver and kidneys a complete rest, which has flow-on effects for the rest of your body – everything from your circulation to your sleep, to your immune function. I should point out, however, that you will feel pretty feral for the first few days – you'll probably be very hungry and will be fighting cravings (especially for things like coffee and sugar). If you drink lots of coffee you'll probably have a headache for the first 2–3 days and feel more emotionally sensitive. This is where the yoga and meditation can really help. Try to remember that you are doing this for you, and that the bigger the challenge, the greater the opportunity for growth.

Get organised

Before you start the cleanse, I recommend giving away foods that you know are unhealthy and that might tempt you to stray from healthy eating. I'm talking highly processed foods, such as sweet or savoury biscuits, chips, sugary drinks or anything in a container or packet with an ingredients list that you need a chemistry degree to understand. (See Tips for Clean Eating on pages 65–81 for further information.)

Also, it's best to buy the food you need for the week ahead and prepare as many of the ingredients as you can before you start. That way, you are less likely to fall off the wagon.

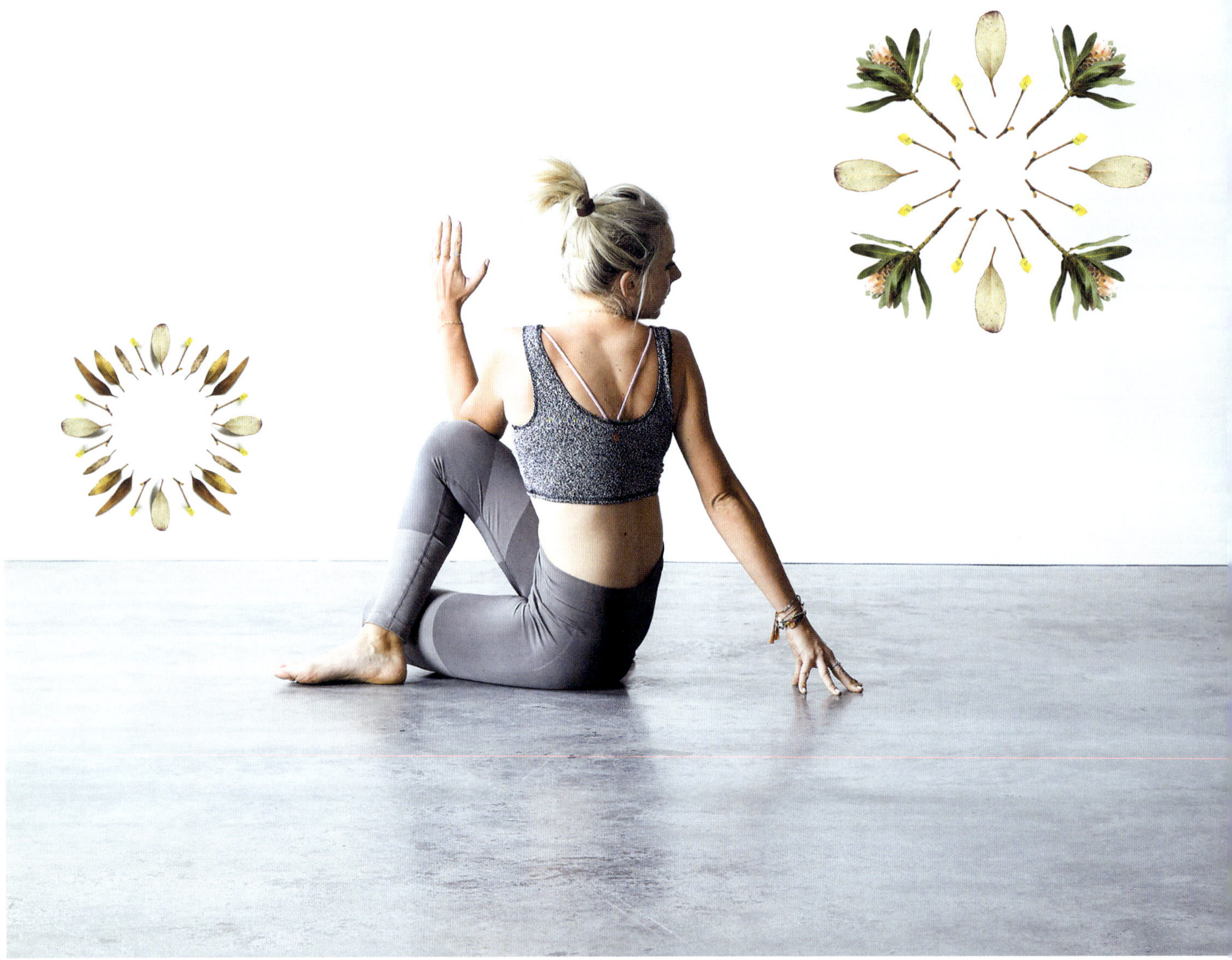

Shopping list

- 2 asparagus spears
- 30 g basil leaves
- 1 head of broccoli
- ½ head red cabbage
- 1 carrot
- 1 continental cucumber
- 2 garlic cloves
- 1 packet mung bean (or chickpea) sprouts
- 2 mushrooms
- handful of rocket
- 225 g baby spinach
- 1 bunch of spring onions
- 3–4 sweet potatoes
- 1 large zucchini
- 1 apple
- 4 avocados
- 4 bananas (peel, halve and freeze 2)
- 2 punnets blueberries
- 2 punnets cherry tomatoes
- 4–5 lemons
- 1 punnet strawberries
- 310 g almonds
- 155 g brazil nuts
- 120 g cashew nuts
- 160 g macadamia nuts
- 115 g pine nuts
- handful of pistachio nuts
- black pepper
- ground cinnamon
- ground nutmeg
- salt flakes
- sweet paprika
- ground turmeric
- herbal teas (nettle, detox, liquorice, chamomile, fennel)
- stevia (liquid)
- 1 small jar of almond butter
- 1.5 litres almond milk
- 1 small bottle of apple cider vinegar
- 1 small jar of coconut oil
- 500 ml coconut water
- 200 ml extra-virgin olive oil
- 1 small jar of tahini
- 600 g quinoa
- 100 g rolled oats

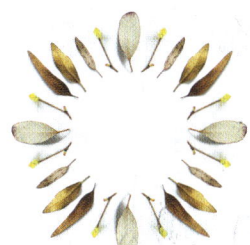
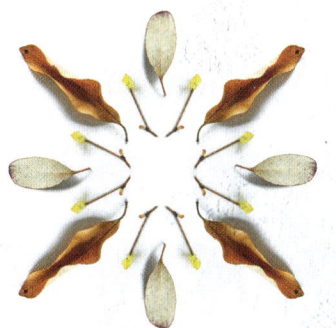

PREP DAY RECIPES

You can prepare these recipes the night before starting the cleanse. It will really help you stay on track if you have these ingredients ready to go in the fridge.

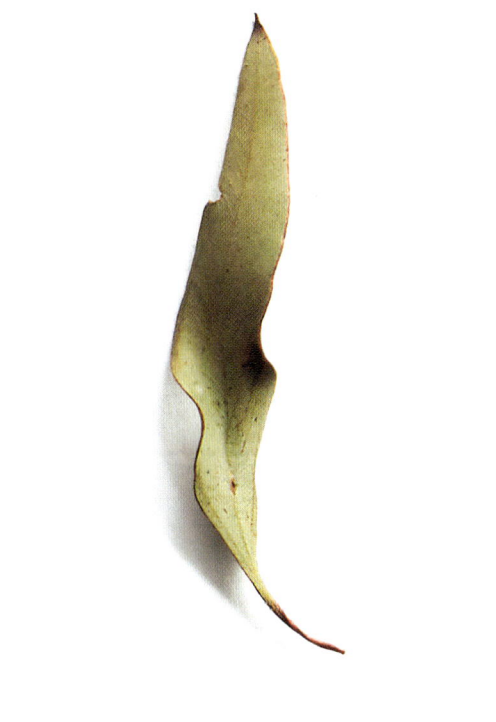

ROASTED SWEET POTATO

Sweet potato is one of my favourite veggies. It is also high in fibre and an excellent source of vitamins A and C.

SERVES 4

2–3 sweet potatoes, scrubbed, cut into 2 cm cubes

2 teaspoons sweet paprika

salt flakes

2–3 tablespoons coconut oil

Preheat the oven to 180°C.

Place the sweet potato in a roasting tin. Sprinkle over the paprika and salt. Add the coconut oil and use your fingers to toss the potato until all the pieces are well covered. Roast for 15–20 minutes, or until the potato is soft and the edges are browned and caramelised.

Allow to cool, then store in the fridge in a sealed container for up to 4 days.

VEGAN BASIL PESTO

Pesto sauces are an easy way to liven up a simple meal with loads of fresh herbs – in this case, delicious basil.

SERVES 4

¾ cup (115 g) pine nuts, toasted

3 tablespoons cashew nuts (activated if possible, see page 108)

1 loosely packed cup (30 g) basil leaves

2 garlic cloves

zest and juice of 1 lemon

3 tablespoons extra-virgin olive oil, plus extra if needed

salt flakes and freshly ground black pepper

Place all the ingredients in a food processor or blender and blitz to your desired consistency (you may need to add some extra oil). Season to taste and store in an airtight container in the fridge for up to 5 days.

BASIC COOKED QUINOA

You can either cook your quinoa ahead of time or make it as you go. I use a mixture of black, red and white quinoa as I love the colours and the nutty flavours, but you can use whatever you prefer. This makes about six cups of cooked quinoa, which you can store in the fridge in a sealed container for up to 1 week and use as you need.

SERVES 4

2 cups (400 g) quinoa, rinsed and drained

Place the quinoa in a saucepan with 1 litre of water. Cover and bring to the boil over a medium heat. Reduce the heat to low and cook, uncovered, for 10–15 minutes or until the water is absorbed and the quinoa has sprouted little tails. Drain, fluff with a fork and allow to cool. Either use some of the cooked quinoa to make up a big salad, or transfer it to a sealed container and keep in the fridge, ready to use as you need it.

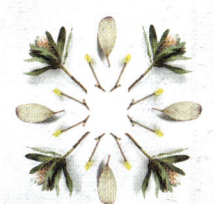
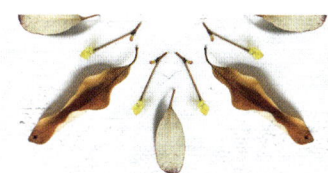
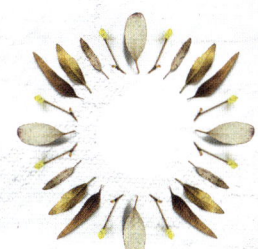

THE RECIPES

I want you to know that leafy greens are all-you-can-eat! So if you want to use more broccoli or spinach than the amounts I suggest, please go for it; or if you want to add in some kale, beet greens or any fresh herb such as coriander, basil or parsley, please do (fresh herbs give any dish an amazing lift). Also, be creative with the ingredients. If it's winter, roast your veggies or turn them into soups. If it's spring or summer, make the most of seasonal berries or other fresh veggies like asparagus, and add them to your salads.

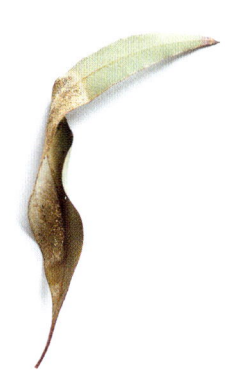

DETOX GREEN SMOOTHIE

This is my go-to green smoothie. It's full of greens and antioxidants, as well as enough energy from the banana and cashews to keep you going all morning or afternoon.

SERVES 1

2 handfuls of baby spinach

3 tablespoons blueberries, or other fresh berries

½ banana (frozen)

3 tablespoons cashew nuts (activated if possible, see page 108)

pinch of ground cinnamon

2 cups (500 ml) almond milk or coconut water

Place all of the ingredients in a blender and pulse until well combined.

CREAMY ALMOND OATS

I love to serve my oats with banana, but they're also delicious with fresh berries.

SERVES 1

½ cup (50 g) rolled oats

1 cup (250 ml) almond milk

½ banana, sliced

pinch of ground cinnamon

Place the oats and almond milk in a saucepan over a medium heat and bring to a simmer. Cook, uncovered, stirring frequently, until the oats are soft (about 5 minutes). You may need to add a splash of water to reach your desired consistency. Transfer to a serving bowl with the banana and sprinkle over the cinnamon.

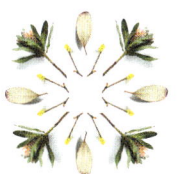

SPICED TURMERIC OATS

The addition of fragrant nutmeg and cinnamon, and earthy turmeric with its golden glow, makes this brekkie extra special.

SERVES 1

½ cup (50 g) rolled oats

1 cup (250 ml) almond milk

½ teaspoon ground turmeric

½ banana, sliced

5 macadamia nuts (activated if possible, see page 108), chopped

pinch of ground nutmeg

pinch of ground cinnamon

Place the oats, almond milk and turmeric in a saucepan over a medium heat and bring to a simmer. Cook, uncovered, stirring frequently, until the oats are soft (about 5 minutes). You may need to add a splash of water to reach your desired consistency. Transfer to a serving bowl, then add the banana, macadamias and spices.

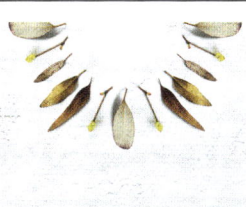

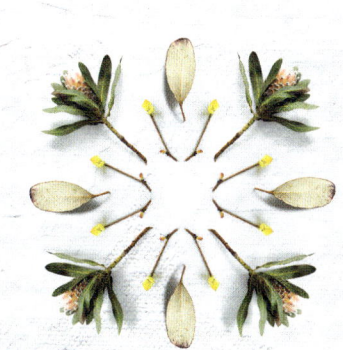

QUINOA PORRIDGE

This nourishing bowl of goodness will well and truly set you up for the day. And it's so quick to make when you've cooked your quinoa in advance.

SERVES 1

½ cup Basic Cooked Quinoa (see page 89)

1 cup (250 ml) almond milk

½ cup (75 g) fresh blueberries

1 teaspoon coconut oil

2–3 drops of stevia

Place the quinoa, almond milk, blueberries, coconut oil and stevia in a saucepan over a medium heat and bring to a simmer. Cook, uncovered, stirring frequently, until creamy (about 5 minutes). You may need to add a splash of water to reach your desired consistency. Transfer to a serving bowl.

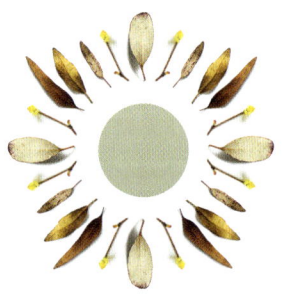

SIMPLE VEGGIE BOWL

Simplicity is the name of the game here: lightly dressed and seasoned veggies with some nice healthy fats from the avocado. Yum!

SERVES 2

1–2 cups (90–180 g) chopped broccoli florets

½ cup Roasted Sweet Potato (see page 88, or cook it fresh if you prefer)

½ avocado, cubed

DRESSING

2 tablespoons extra-virgin olive oil

juice of ½ lemon

salt flakes and freshly ground black pepper

Place the dressing ingredients in a jar and shake to combine.

Place the broccoli in a small saucepan with 2 cm of water. Cover and bring to the boil over a medium heat. Simmer for 2–3 minutes, or until the broccoli has softened but still has crunch. Drain, place in a serving bowl with the sweet potato and toss (this will warm the sweet potato). Add the avocado and the dressing and toss gently until everything is coated.

ZUCCHINI PASTA SALAD

This is a favourite meal of mine. It's so clean and satisfying.

SERVES 2

1 large zucchini, sliced into long, thin strips with a spiraliser or veggie peeler

½ carrot, sliced into long, strips with a spiraliser or veggie peeler (or grated)

2 mushrooms, chopped

1 spring onion, sliced

small pinch of salt flakes

½ punnet (125 g) cherry tomatoes, quartered

½ continental cucumber, chopped

3 tablespoons Vegan Basil Pesto (see page 89)

Gently toss all the ingredients together with the pesto. Serve immediately.

Alternatively, sauté the zucchini, carrot, mushrooms, spring onion and salt in 2 teaspoons of extra-virgin olive oil for 1 minute. Mix through the cherry tomatoes, cucumber and pesto and serve.

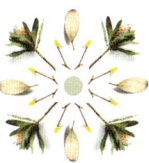

SUPERFOOD SALAD

Make a double batch of this salad and the dressing and store them separately in the fridge for up to three days. Simply combine and toss before you eat.

SERVES 2

handful of baby spinach

handful of finely shredded red cabbage

½ cup mung bean (or chickpea) sprouts

½ spring onion, finely sliced

½ punnet (125 g) cherry tomatoes, quartered

½ cup (75 g) blueberries

½ cup (80 g) almonds, (activated if possible, see page 108), roughly chopped

½ cup Basic Cooked Quinoa (see page 89)

basil leaves, torn

DRESSING

3 tablespoons extra-virgin olive oil

juice of 1 lemon

2 tablespoons tahini

salt flakes and freshly ground black pepper.

Place the dressing ingredients in a jar and shake to combine. Combine the salad ingredients in a large bowl. Add the dressing and toss well.

QUINOA SALAD

Using your pre-cooked quinoa, this fuss-free salad is as simple as tossing everything together in a bowl.

SERVES 2

1 cup Basic Cooked Quinoa (see page 89)

½ punnet (125 g) cherry tomatoes

handful of baby spinach, roughly chopped

small handful of rocket, roughly chopped

½ avocado, sliced

2 asparagus spears or ¼ cup (45 g) chopped broccoli florets, steamed

½ cup fresh berries (any kind)

2 tablespoons extra-virgin olive oil

1 tablespoon apple cider vinegar

Combine all of the ingredients in a serving bowl and toss gently.

TURMERIC LATTE

This warming drink is the easiest way to get some medicinal spices into your diet.

SERVES 1

1 cup (250 ml) almond milk

¼ teaspoon ground turmeric

pinch of ground nutmeg

pinch of ground cinnamon, plus extra to serve

2–3 drops of stevia

Place all the ingredients in a small saucepan and heat gently for 3–5 minutes, stirring occasionally. Pour into a mug and top with an extra sprinkle of cinnamon.

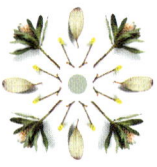

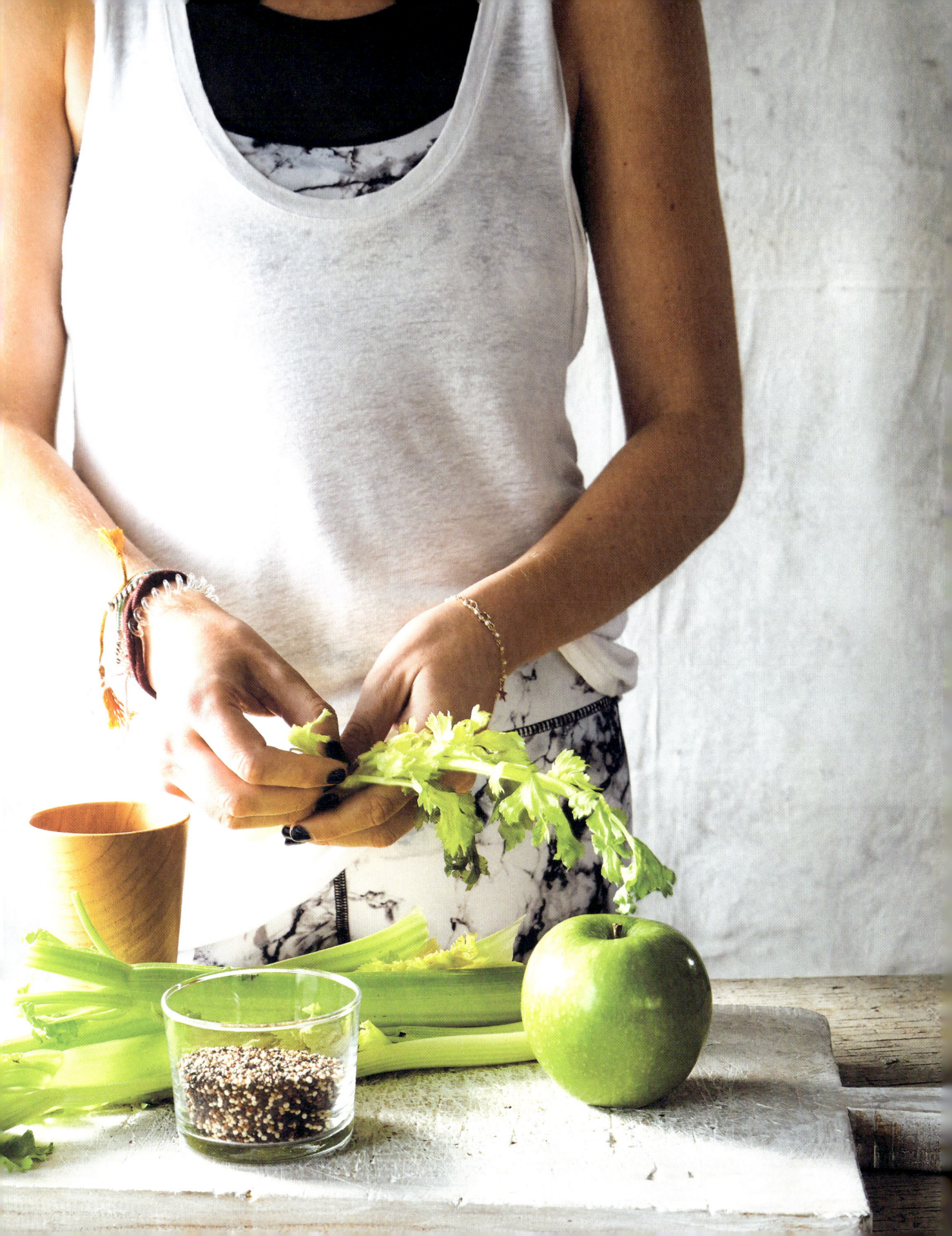

COPING WITH CRAVINGS

If this is your first cleanse, I have to be honest – you will be VERY hungry on the first day, and you will probably feel pretty rough as you withdraw from caffeine and/or sugar. Try to remember that the first two days are always the hardest and that you will feel amazing by the end.

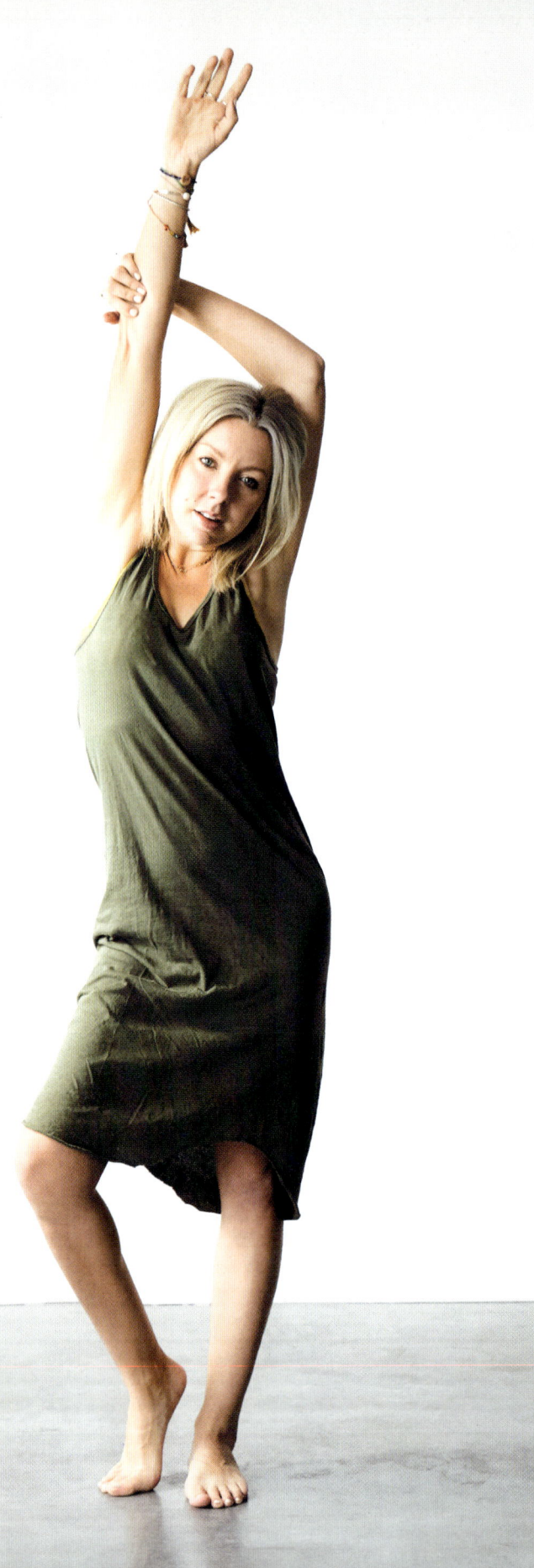

I have a saying when I'm on a cleanse: 'Flick the switch.' What I mean by that is do something that changes the channel: go for a walk, see a mate, go to the movies, anything to get your mind off food! And if you're really craving sweet foods, snack on banana slices topped with raw almonds or apple slices spread with almond butter (try to have half a banana and half an apple for each snack if you are having these in addition to your normal daily snacks). The sweetness of the fruit is balanced by the satisfying healthy fats in the almonds.

Breathe deeply

If you are struggling with cravings, and the tips I mentioned earlier aren't working, try focusing on taking a few deep breaths. I know it sounds weird, but you can actually influence your whole mental state by breathing in this way. Think about it. When you're anxious, your breathing is fast and shallow (which means you're only using the top part of your lungs). But when you're calm and centred, your breathing is slow and deep (your diaphragm lifts up to allow your lungs to fill with air). To practise deep breathing, simply sit down and clasp your hands behind your head – this opens your chest and allows your diaphragm to do its job. Or you could just place your hands on your belly and take ten slow breaths – your hands should rise slightly with each inhalation. Considering that you take a breath about 21,600 times per day, it makes sense that the more relaxed your breathing is, the more relaxed you'll be feeling.

Drink water

Please drink at least 2 litres of water every single day. This is especially important when you are on a cleanse, as the idea is to flush your kidneys and other organs of elimination, and there's no flushing without plenty of water!

Did you know that the first sign of dehydration is actually hunger? Headaches, moodiness and feeling tired are also signs of dehydration. In fact, by the time you are actually feeling thirsty you are already dehydrated. So think about having a big bottle or glass on your desk so it's in front of you all day long.

Eat mindfully

Mindfulness is about observing your thoughts and letting them go rather than attaching to them and letting them take you down a rabbit hole of worry. It's about bringing your attention to the present moment – to what you are noticing with your senses. When it comes to food, you want to taste the flavours, feel the textures and smell the different aromas. To do this, make sure you are seated for every meal and that there are no distractions (no screens, no loud music). Smile before you take your first bite and thank yourself for taking such good care of your body. Then really chew each mouthful rather than just gulping it down. This is great for your digestion, plus it helps to trigger satiety hormones, so you will feel much fuller.

Morning yoga
Several rounds of sun A (see page 36) followed by the warrior poses (see page 41) and triangle pose (see page 60).

Evening yoga
Run through the Sleep sequence on page 58. Finish up with knees to chest pose (see page 61).

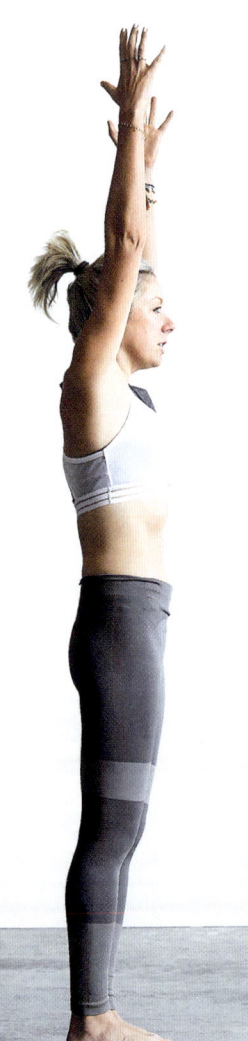

DAY 1

<u>Morning yoga</u>

<u>Digestion starter</u>
1 tablespoon lemon juice in 1 cup warm water

<u>Breakfast</u>
Detox Green Smoothie (see page 90)

<u>Snack</u>
10 x raw almonds + detox tea

<u>Lunch</u>
Simple Veggie Bowl (see page 92)

<u>Snack</u>
5 x brazil nuts

<u>Dinner</u>
Zucchini Pasta Salad (see page 93; make enough for tomorrow's lunch)

<u>Evening yoga</u>

DAY 2

<u>Morning yoga</u>

<u>Digestion starter</u>
1 tablespoon lemon juice in 1 cup warm water

<u>Breakfast</u>
Creamy Almond Oats (see page 91)

<u>Snack</u>
10 x macadamia nuts + nettle tea

<u>Lunch</u>
Zucchini Pasta Salad (leftovers)

<u>Snack</u>
Sliced ½ banana (left over from breakfast), sprinkled with cinnamon

<u>Dinner</u>
Simple Veggie Bowl (see page 92; steam enough greens for tomorrow's lunch)

Chamomile tea

<u>Evening yoga</u>

Midweek motivation
You may start craving sugary things around days 2 and 3. Stay strong! Know it will pass, and go for berries or liquorice tea to help with the sweet cravings.

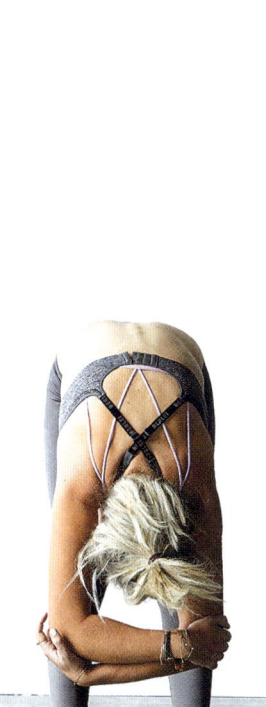

DAY 3

Morning yoga

Digestion starter
1 tablespoon lemon juice in 1 cup warm water

Breakfast
Spiced Turmeric Oats (see page 91)

Snack
1 apple sliced and spread with 2 tablespoons almond butter and sprinkled with cinnamon + detox tea

Lunch
Leftover greens with Vegan Basil Pesto, pistachios and ½ an avocado

Snack
10 x raw almonds

Dinner
Superfood Salad (see page 93; make enough for tomorrow's lunch)

Turmeric latte (see page 94)

Evening yoga

DAY 4

Morning yoga

Digestion starter
1 tablespoon lemon juice in 1 cup warm water

Breakfast
Detox Green Smoothie (see page 90)

Snack
10 x raw almonds + liquorice tea

Lunch
Superfood Salad (leftovers)

Snack
handful of strawberries

Dinner
Quinoa Salad (see page 94; make enough for tomorrow's lunch)

Fennel tea

Evening yoga

DAY 5

__Morning yoga__

__Digestion starter__
1 tablespoon lemon juice
in 1 cup warm water

__Breakfast__
Spiced Turmeric Oats (see page 91)

__Snack__
10 x raw almonds
+ nettle tea

__Lunch__
Quinoa Salad (leftovers)

__Snack__
5 x brazil nuts

__Dinner__
Zucchini Pasta Salad
(see page 93; make enough
for tomorrow's lunch)

Chamomile tea

__Evening yoga__

DAY 6

__Morning yoga__

__Digestion starter__
1 tablespoon lemon juice
in 1 cup warm water

__Breakfast__
Quinoa Porridge (see page 92)

__Snack__
handful of berries + detox tea

__Lunch__
Zucchini Pasta Salad
(leftovers, with extra greens)

__Snack__
10 x raw almonds

__Dinner__
Simple Veggie Bowl (see page 92;
make enough for tomorrow's lunch)

Fennel tea

__Evening yoga__

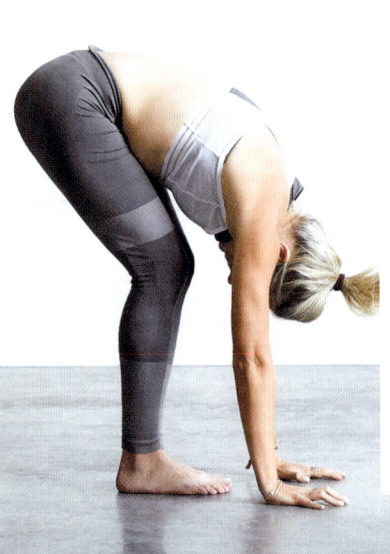

DAY 7

Morning yoga

Digestion starter
1 tablespoon lemon juice in 1 cup warm water

Breakfast
Detox Green Smoothie (see page 90)

Snack
10 x almonds + nettle tea

Lunch
Leftover or fresh steamed greens with avocado, almond butter, sprouts and nuts

Snack
handful of berries

Dinner
Zucchini Pasta Salad (page 93)

Turmeric Latte (page 94)

Evening yoga

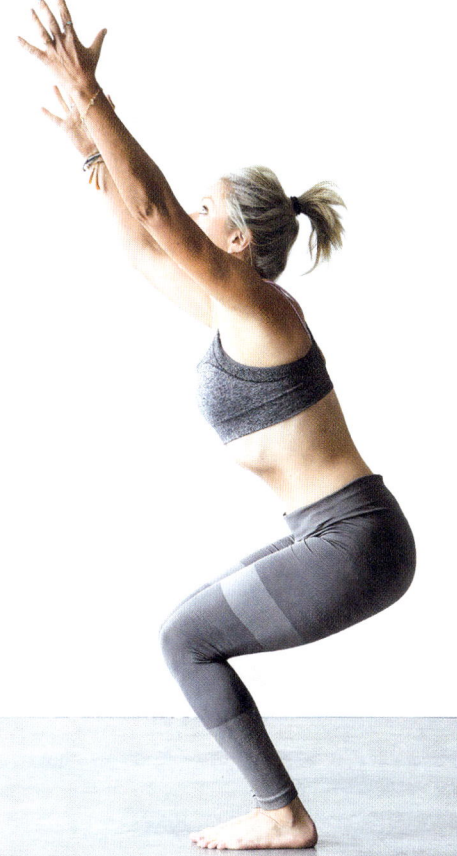

Congratulations!
If you have been able to stick to the cleanse for the whole week, you will be feeling amazing! Your tastebuds will be changing and you will feel bright, clear and connected. Notice this feeling and how much good stuff happens from this space.

Now that you're familiar with the principles of clean eating and some of the traditional concepts around yoga and food, such as vegetarianism and the Ayurvedic style of eating, you can choose recipes from the following pages to best suit your diet and lifestyle. The drinks, breakfasts and savoury and sweet dishes in this section are all designed to go hand in hand with your yoga practice, being high in nutrients and based around good-quality, unrefined wholefoods. Enjoy the healthy-eating journey!

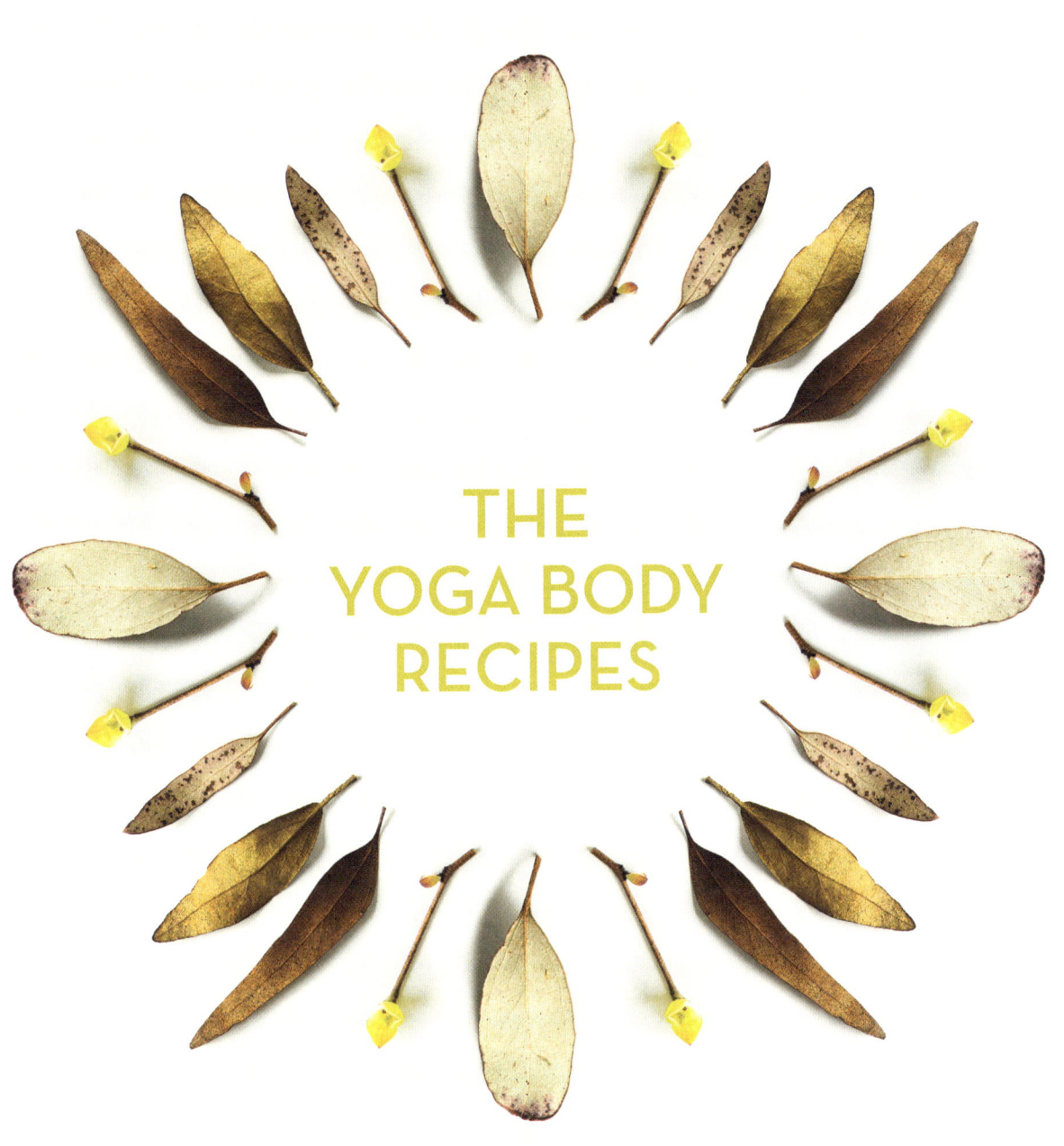

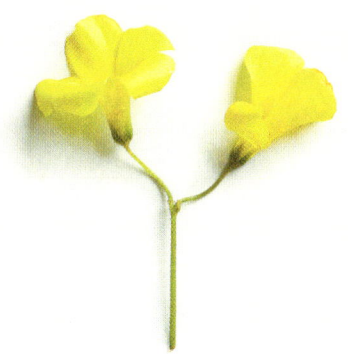

NOTES ON THE RECIPES

Wherever possible, all the foods I use in my recipes are whole, raw, organic, seasonal, unprocessed and as close to their natural state as possible. If you can, do the same. The following ingredients appear in lots of my recipes, and I want to share a couple of tips here just in case you're not familiar with their preparation or use.

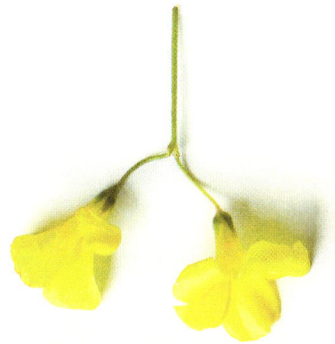

Cooking temperatures in my recipes are for a conventional oven. If you are using a fan-forced oven, you'll need to drop the temperature by 10–20°C (check your oven manual).

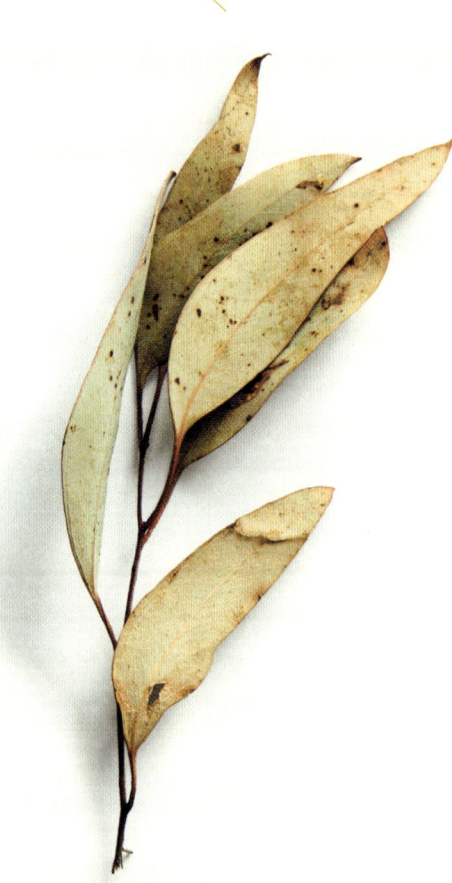

Assume that any fresh fruits (bananas, mangoes, avocados etc.) are ripe, unless I say otherwise.

Almond butter

This ground almond paste, with all its lovely oils, is a wonderful butter substitute. I prefer mine raw (not roasted) because it's the healthier option. Almonds are loaded with fibre, good fats and protein, plus they've got a fair bit of magnesium and calcium, too.

Almond meal (almond flour)

This grain-free flour is another kitchen staple. Whole almond meal has a coarse texture and is great in brekkie creations, for crumbing meats and fish, and even in desserts and raw treats. Blanched almond meal (often called almond flour) is more refined, as the almond skin is removed before grinding.

Bee pollen

Bee pollen is the soft yellow 'dust' from flowers that bees brush into the pollen sacs on their back legs. It's very high in protein and other nutrients. People with pollen allergies should avoid bee pollen; vegans might prefer to leave it out, too. I sprinkle it on pancakes, porridge and smoothies.

Buckwheat

Despite its name, buckwheat is not a grain but the fruit of a plant related to sorrel and rhubarb. It's sold as groats or flour. Groats are the light-coloured kernels that you can buy whole or ground (cracked) and either raw or roasted (called kasha). Buckwheat flour is available in light and dark versions. The darker type contains more of the hull, and therefore more fibre and other nutrients, and has a stronger, nuttier flavour. I love to use buckwheat groats for porridge or as a replacement for burghul (cracked wheat) in tabouli. Buckwheat flour makes delicious pancakes and slices, and I often add it to gluten-free recipes.

Cacao

Technically, cacao and cocoa are the same thing, but in everyday use, cacao usually refers to the raw, unprocessed beans, and cocoa to the beans that have been roasted and processed (and usually combined with milk and sugar to make chocolate). Raw cacao powder is the healthiest way to get a chocolate hit; add it to a smoothie, or make hot chocolate, energy balls or a raw choccy cake. It's delicious and full of health benefits, especially for our brains. It's high in magnesium (great for our muscles and heart) and phenylalanine, a precursor to two brain chemicals that make us feel good (norepinephrine and dopamine) – maybe that's why we love chocolate so much!

Chia seeds

Chia seeds provide an amazing hit of nutrients, especially protein, calcium and omega-3 fatty acids. To get the full benefits, soak the seeds – even 5 minutes is enough. They're quite gelatinous, so people use them to thicken sauces and as a substitute for eggs. I add them to my brekkie every day, and sprinkle them on smoothies and salads. Don't boil or bake them at high temperatures as this will reduce their nutrients.

Chilli

When I mention red chillies in a recipe, I'm usually referring to the long, thin cayenne chillies that you can get at any supermarket. These are quite mild compared with other varieties, but they are still very spicy. Simply trim the stem and slice them finely, using the seeds and all. (Make sure you wash your hands after chopping them, and don't get the juice in your eyes.) If you're not big on chillies, use less than I suggest, or if you love them, by all means add more, or use the hotter varieties. I'm a big fan of bird's eye chillies (which are very hot!).

Coconut flour

Coconut flour is quite dense and needs help sticking together, so if I'm making coconut flour pancakes, for example, I will add an extra egg to help bind the mixture. But it tastes amazing!

Coconut milk and coconut cream

Coconut milk and cream are made the same way, just using different amounts of water. You can make them yourself or buy them ready-made. If possible, buy organic coconut milk and cream packed in BPA-free tins (BPA is a toxic chemical that works like oestrogen and can affect your hormones).

Coconut oil

Coconut oil is solid at cooler temperatures, so can be tricky to measure. I pop the jar into a pot of hot water to melt it. Unlike regular olive oil (not extra-virgin), coconut oil doesn't break down or go rancid when cooked at high temperatures – making it a winner. People worry about coconut oil making them fat. It *is* a saturated fat, but it's a medium-chain fatty acid, which means the body can use it quickly (rather than having to store it). It's awesome used topically, too – I use it to moisturise my face and body. It's also thermogenic, meaning it helps to speed up your metabolism.

Coconut sugar

Also known as coconut sap sugar or coconut palm sugar, this is coconut nectar that has been dried. Its granulated texture makes it easy to use in place of raw sugar in baking. It has a delicious molasses flavour.

Coconut water

Coconut water is the liquid from young coconuts, and is naturally sweet. It makes a fantastic base for smoothies and, if you're a cocktail fan, then it's great mixed with your favourite alcohol (and the electrolytes will help to prevent a hangover!).

Dates, medjool

Dates are a great source of the electrolyte potassium, which is a key player for heart health. Plus, they're full of fibre and will keep you regular. Medjool dates are bigger, sweeter and squidgier than regular dried dates. They're very sweet, though, so to avoid a sugar rush when snacking on them I pop the seed out and replace it with a brazil nut. The protein and fat from the nut help to lower the glycaemic load and make for a slower release of energy.

Honey, raw

I always use raw honey in my cooking. Raw honey has been filtered, but in a way that doesn't destroy its nutrients. It is not pasteurised (the heating and filtration process that makes it clear), so all its beneficial enzymes are still present. Raw honey can be solid at room temperature (depending on how cold it is), and is milky (not clear). It's about twice as sweet as sugar, so you don't need to use as much. Plus, local honey is now a big thing as more and more people are setting up 'rooftop' hives, which means the bees will be feeding off local pollens. Having locally made honey can help decrease the symptoms of hay fever, so it's a great choice.

Maple syrup

Maple syrup is a wonderful sweetener: it has a great flavour, is full of minerals and has less fructose than honey, dates and agave. Make sure you choose 100 per cent syrup, not the imitation stuff. It costs more, but it's so much healthier.

Millet

This is an ancient seed that we use like a grain. It's gluten free so is great for any paleo recipe. Rinse millet before using. I love to add a little to a mash to give it more depth, use it to make a creamy coconut porridge, or just cook it the same way I would rice or quinoa.

Non-dairy milks

I often use almond milk in my recipes as an alternative to cow's milk, but there are heaps of others you could use in its place, such as milk made from oats, rice, cashew nuts, macadamia nuts, quinoa or hazelnuts. It's easy to make your own nut milk if you have a really good food processor. The ratio is 1 cup of nuts to 2 cups of water. (You'll need to soak the nuts overnight first, and give them a good rinse.) Strain the nut puree through a fine mesh sieve and you're done! (You can save the fibrous bits and use them in raw treats, or simply add them to a granola mix.) If you don't have time to make your own nut milk, you can buy it off the shelf. Just read the label and stay away from the stuff with loads of sugar or sweeteners, and watch out for preservatives. There should be about four ingredients and you should be able to pronounce all of them.

Nuts and seeds, activated

Nuts and seeds are brilliant sources of good fats. When my recipes refer to activating nuts, this means to soak them in water for 2–3 hours (or overnight if possible), then rinse. This removes enzyme inhibitors and makes them easier to digest. After rinsing (unless you're about to blend them up for a smoothie or raw treat), spread the nuts out on a baking tray and place in a 50°C oven or dehydrator to dry out (this will take anywhere from 6 to 24 hours depending on the type of nut). Store your activated nuts in sealed glass jars in the pantry.

Oats

I like to cook with oats, and often use them in my recipes. Although oats themselves don't contain gluten, because of the way we process them, most oatmeal brands have been cross-contaminated with minuscule amounts of wheat, barley and/or rye, so we can't call them 'gluten free'. About 30 per cent of people who have coeliac disease cannot tolerate oats (even when the cross-contamination is almost eliminated), so if you have coeliac disease or a particularly severe gluten allergy, proceed with caution.

Olive oil

Olive oil in my recipes is almost always extra-virgin (unless I'm deliberately trying to avoid the peppery taste it can have) – this means that it's the first pressing with no chemicals or additives, so it's going to be super fresh. Regular olive oil becomes unstable and rancid when used in cooking at high temperatures, but good-quality extra-virgin varieties are much higher in polyphenols (that's the antioxidant part of the olive oil) and this prevents the double bond in the monounsaturated fat from breaking.

Quinoa

This seed is packed with nutrients and is very high in protein, so it's excellent if you're vegetarian or vegan. It's also versatile: you can get quinoa seeds, quinoa flakes, puffed quinoa, and even quinoa milk and quinoa flour. There is white quinoa, red and a royal black, though they're pretty much on par nutrient-wise (the coloured ones may have a slightly higher mineral content). I find the white has the mildest flavour. You cook it in a similar way to rice and it suits both sweet and savoury dishes.

Salt

When I talk about seasoning with salt in my recipes I'm not referring to table salt, which is highly processed. I love to use pink salt – it tastes just like normal salt but has loads more minerals (about 84 trace minerals, in fact). I use Murray River or Himalayan. Celtic salt and rock salt are healthy options, too. Use salt sparingly, though, and stay away from the bleached stuff.

Stevia

Stevia, which is made from the leaves of a South American herb, is about 300 times sweeter than sugar. It has no calories and no impact on blood-sugar levels. You can buy stevia in powder or liquid form. Use it sparingly – if you use more than a couple of drops of liquid you'll get a pretty nasty aftertaste. It doesn't taste quite the same as sugar, but once you're used to it, you'll be converted. I love it!

Tahini

Tahini is a paste made from crushed sesame seeds. You can buy hulled (where the seed casing has been removed) and unhulled (made from the whole seed). Both are high in protein and good fats. Hulled tahini is lighter in colour and has a milder taste; unhulled has more calcium and fibre. You can also get black tahini, which tastes similar to hulled tahini. Tahini is great in salad dressings, dips and energy balls.

Tamari

Instead of soy sauce in my recipes I like to use tamari – a Japanese fermented soy sauce with a darker colour and richer flavour than traditional soy sauce. It contains much less salt and is a good source of vitamin B3, protein and manganese. It is also made with far less wheat than normal soy sauce, if any, and is therefore a good low-gluten or gluten-free alternative. Look for 'gluten free' on the label.

Vanilla pods

Vanilla pods, like honey and cinnamon, are a great libido enhancer. Wrap the pods in foil, seal in a zip-lock bag, and store them in a cool, dark place so they don't dry out. Vanilla pods can be pricey, but you can always use powdered vanilla (make sure it's 100 per cent vanilla) or vanilla extract (not the chemically produced essence) instead.

Yoghurt

Some people who react badly to cow's milk can tolerate yoghurt as it's partially fermented and is a little easier to digest. Choose organic or biodynamic full-cream options, as they're more nutritious than low-fat yoghurt. If you can't handle cow's milk yoghurt, try sheep or goat's milk yoghurt – they have a slightly stronger flavour. Then there are coconut or nut milk yoghurts for a vegan option. Always read the label carefully; you don't want any added sugar or gelatine. We're after real foods, as close to their natural state as possible.

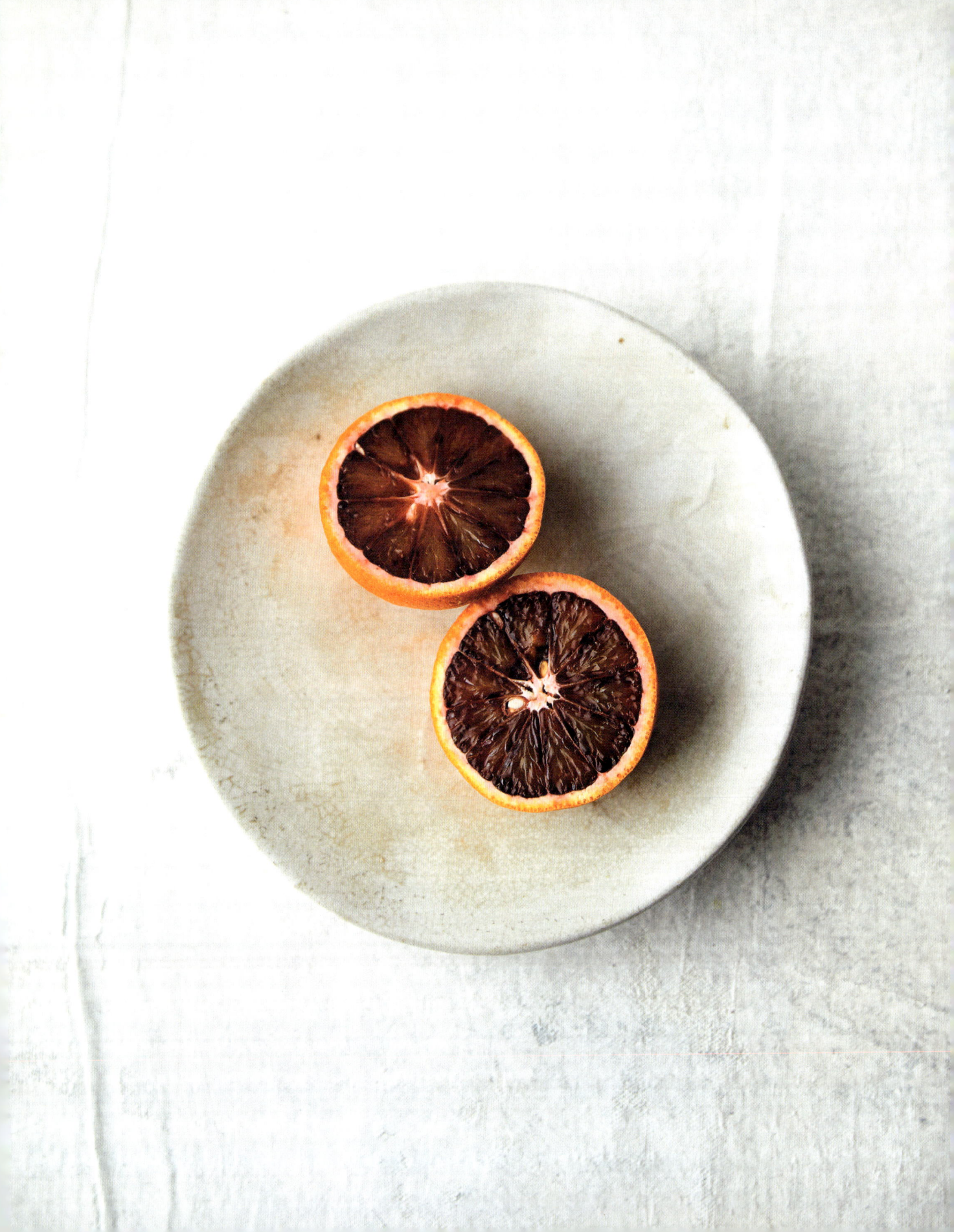

DRINKS

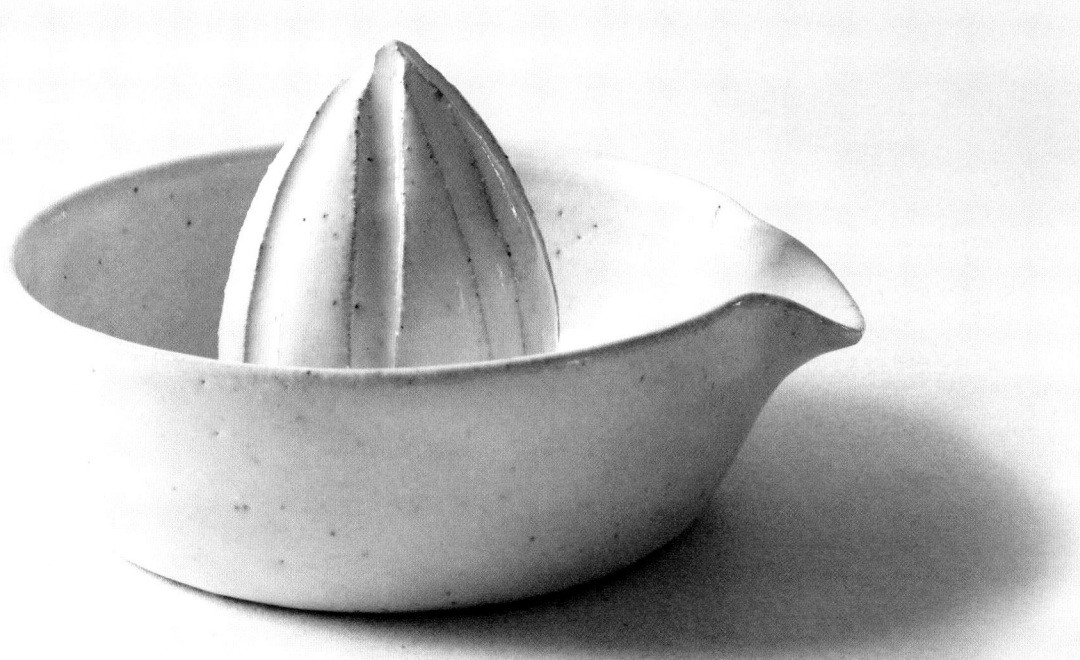

CHAKRA-BALANCING JUICE

Juices are a great way of getting a hit of nutrition in without filling you up too much, and this one has the perfect balance of flavours. I love to have it as a post-yoga snack with a Cookie Dough Ball (see page 202).

SERVES 2

3 carrots

2 small–medium beetroot, roughly chopped

2 celery stalks

1 apple

½ cup (80 g) roughly chopped pineapple, plus extra to serve

Pop everything through a juicer, pour into glasses and enjoy. Sometimes I love to pop a triangle of pineapple on the rim of the glass to finish things off, 1980s style!

DAIRY FREE GLUTEN FREE GRAIN FREE PALEO RAW VEGAN VEGETARIAN

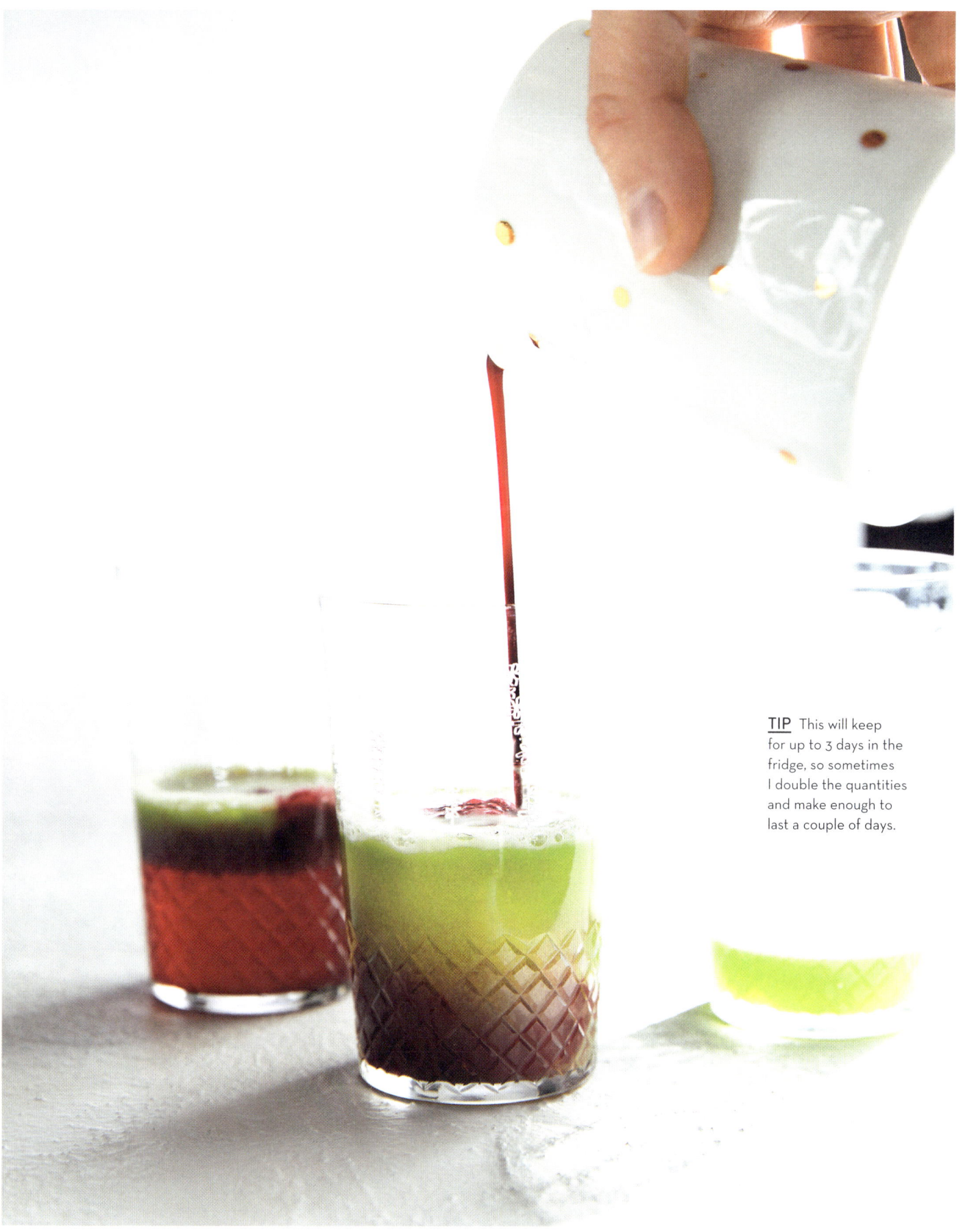

TIP This will keep for up to 3 days in the fridge, so sometimes I double the quantities and make enough to last a couple of days.

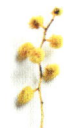

TROPICANA SMOOTHIE BOWL

This recipe just feels like summer to me. It's got that sweet tropical tang of mango and banana, but also contains a nice whack of ground turmeric, which is prized in Ayurvedic medicine for its healing benefits. Turmeric is a powerful antioxidant, and is said to aid digestion and promote the immune system as well as helping with the healthy function of the brain and nervous system.

SERVES 2

2 frozen mango cheeks

1 frozen banana

½ cup (80 g) macadamia nuts (activated if possible, see page 108)

½ teaspoon ground turmeric

1 tablespoon coconut oil, melted

3 tablespoons honey (or sweetener of your choice)

1½ cups (375 ml) coconut milk

TO SERVE

edible flowers

bee pollen

shredded coconut

Pop everything into a blender and whiz it up until thick and smooth (the longer you let it go, the better the consistency will be). Top with edible flowers, bee pollen and shredded coconut, take a snap for social media, then tuck on in!

<u>TIP</u> If you don't have time to activate the macadamia nuts, don't worry - this recipe will still work perfectly. The reason we soak nuts and seeds to activate them before use is to help remove the phytic acid that can bind minerals in the digestive tract and make them more difficult for our bodies to absorb.

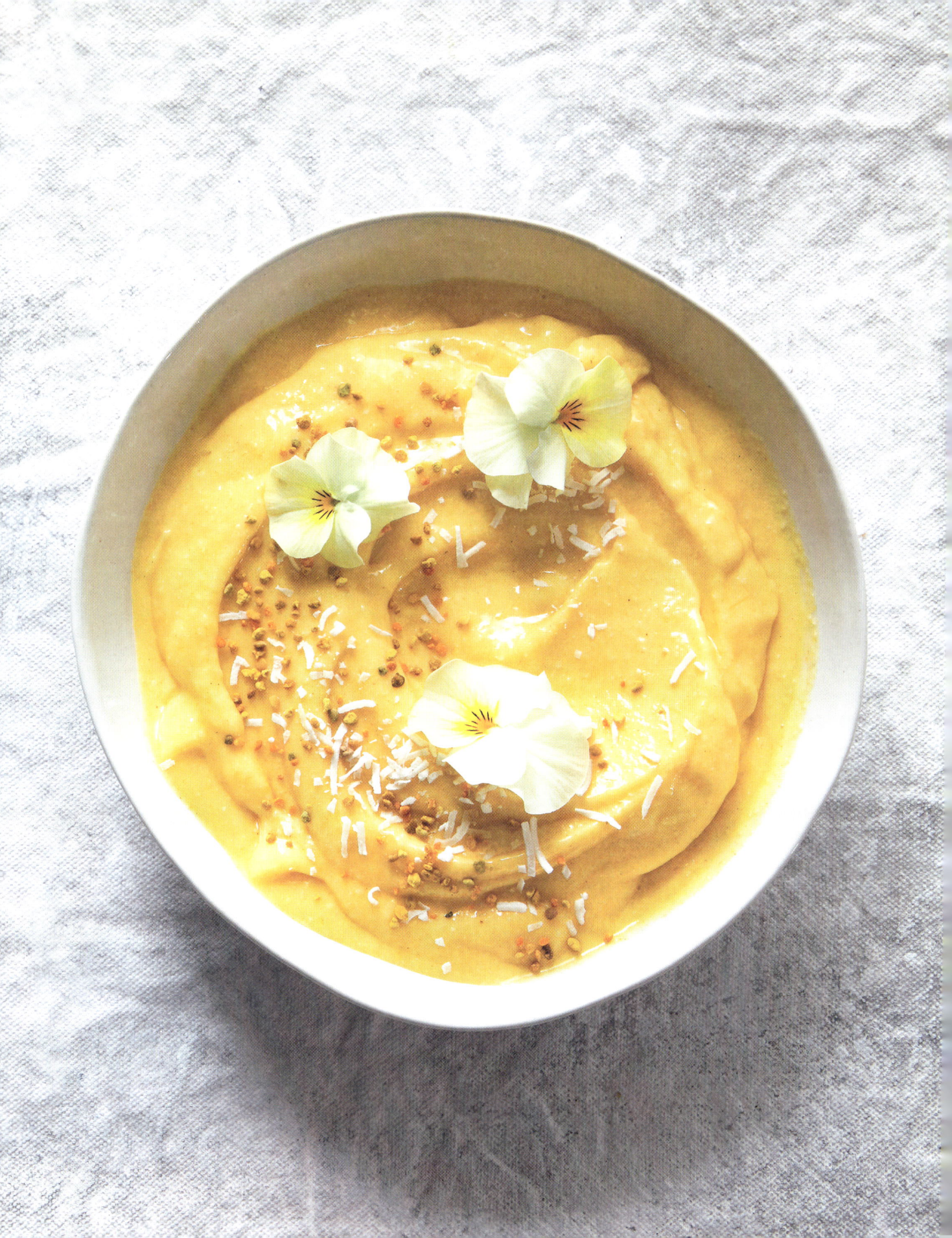

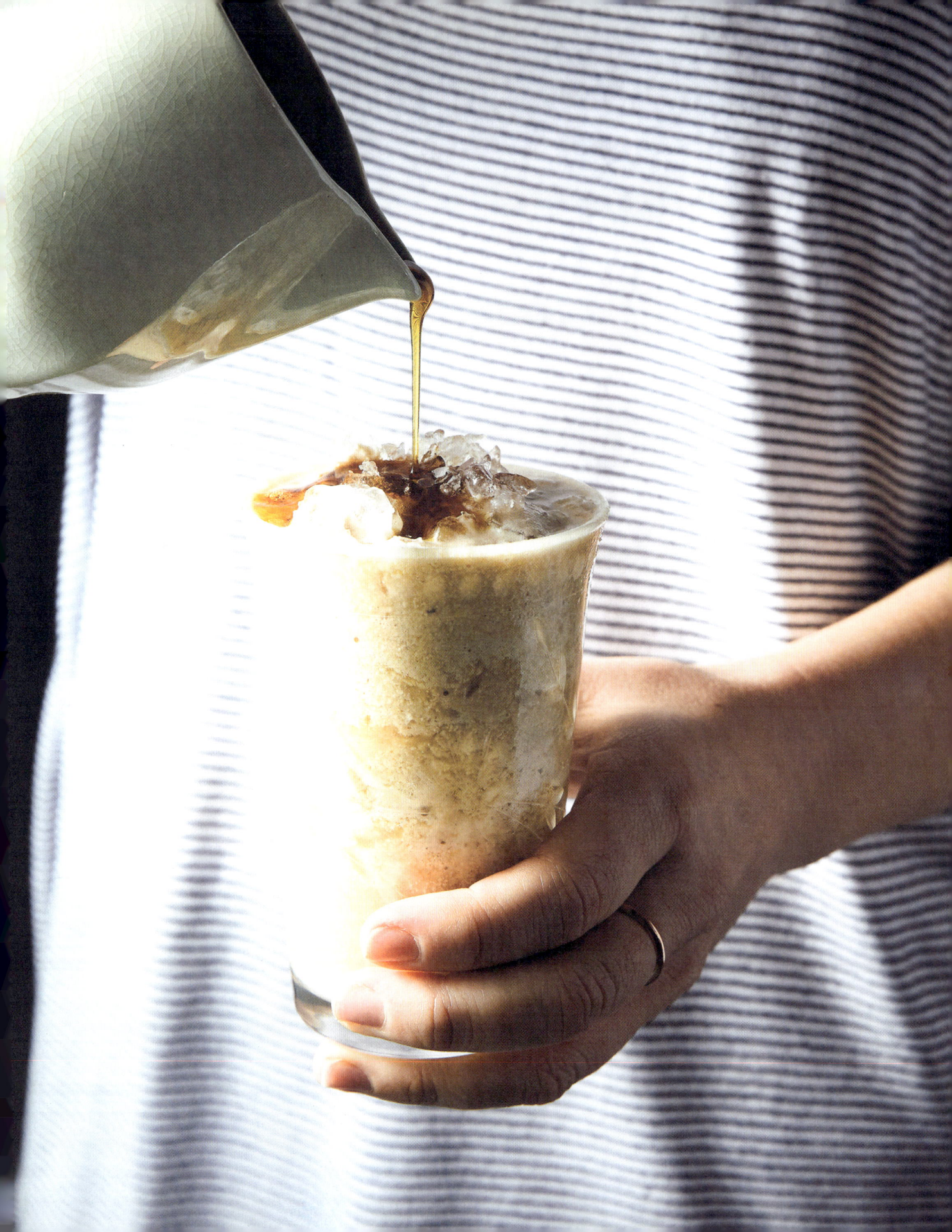

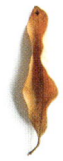

ICED MAPLE-CASHEW LATTE

Maple syrup is one of my all-time favourite flavours, and though coffee may be best known for the caffeine hit it delivers, it's also full of antioxidants that provide the body with tons of health benefits. Combined here they make the perfect summertime drink.

SERVES 2

1 shot (30 ml) espresso coffee

1 cup (150 g) cashew nuts (activated if possible, see page 108)

1 cup (135 g) ice cubes

2 tablespoons maple syrup, plus extra to serve

pinch of salt flakes

Pop everything into a blender with 1 cup (250 ml) of water and blitz together until it looks like a slushie (you don't want it silky smooth). Pour into glasses, top with a few extra drops of maple syrup and enjoy this summery delight.

TIP You can use instant coffee here if you'd rather; just mix a few teaspoons with a tablespoon of boiling water to dissolve before adding to the blender with the rest of the ingredients. If you're not a coffee fiend, try whipping this one up without it – it tastes delish both ways.

DAIRY FREE GLUTEN FREE GRAIN FREE
PALEO VEGAN VEGETARIAN

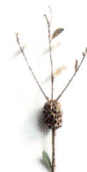

GREEN TEA AND COCONUT BUBBLE TEA

While I've always been fascinated by this creation, I only tried it recently in Mauritius for the very first time. I loved it (of course). This is my healthy take on a bubble tea, using coconut milk as a dairy alternative, which gives you all of the health benefits of the medium-chain fatty acids coconut milk contains while also helping you to feel full for longer.

SERVES 2

½ cup (75 g) tapioca balls

2 green tea bags

1 cup (250 ml) coconut milk

½ teaspoon matcha green tea powder

1 tablespoon honey (or sweetener of your choice)

Add the tapioca balls to a saucepan of boiling water, reduce the heat to a simmer and cook for 30 minutes. Turn off the heat and leave to stand for 15 minutes, then drain.

Add the tea bags, 1 cup (250 ml) of water and the coconut milk to a saucepan over a medium heat. Bring to a simmer, then stir through the matcha green tea powder, honey and tapioca balls. Remove from the heat and pour into glasses, then give everything a good old stir together. Enjoy warm or chilled with a wide straw for sucking up those lovely little tapioca 'bubbles'.

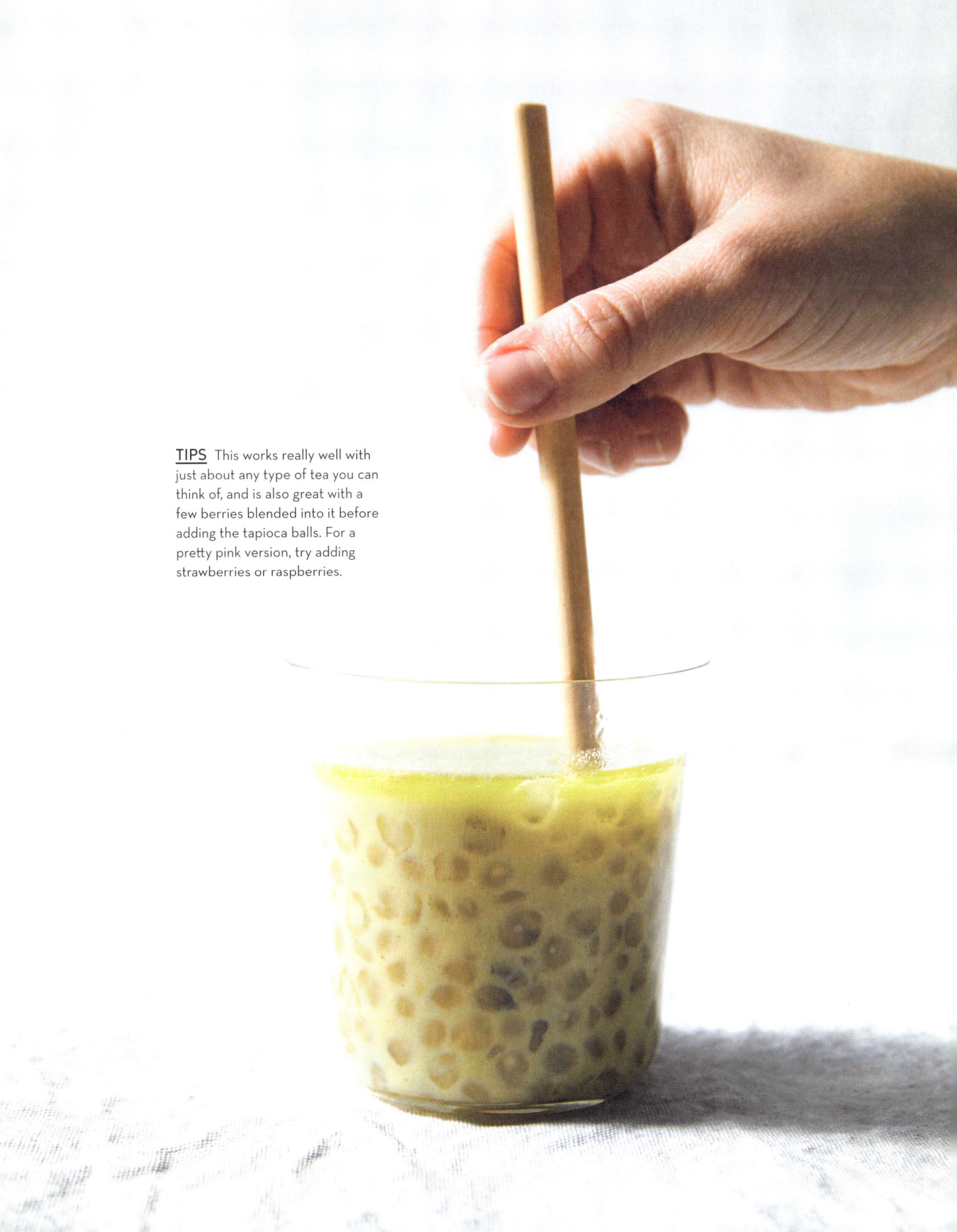

TIPS This works really well with just about any type of tea you can think of, and is also great with a few berries blended into it before adding the tapioca balls. For a pretty pink version, try adding strawberries or raspberries.

WARM BANANA-CHAI SMOOTHIE

Chai spices happen to be some of my favourite flavours. They have a warming effect on the body, and are rich in antioxidants. They bring some serious health benefits to the table too, helping to improve digestion, fight inflammation and improve circulation. I love using them like this, in my favourite warm smoothie – it's perfect for a winter's day.

SERVES 2

1 banana

½ cup (80 g) macadamia nuts
(activated if possible, see page 108)

½ teaspoon ground cinnamon, plus extra to serve

¼ teaspoon ground nutmeg

¼ teaspoon ground ginger

2 cups (500 ml) coconut milk

Pop everything into a blender and whiz it to your preferred consistency. Transfer the mix to a saucepan and warm it through over a medium heat. Pour into cups, top with an extra pinch or two of cinnamon, then tuck on in.

DAIRY FREE   GLUTEN FREE   GRAIN FREE
PALEO   VEGAN   VEGETARIAN

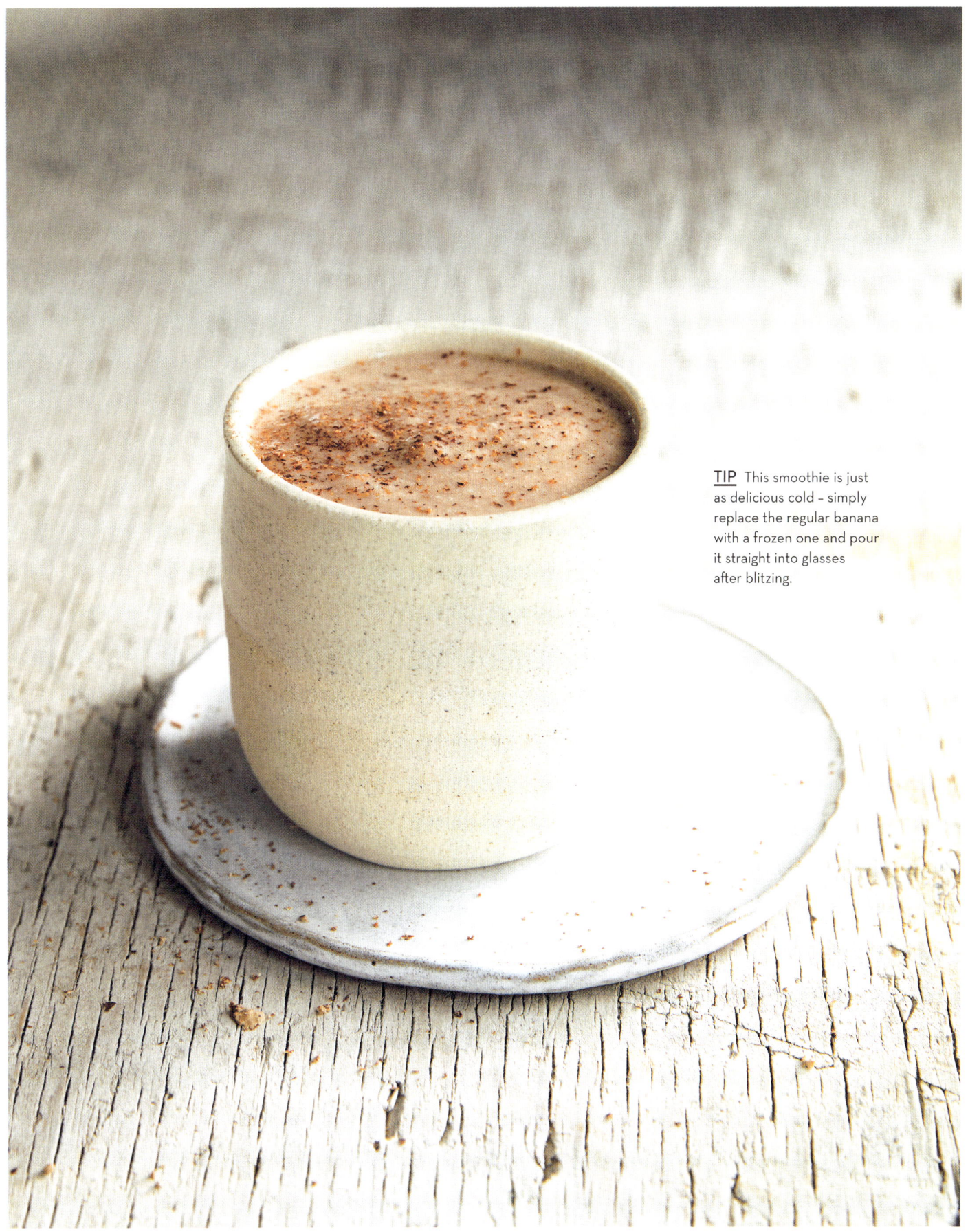

TIP This smoothie is just as delicious cold – simply replace the regular banana with a frozen one and pour it straight into glasses after blitzing.

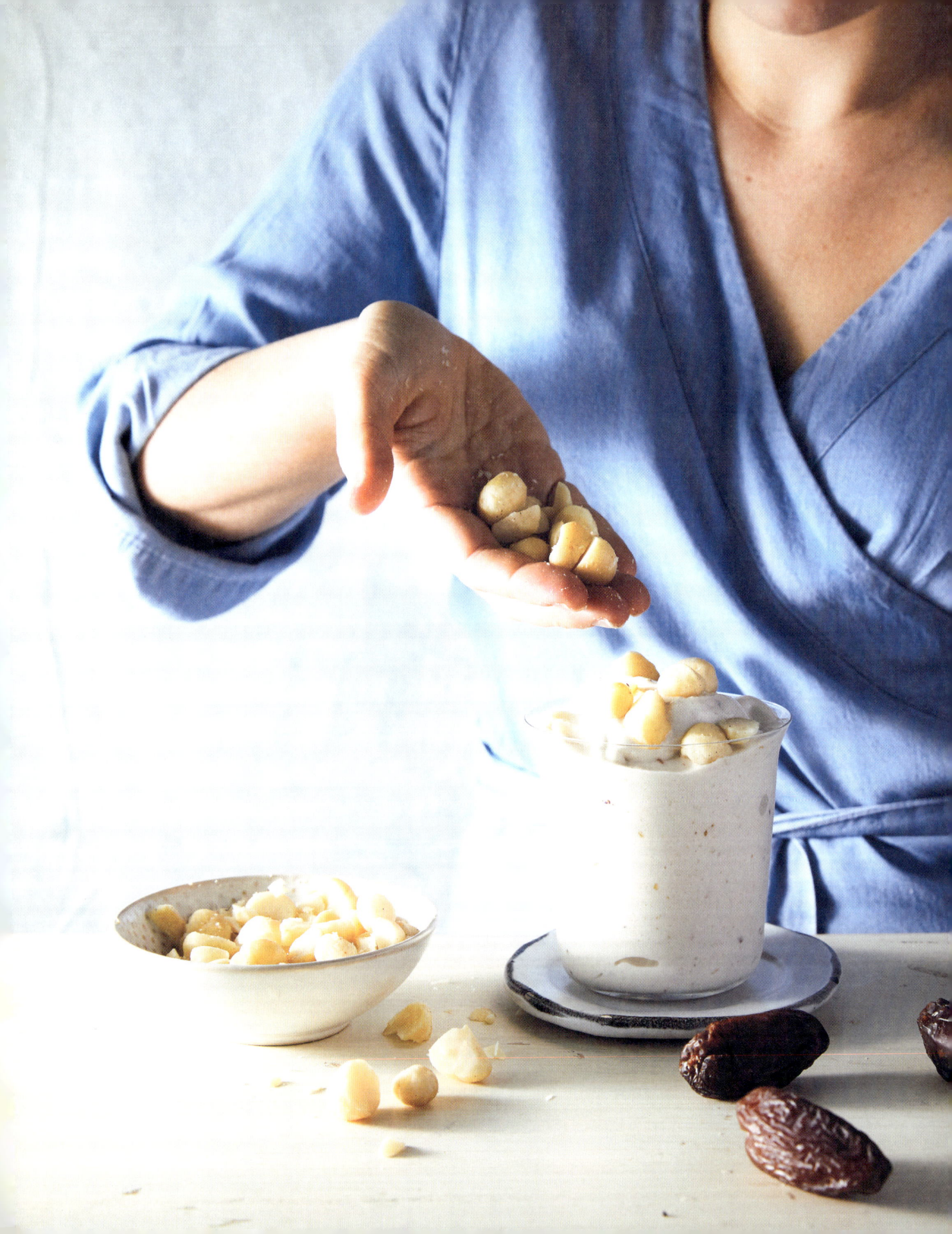

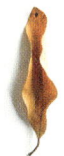

SALTED CARAMEL BONE BROTH SMOOTHIE

I tried my first sweet bone broth smoothie at a whole foods mecca in Bondi called The Health Emporium. I eyed it off a few times before I actually had the courage to try it, as the thought of it seemed so strange to me! I tried it and, needless to say, loved it, so this recipe takes inspiration from that experience. It's super easy to make – when you whip up your next batch of bone broth, just pour a little of it into ice-cube trays and store them in the freezer so you're good to go.

SERVES 2

2 beef bone broth ice cubes (see page 188)

1 frozen banana

3 tablespoons macadamia nuts (activated if possible, see page 108), plus extra, chopped, to serve

2 pitted medjool dates

1½ cups (375 ml) coconut milk

pinch of salt flakes

Pop everything into a blender and whiz together until silky smooth. Pour into glasses, sprinkle with the extra macadamias, then sip away. Cheers, big ears!

TIP Adding a scoop of vanilla protein powder to this recipe works a treat when you need a bit of a protein boost. If you're using protein powders, try to steer clear of those filled with artificial colours, flavours and other nasties, and find one that's naturally sweetened instead.

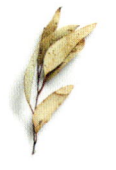

'SHROOM COFFEE

My naturopath, Jad, got me onto this drink and it's become part of my daily ritual, as it's really simple but full of health benefits. Lion's mane is a mushroom that has been used for thousands of years in traditional Chinese medicine as a restorative. It is also said to improve brain function – when I add it to my coffee I definitely feel clearer and more focused a short time after drinking it. I've added another mushroom, chaga, to this creation for its immune-boosting properties. Give it a go and don't be too worried about the flavour of your morning cuppa, as these 'shrooms team really well with coffee.

SERVES 2

2 heaped tablespoons ground coffee

2 cups (500 ml) boiling water

1 teaspoon lion's mane powder

½ teaspoon chaga powder

Place the coffee in a coffee plunger and pour over the boiling water. Add the mushroom powders and give everything a good stir, then plunge and enjoy.

TIP If you don't have a coffee press, this is still super easy to make. Just switch out the ground coffee for 1 teaspoon of instant coffee powder, divide the ingredients between cups and give everything a good mix before tucking in.

DAIRY FREE FRUCTOSE FRIENDLY GLUTEN FREE
GRAIN FREE PALEO VEGAN VEGETARIAN

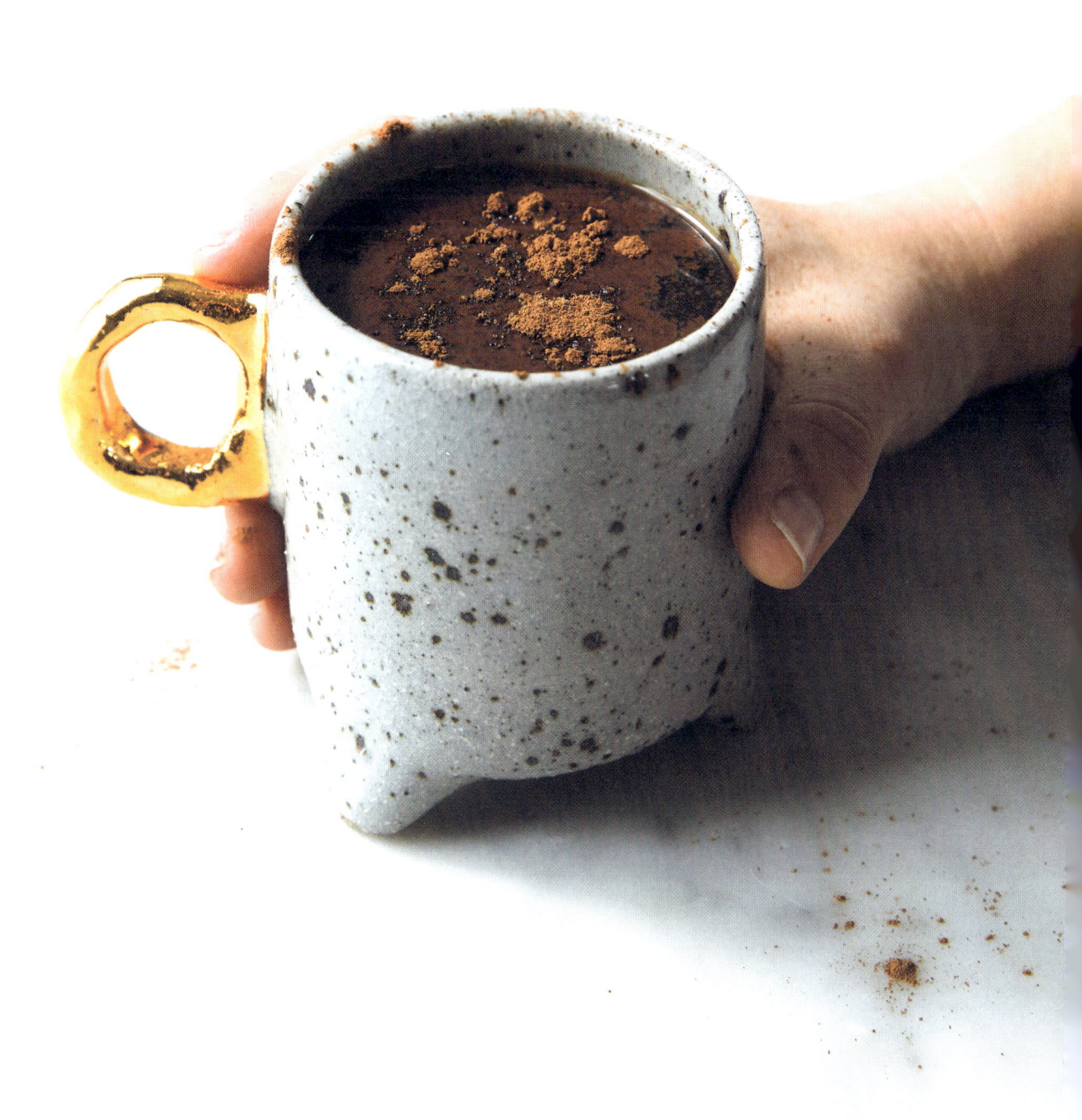

HORCHATA

This Mexican spiced drink is traditionally made with rice milk, but I liked the idea of a quinoa version instead. This gives it a lovely nutty flavour and a hefty whack of protein as well as keeping it dairy free. Give it a go – I promise you won't be disappointed.

SERVES 3–4

1 cup (200 g) quinoa, soaked overnight and rinsed

½ cup (80 g) almonds
(activated if possible, see page 108)

4 pitted medjool dates
(or sweetener of your choice)

1 teaspoon ground cinnamon,
plus extra to serve

¼ teaspoon ground nutmeg,
plus extra to serve

pinch of ground allspice

ice cubes, to serve

Add everything to a blender with 2 cups (500 ml) of water and whiz it up until thick and silky. Pour into large ice-filled glasses and top with an extra sprinkle or two of cinnamon and nutmeg.

DAIRY FREE GLUTEN FREE GRAIN FREE PALEO RAW VEGAN VEGETARIAN

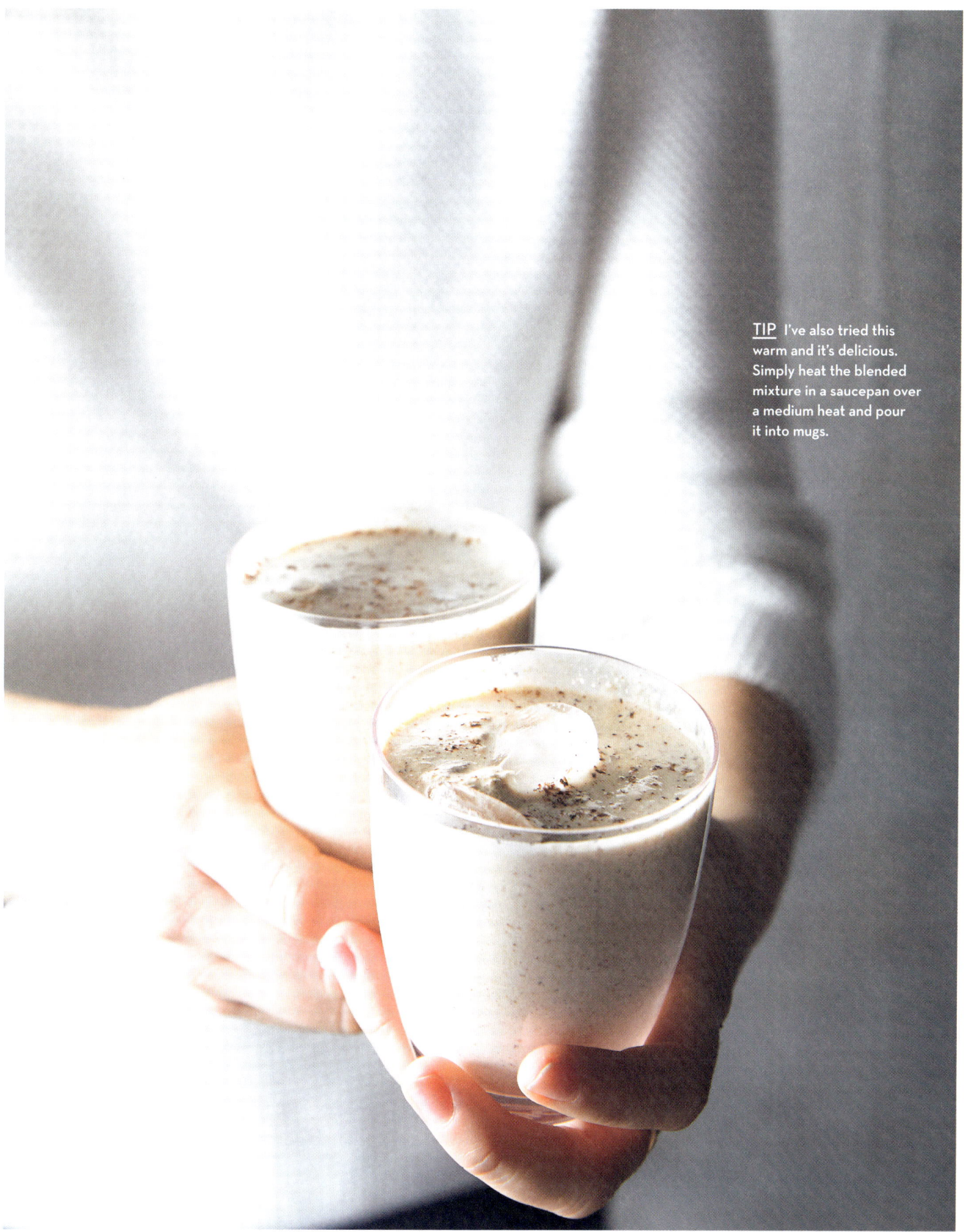

TIP I've also tried this warm and it's delicious. Simply heat the blended mixture in a saucepan over a medium heat and pour it into mugs.

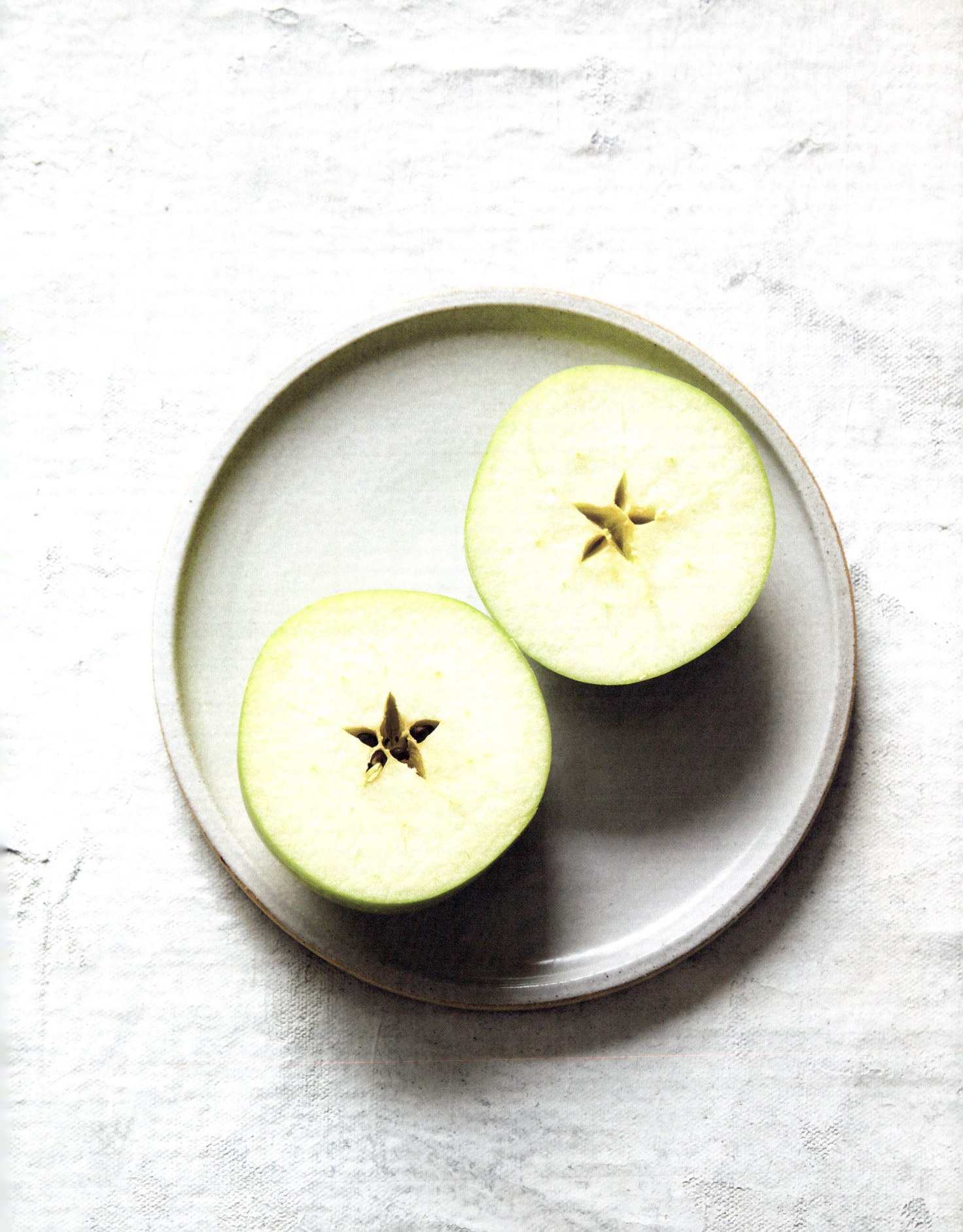

BREAKFAST

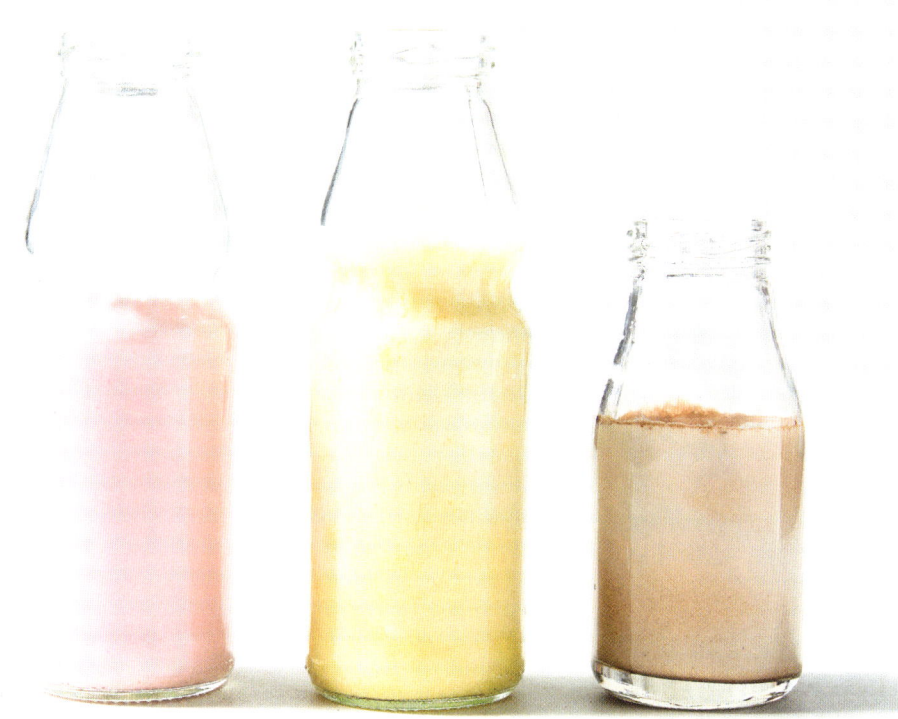

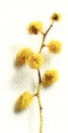

WARM TURMERIC KARMA OATS

I love this recipe because if you have it first thing it really helps to keep you warm all day long. Curcumin is the active ingredient in turmeric that gives it its lovely colour and potent anti-inflammatory properties, which it lends to this lovely bright bowl of goodness.

SERVES 2

1 tablespoon coconut oil

1 cup (100 g) rolled oats

2 cups (500 ml) coconut milk or almond milk

¼ teaspoon ground turmeric

pinch of ground cinnamon

pinch of salt flakes

TO SERVE

2 tablespoons macadamia nut butter

1 banana, sliced

handful of edible flowers

1 teaspoon rolled oats

2 tablespoons maple syrup

Melt the coconut oil in a saucepan over a medium heat, then add your oats, coconut or almond milk, turmeric, cinnamon and salt. Give everything a good mix together and cook, stirring, for 5–6 minutes until lovely and creamy.

To serve, divide the creamy oat mixture between bowls and top with the macadamia nut butter, banana slices, edible flowers, oats and maple syrup. It's as pretty as a picture and smells delicious, so take a moment to enjoy the look and aroma before mindfully enjoying your nourishing brekkie.

TIP While I reckon macadamia nut butter tastes the best, any nut butter will do the trick here. Pop your favourite on top and make the recipe yours.

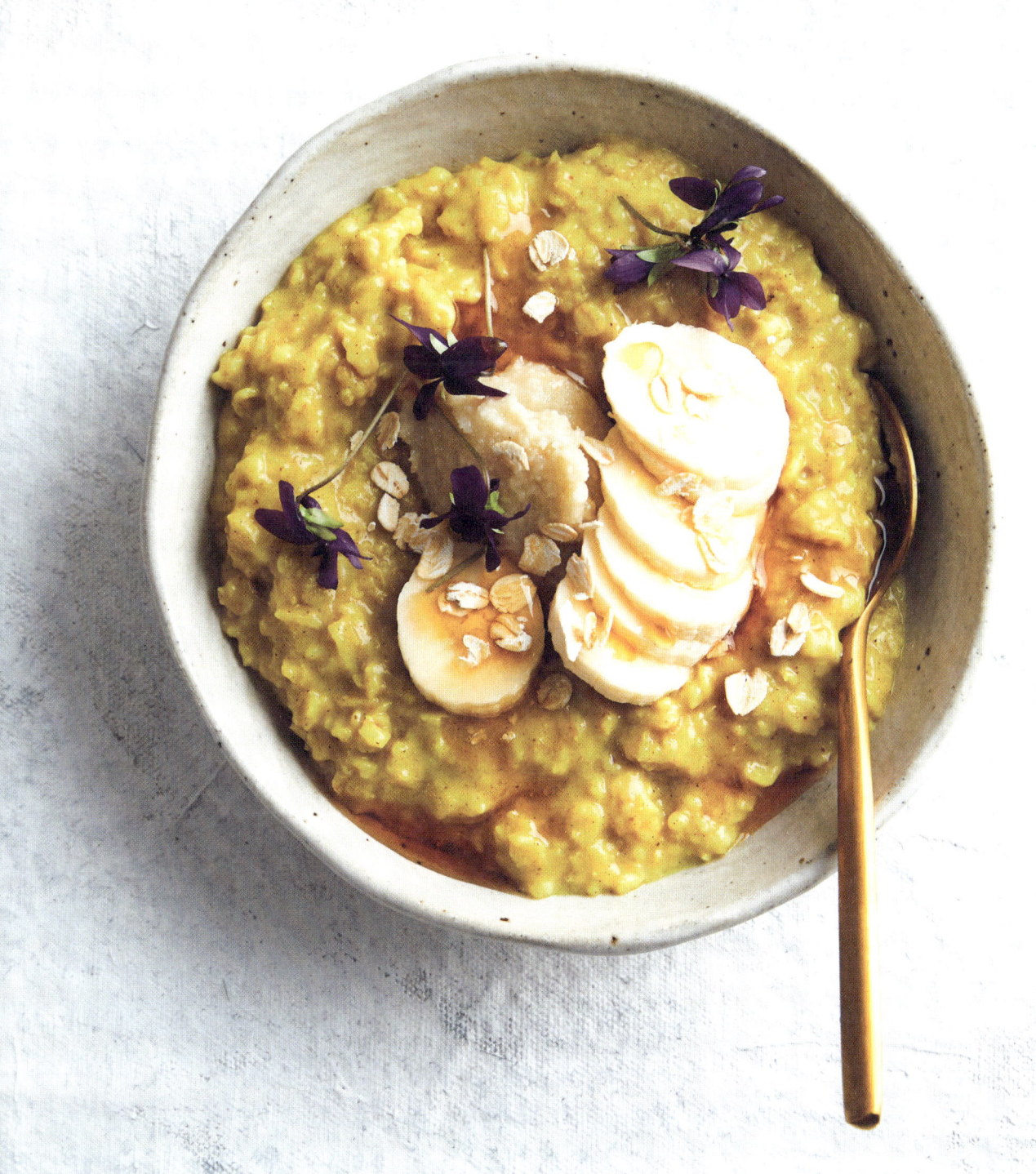

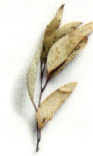

GINGER GRANOLA WITH PEACH

This is a healing ginger granola served with fresh peaches and coconut yoghurt, and I can't think of a more perfect brekkie. The granola makes the most amazing dessert ingredient, too – I love to sprinkle it over coconut ice cream and fresh fruit. It also makes a great crunchy topping for pancakes (or pretty much anything sweet), adding loads of lovely texture. I even like to eat a handful on its own as a snack.

SERVES 6

4 cups (400 g) rolled oats

3 tablespoons honey

3 tablespoons coconut oil, melted

1 tablespoon roughly chopped crystallised ginger

½ cup (125 ml) freshly squeezed orange juice

½ cup (60 g) roughly chopped pecans (activated if possible, see page 108)

½ cup (60 g) sunflower seeds (activated if possible, see page 108)

½ cup (60 g) roughly chopped walnuts (activated if possible, see page 108)

zest of ½ orange

½ cup (30 g) shredded coconut

pinch of salt flakes

TO SERVE

peach wedges

coconut yoghurt

Preheat the oven to 180°C. Line a large baking tray with baking paper.

Pop everything into a large bowl and mix together really well. Spoon the mixture onto the baking tray and press evenly over the base.

Bake for 20 minutes until nicely toasted, giving everything a little mix halfway through cooking to make sure that it cooks evenly and doesn't burn in places. Allow to cool (though I like to sneak my first portion in while it's still lovely and warm!), then store in an airtight container and enjoy all week long for brekkie with juicy peaches and coconut yoghurt.

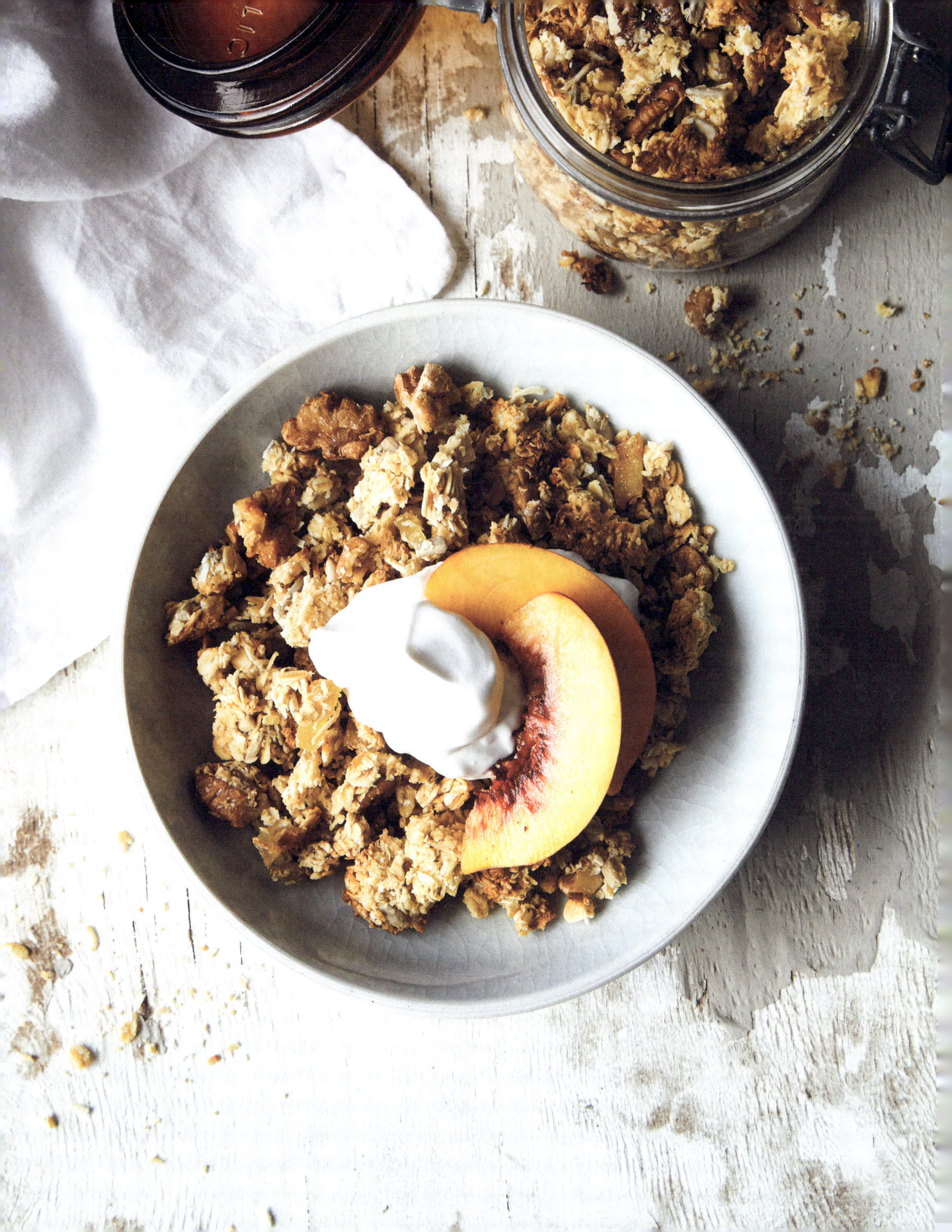

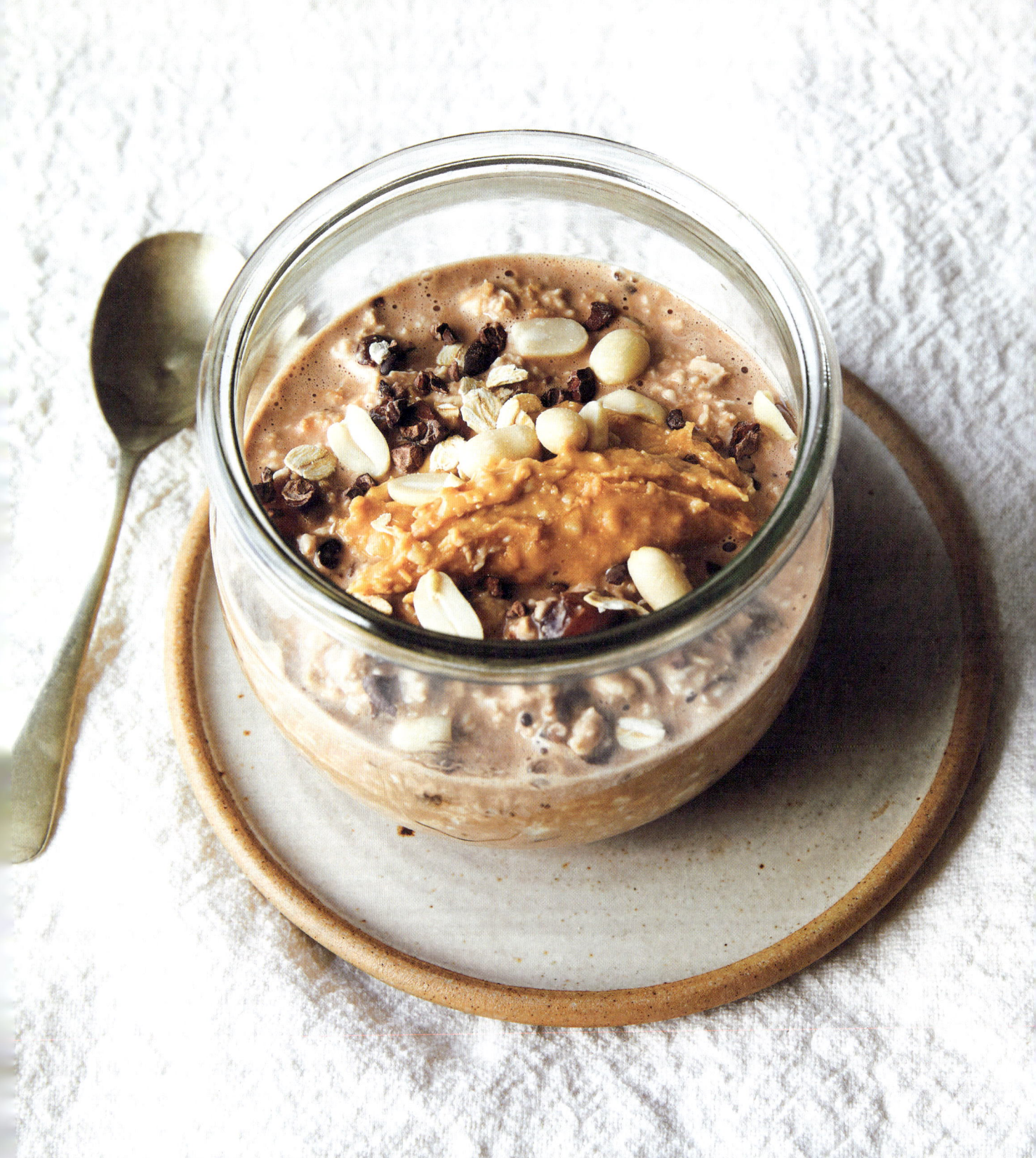

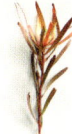

'SNICKERS' BIRCHER

Who doesn't love a Snickers bar (or a Snickers ice cream, while I'm on the subject)? My aim is always to create healthier versions of favourite (unhealthy) treats. So, meet this Snickers-inspired recipe. The cacao powder and nibs give you a lovely chocolatey, antioxidant-packed hit and will get your brain buzzing, while the oats will help power you up and keep you feeling fuller for longer. Chocolate for breakfast? You bet!

SERVES 2

1 cup (100 g) rolled oats

2 cups (500 ml) almond milk

2 tablespoons good-quality peanut butter

1 tablespoon maple syrup

1 tablespoon cacao powder

1 tablespoon cacao nibs

1 tablespoon chopped peanuts

4 pitted medjool dates, roughly chopped

TO SERVE

rolled oats

cacao nibs

peanuts

peanut butter

First up, give your oats a good rinse, then drain them and pop them into a large bowl.

Place the almond milk, peanut butter, maple syrup and cacao powder in a blender and whiz together until the mixture looks (and tastes) like chocolate nut milk. Pour the milk mixture over the oats and mix together well, then stir through the cacao nibs, transfer to the fridge and leave to soak for at least 2–3 hours, but ideally overnight (it'll taste better if you give it longer to soak).

When you're ready to serve, just pull the bircher out of the fridge, stir through the peanuts and dates and top with a few extra oats, cacao nibs and peanuts and a dollop or two of peanut butter. Dig in.

<u>**TIPS**</u> This creation makes a perfect gift – pop it in little jars topped with cute fabric and tied with ribbons, then share the love! And any nut milk or nut butter works a treat here, too – I like to use organic, good-quality peanut butter and nuts, but try it with almonds if peanuts aren't your bag.

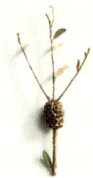

PALEO CHAMOMILE AND LEMON LOAF

This loaf is pretty delish. Made with almond meal and coconut flour, it's also quite filling, so one or two slices will go a long way. Chamomile is great for calming both the nervous and digestive systems, making this my go-to post-yoga brekkie if I have a full-on day ahead.

MAKES 1 LOAF

250 g butter, plus extra for greasing

2 tablespoons chamomile tea leaves

2 cups (200 g) almond meal

½ cup (70 g) coconut flour

2 teaspoons baking powder

½ cup (100 g) coconut sugar

pinch of salt flakes

1½ cups (375 ml) almond milk

3 eggs, whisked

⅓ cup (80 ml) maple syrup

juice of 1 lemon, plus zest of ½

TO SERVE (OPTIONAL)

coconut yoghurt

dried chamomile flowers

Preheat the oven to 180°C and grease a loaf tin with a little butter.

Melt the butter in a saucepan over a medium heat. Add the chamomile tea leaves, remove the pan from the heat and leave to steep for 5 minutes.

Meanwhile, add the almond meal, coconut flour, baking powder, coconut sugar and salt to a large bowl and mix together well. Make a well in the centre, add the chamomile-infused butter mixture and mix well, then stir in the almond milk, eggs, maple syrup, lemon juice and zest to form a batter.

Pour the batter into the prepared tin and bake for 1 hour 15 minutes to 1 hour 30 minutes, or until a skewer inserted into the centre of the loaf comes out clean. Remove from the oven and leave to cool, then transfer to the fridge to chill and firm. Slice and serve either as is or toasted and topped with a dollop of coconut yoghurt and a few chamomile flowers. Yum!

TIPS This recipe is designed for brekkie, but it also makes a sweet post-dinner treat, as it is completely caffeine free. If you can't get your hands on coconut sugar, then raw sugar, muscovado or panela cane sugar will all work well here, too. And if you can get hold of chamomile flowers for decoration, try steeping a few in the butter mixture along with the tea (being sure to give it a strain before use) to give it even more chamomile flavour.

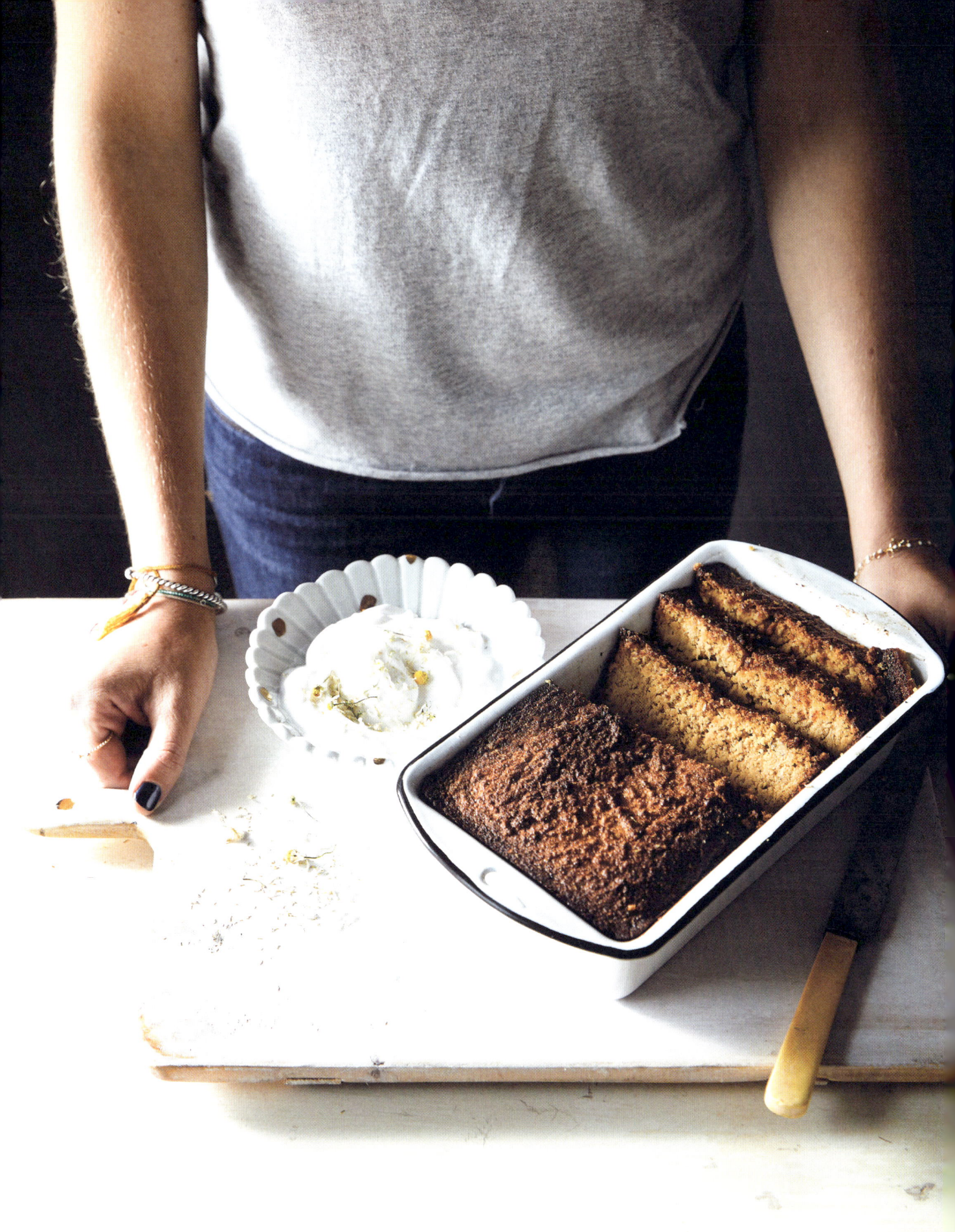

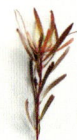

NECTARINE AND STRAWBERRY BRUSCHETTA

This dish is very, very quick to make, so it's an awesome one to impress your mates with for brunch. It's also a great source of protein, meaning it will keep you feeling fuller for longer.

SERVES 2

⅓ cup (90 g) ricotta

4 slices of paleo, gluten-free or regular good-quality bread, toasted

2 nectarines, sliced into thin wedges

5 strawberries, halved

2 teaspoons honey

1 teaspoon balsamic vinegar

salt flakes and freshly ground black pepper

handful of basil leaves

Spread the ricotta over the toast slices in a generous, even layer.

Mix the nectarine and strawberry pieces together in a bowl, then top the toast with the mixed fruit. Drizzle over the honey and balsamic vinegar, season with salt and pepper and scatter over the basil leaves to finish. Now enjoy this colourful creation!

TIP You can use any kind of bread you like here. Personally, I have a gluten-free buckwheat loaf that I like to use, but go ahead and choose what you like to make this your own.

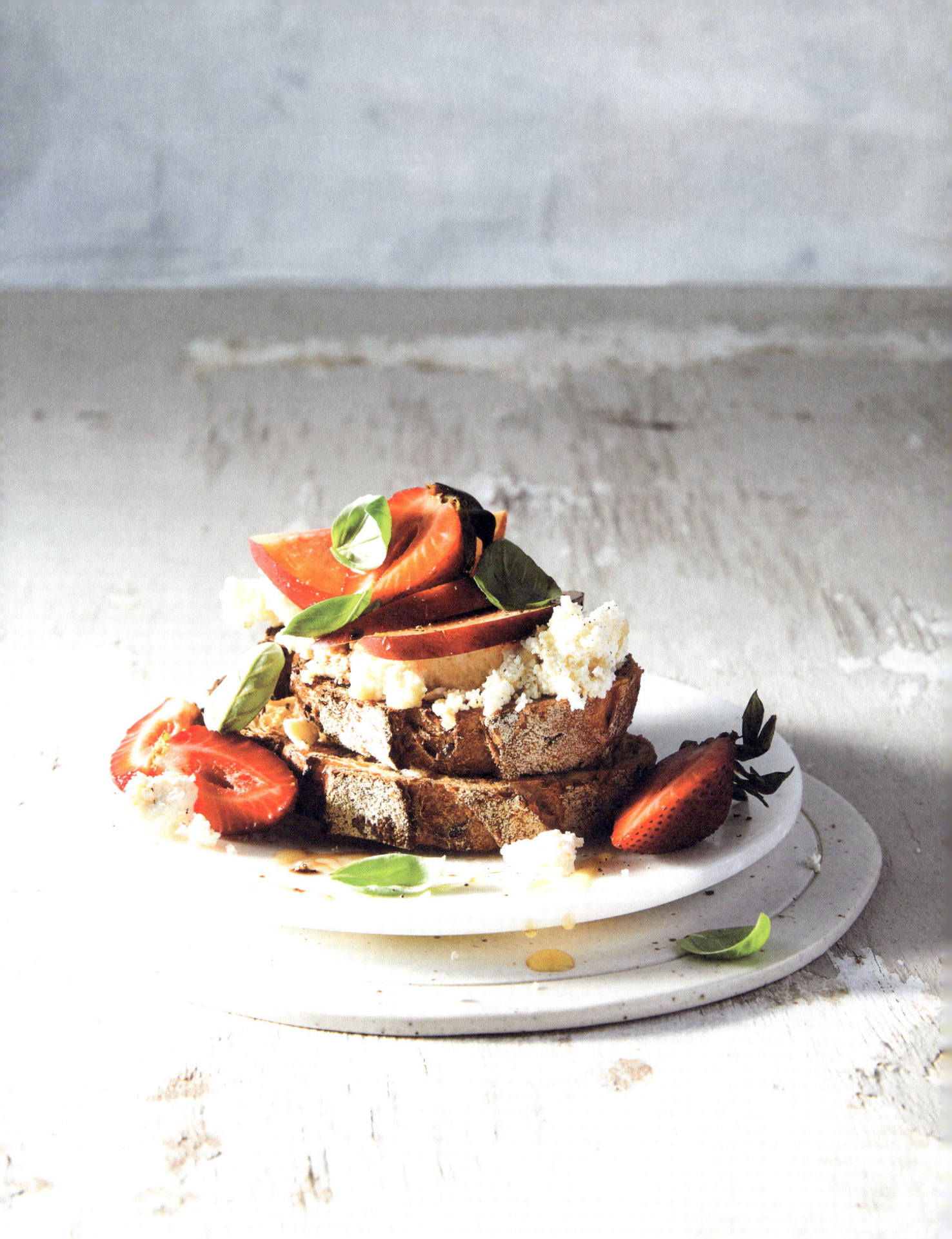

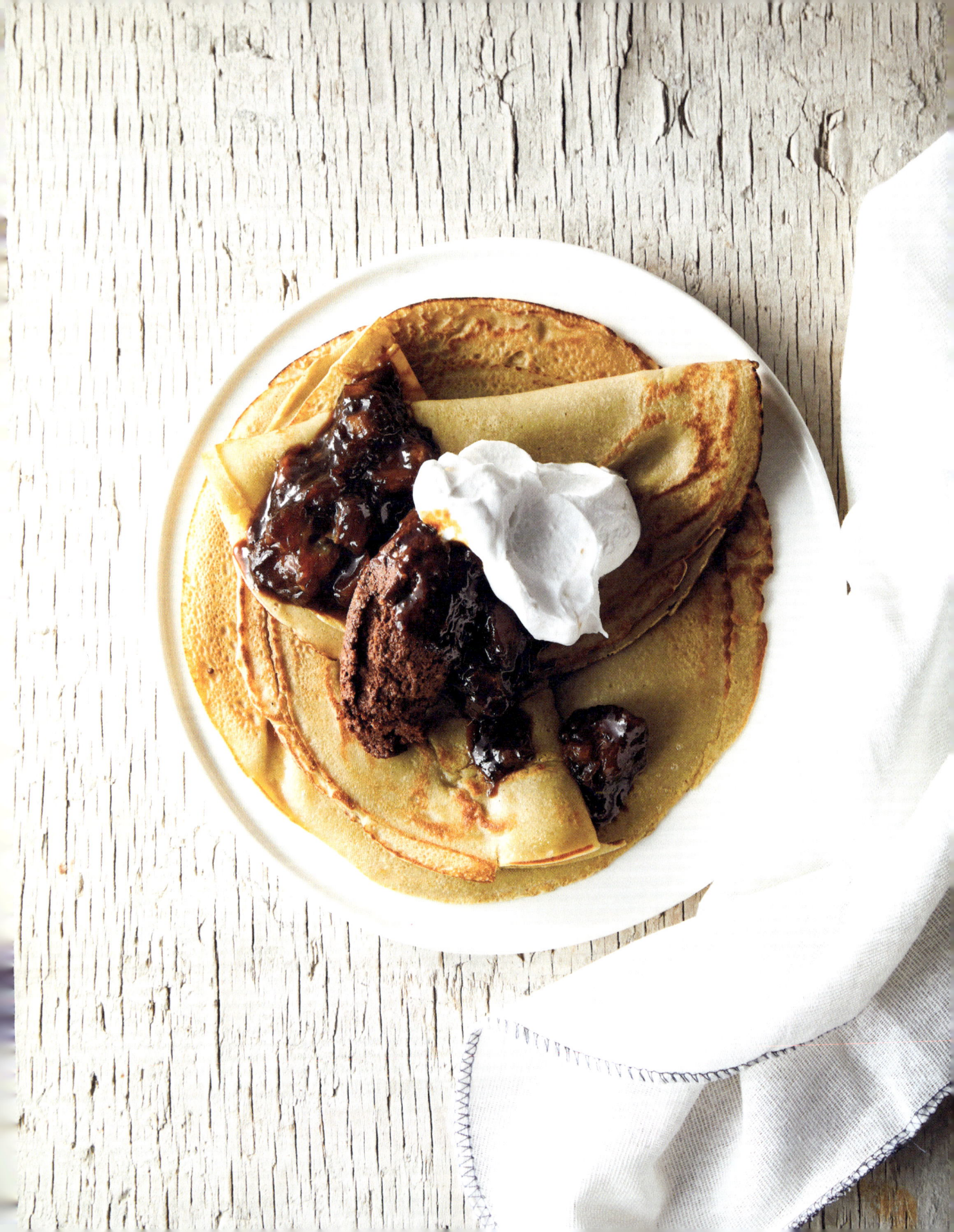

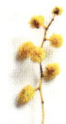

CREPES WITH 'NUTELLA' AND BANANA JAM

This recipe is inspired by a trip I took to Mauritius. The food there is incredible and has a huge French influence – hence the 'Nutella' crepe part of this creation – but something else I discovered there that tasted amazing was banana jam. This banana jam recipe is a super-healthy take on the one that I had in Mauritius. It is also lovely served with granola and yoghurt.

SERVES 2

1 cup (130 g) buckwheat flour

2 eggs

1 cup (250 ml) almond milk

pinch of salt flakes

butter or coconut oil, for frying

coconut yoghurt, to serve

'NUTELLA'

1 cup (140 g) hazelnuts (activated if possible, see page 108)

2 tablespoons cacao powder

½ cup (125 ml) maple syrup

3 tablespoons almond milk, plus extra if needed

pinch of salt flakes

MAURITIAN BANANA JAM

1 cup (200 g) coconut sugar

juice of ½ lime

½ tablespoon butter

small pinch of salt flakes

2 large bananas, sliced

Start with the toppings so the crepes can be served hot. To make the 'Nutella', whiz everything together in a blender, adding an extra splash of almond milk if necessary, until smooth. Set aside.

For the banana jam, add the coconut sugar, lime juice, butter, salt and 1½ tablespoons of water to a saucepan set over a medium heat. Stir to dissolve the sugar, then add the bananas, bring to a simmer and cook for 10 minutes until nice and jammy. Spoon into a bowl and set aside.

Now it's time to make the crepes and bring this party together. Combine the buckwheat flour, eggs, almond milk and salt in a large bowl and whisk together to form a lovely, lump-free batter.

Heat a knob of butter or coconut oil in a frying pan over a medium heat. Add 3 tablespoons of batter and swirl the pan to spread it over the base. Cook for 1–2 minutes, or until you see air bubbles in the centre of the crepe and the edges are starting to crisp. Flip and cook for another 1 minute. Set aside and keep warm, then repeat with the remaining batter.

Divide the crepes between serving plates and slather with the 'Nutella' and banana jam. Finish with a dollop of coconut yoghurt. Delishimo!

TIP This recipe makes more jam and 'Nutella' than you'll need, so store the leftovers in sterilised jars in the fridge (where they will keep for yonks) for next time around. The 'Nutella' is also great spooned over strawberries or slathered over gluten-free bread and topped with banana slices.

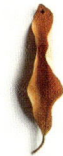

BANANA BREKKIE CAKE

A cross between a cake and a pudding, this tastes unreal! And, thanks to the eggs, it's a great way of getting some complete protein into your morning meal, which is not always an option when you start the day with something sweet.

SERVES 4

½ cup (50 g) rolled oats

½ cup (55 g) almond meal

2 eggs

3 tablespoons maple syrup

3 tablespoons almond milk

3 tablespoons baking powder

½ teaspoon ground cinnamon

¼ teaspoon ground nutmeg

2 bananas, sliced

TO SERVE

maple syrup

almond butter

coconut ice cream

Preheat the oven to 180°C and line a 21 cm square cake tin with baking paper.

This is so, so simple – just pop everything except the banana slices into a big bowl and give it a good old mix together to combine, then spoon the lot into the prepared tin. Arrange the banana slices on top and bake for 25 minutes, or until golden on top.

To serve, cut into four and scoop the pieces out of the tin and into bowls. Enjoy warm topped with a drizzle of maple syrup, a dollop of almond butter and a scoop (or two) of coconut ice cream.

TIP There are no rules here, so feel free to play around with this recipe all you like. You could switch the bananas for apples to make an apple pie version, or add a few spoonfuls of cacao powder and cacao nibs for a chocolate hit. Whatever tickles your fancy!

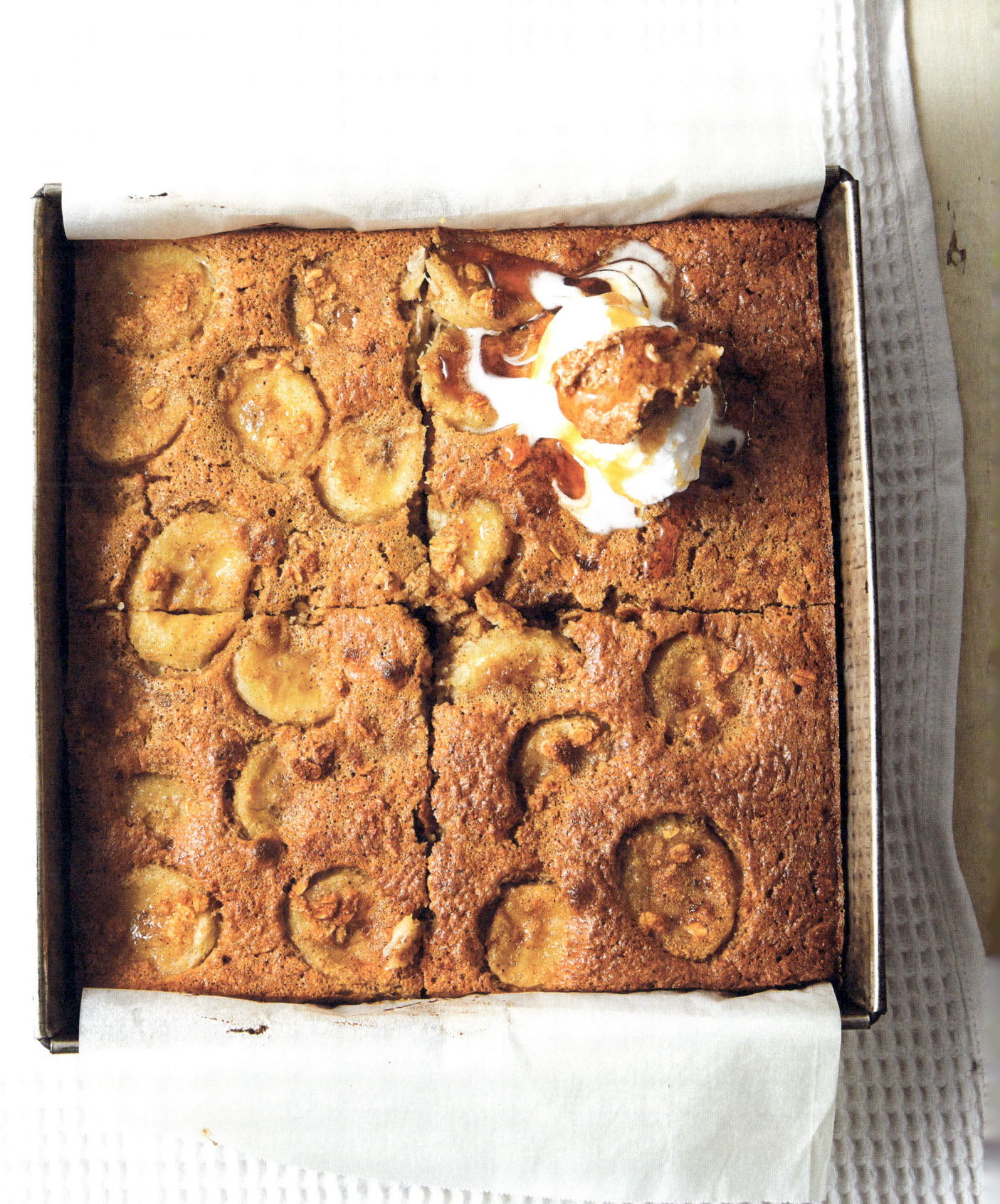

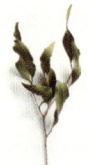

SUPERFOOD EGG WHITE SCRAMBLE

First up, I'm a huge fan of whole eggs - the yolks are loaded with health benefits, so by all means keep them in here if you want a richer meal. I eat this a lot when I'm travelling because it's really easy to have made at a hotel buffet, though I also eat it a lot at home, too. When I do, I never throw out the yolks - I'll use them to make mayonnaise or aioli or I'll add them to my homemade hair and beauty treatments.

SERVES 2

4 egg whites

2 egg yolks

1 bunch of kale, stalks removed and leaves finely chopped

½ cup (45 g) finely chopped broccoli florets

handful of baby spinach, finely sliced

¼ red onion, finely diced

¼ green capsicum, finely diced

½ zucchini, grated

salt flakes and freshly ground black pepper

2 tablespoons butter

TO SERVE

large handful of basil or coriander leaves

chilli flakes (optional)

Add the egg whites and yolks to a bowl and give them a quick, light whisk. Pop in the kale, broccoli, spinach, onion, capsicum and zucchini, whisk everything together really well to combine and season with salt and pepper.

Melt the butter in a saucepan over a medium heat and pour in the scramble mix. Cook, stirring continuously, until the egg is almost set, then remove from the heat and divide between plates or bowls. Scatter over the basil or coriander leaves and a pinch or two of chilli flakes, if you like, and tuck on in!

<u>TIPS</u> You can use any colour capsicum here, but I like to keep everything nice and green. Also, if you don't like cooking with butter, use the same quantity of olive oil instead - it works a treat.

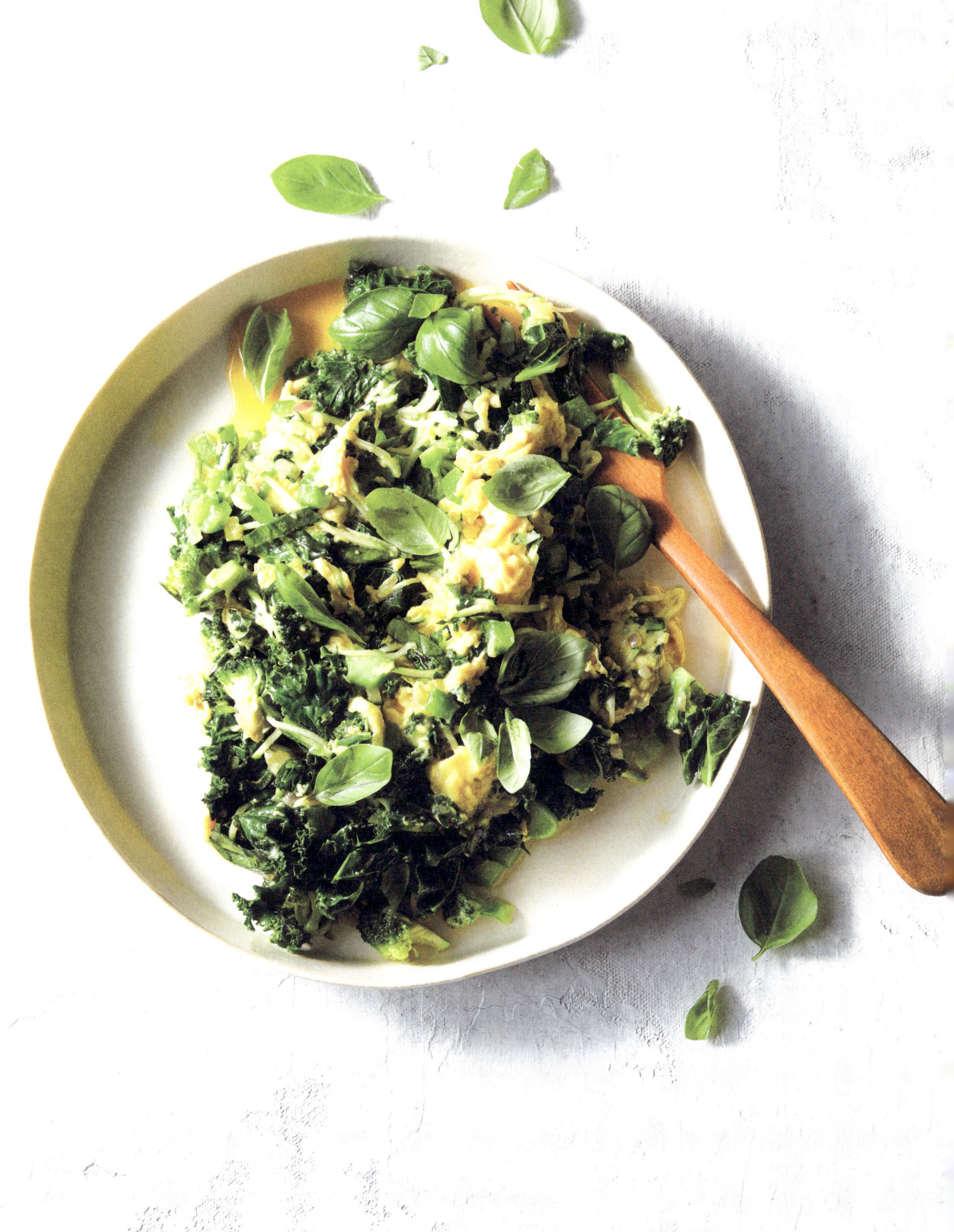

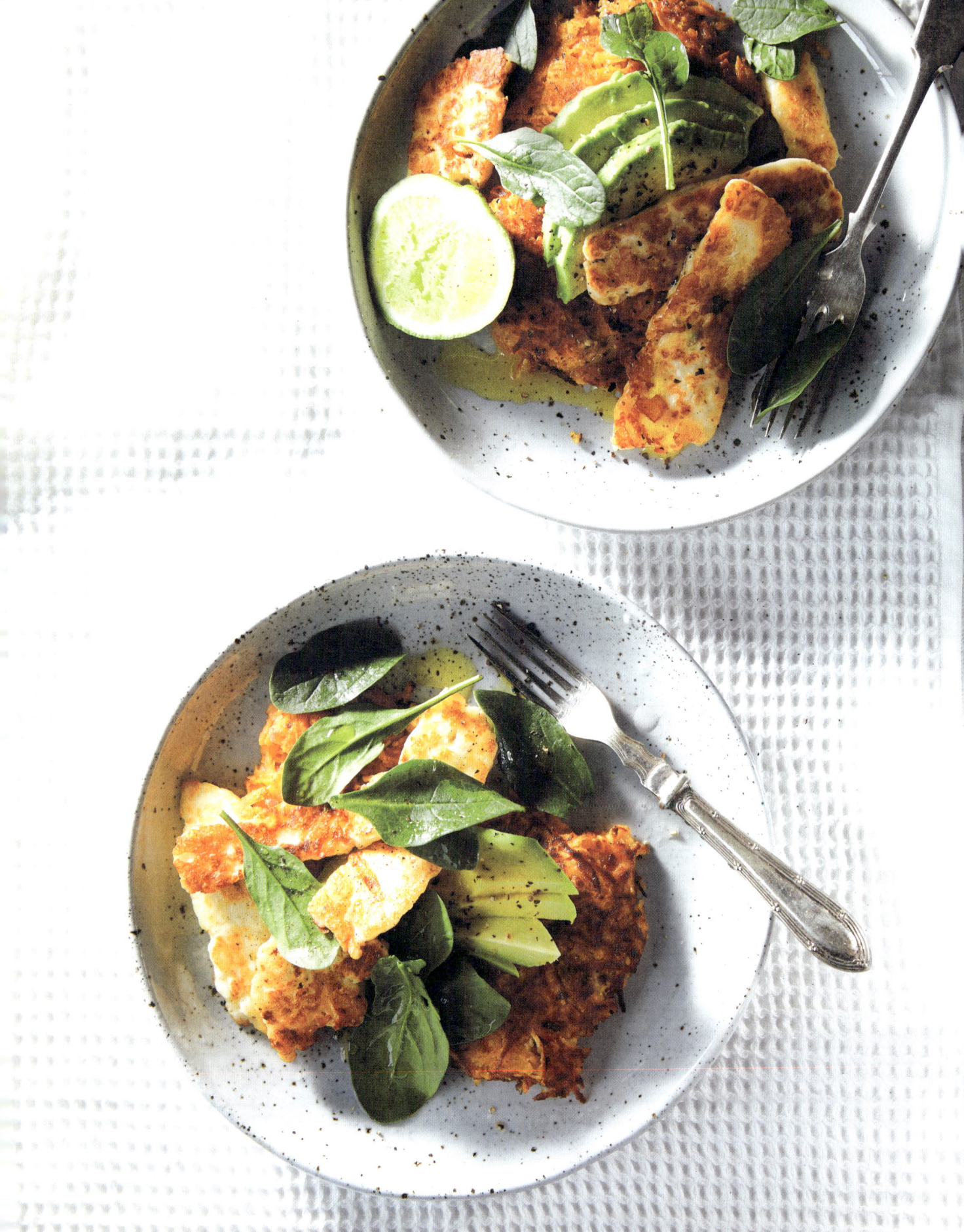

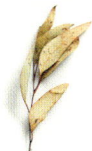

SWEET SPUD HASH BROWNS WITH HALOUMI

These sweet spud hash browns are brilliant because they can be used to add some slow-release complex carbohydrates to almost any savoury dish. I love making them with eggs for dinner – they're pretty speedy and simple to whip up. If you want to make this vegan, just hold the haloumi.

SERVES 2

80 g haloumi, cut into 4 long slices

1 avocado, sliced into thin wedges

baby spinach, to serve

lime cheeks, to serve

SWEET SPUD HASH BROWNS

1 cup (125 g) grated sweet potato

½ red onion, finely chopped

3 tablespoons almond meal

2 tablespoons extra-virgin olive oil, plus extra if needed

salt flakes and freshly ground black pepper

For the sweet spud hash browns, pop the grated sweet potato, onion, almond meal and 1 tablespoon of the olive oil in a bowl. Season with salt and pepper and mix everything together well.

Heat the remaining olive oil in a frying pan over a medium heat. Add the sweet spud mixture to the pan in four even portions, using a spatula to flatten each. Cook the hash browns for 2–3 minutes on each side until golden and crispy, then remove from the pan and keep warm.

Add the haloumi to the pan, together with another splash of oil, if needed, and cook for 2 minutes on one side until nicely golden, then flip and cook for a further 1 minute. Divide the haloumi between plates together with the hash browns and avo pieces, season with salt and pepper and serve with a few baby spinach leaves and some lime cheeks for squeezing.

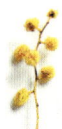

SALMON AND KALE OMELETTE

I love this meal because it not only keeps me full for so long – thanks to the complete protein in the eggs and the salmon – but also because it works so well for brekkie, lunch or dinner. It's one of the most wholesome and nutrient-dense meals in town.

SERVES 2

6 eggs

¼ red onion, sliced

salt flakes and freshly ground black pepper

2 tablespoons extra-virgin olive oil

200 g smoked salmon, sliced into ribbons

2 large handfuls of purple kale, stalks removed and leaves finely sliced (or use kalettes)

1 teaspoon capers

dill fronds, to serve

Combine the eggs and onion in a bowl, season with salt and pepper and give everything a good mix.

Heat 1 tablespoon of the olive oil in a frying pan over a medium heat and pour in half of the omelette mix, then tilt the pan so it covers all of the base. Add half of the smoked salmon, kale and capers and cook for 3–4 minutes, then carefully slide the omelette out onto a plate. Repeat with the rest of the mixture, topping each omelette with a scattering of dill.

<u>TIPS</u> I like to use wild salmon if I can get hold of it, as it's more environmentally sustainable and is less likely to have been fed food dyes and pellets. If you can't find purple kale, any leafy green will do the job here.

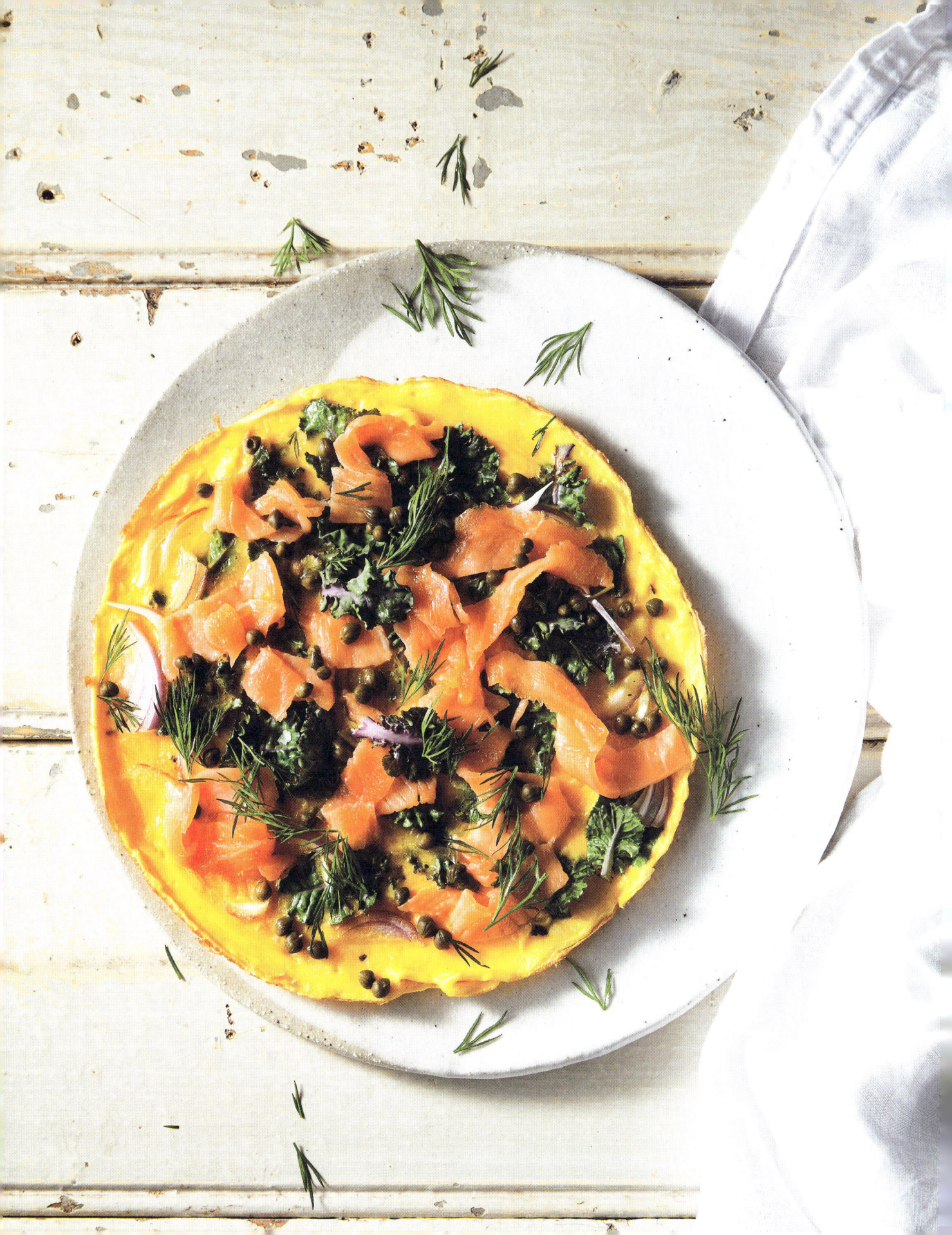

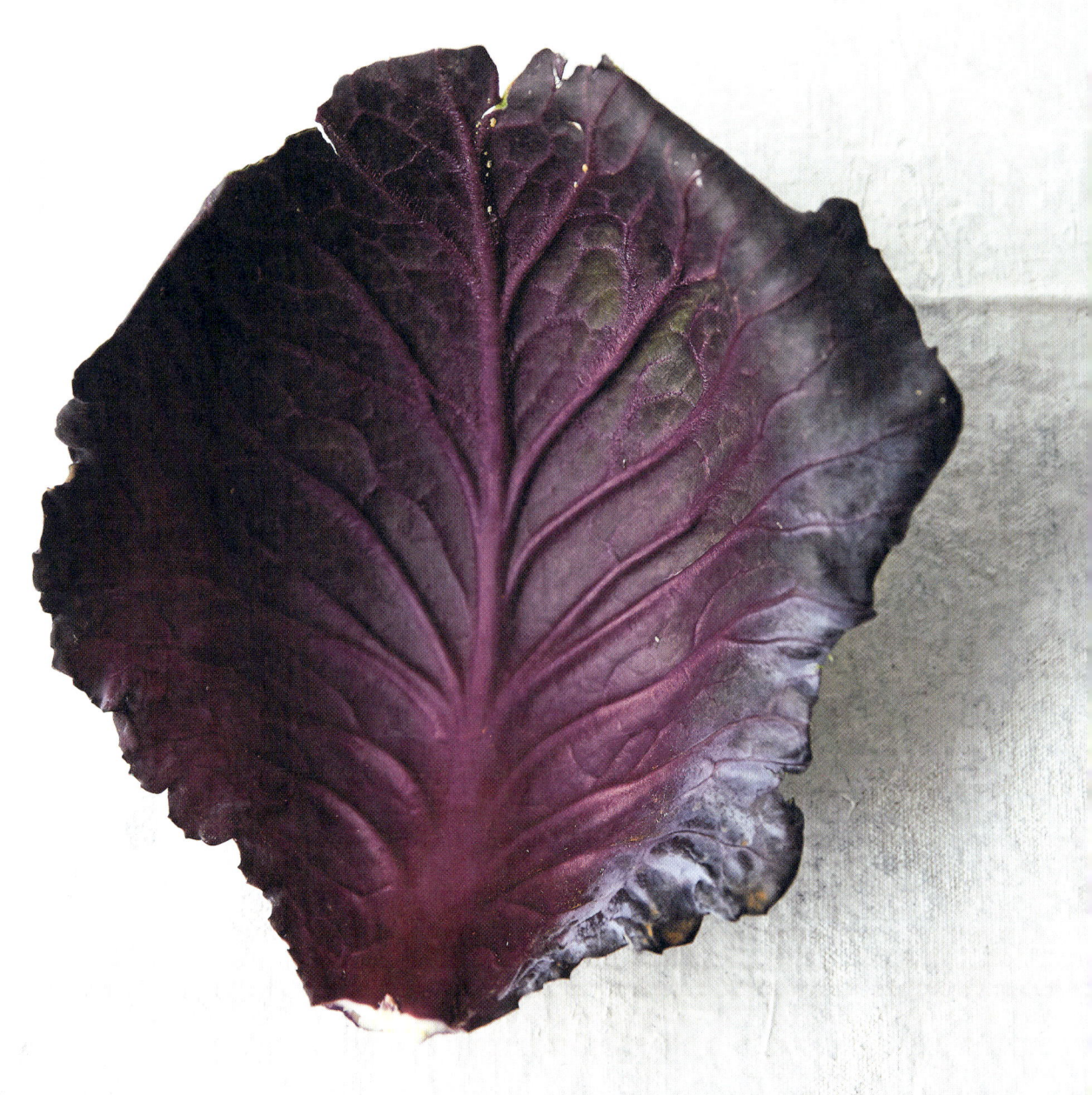

SAVOURY

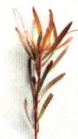

SPICED BEETROOT DIP WITH RAINBOW VEG

This beetroot dip is one of the yummiest things I've eaten, thanks to the sprinkle of garam masala that gives it such an interesting flavour twist. This makes the perfect vegan snack with carrot, cucumber and capsicum sticks, though non-vegans should know that soft goat's cheese used in place of the cashews is very tasty too.

SERVES 4–6

2 large beetroot, roughly chopped

¼ red onion

½ cup (80 g) cashew nuts (activated if possible, see page 108)

½ teaspoon garam masala

3 tablespoons extra-virgin olive oil

zest and juice of ½ lemon

salt flakes and freshly ground black pepper

RAINBOW VEGGIE DIPPERS

baby carrots, fennel, radishes, red and yellow capsicum and Lebanese cucumbers, used whole or sliced into dipping-sized portions

Place all the ingredients, except the veggie dippers, in a blender and whiz together until smooth. Season generously with salt and pepper, spoon into a bowl and use your rainbow veggie dippers to tuck in. Any leftover dip (should you have any!) will keep for up to 4 days in the fridge.

TIP You'll need a pretty sturdy high-speed blender to blend raw beetroot to the desired consistency – if yours isn't up to the job, then use a food processor instead.

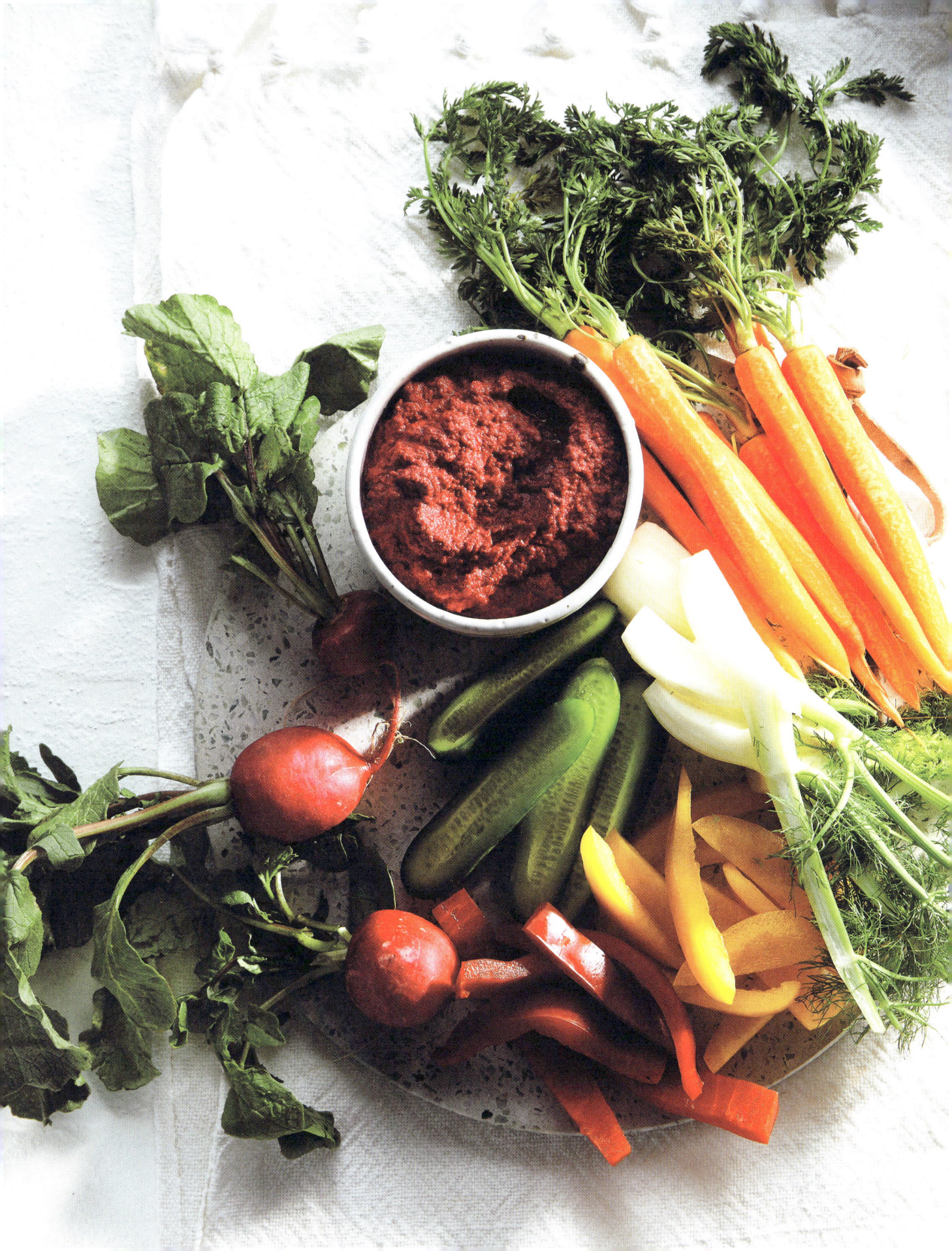

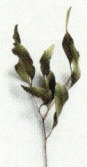

FENNEL AND ORANGE SALAD

This fresh, bright, summery salad is perfect as a light meal before a yoga class, and makes a brilliant side to go with a serve of protein. Fennel is the nutritional bomb – it's a great source of fibre, B vitamins and even vitamin C – and coupling it with oranges makes this salad the perfect immune booster. It's also really pretty and is super fast to prepare, as once you've got everything chopped up it's just a matter of a speedy assemble. That's a win-win in my book.

SERVES 4

1 large fennel bulb, finely sliced

2 oranges, peeled and segmented

2 tablespoons dried cranberries

handful of mint leaves

¼ red onion, finely sliced into rings

salt flakes and freshly ground black pepper

DRESSING

3 tablespoons extra-virgin olive oil

1 tablespoon apple cider vinegar

Pop all of the salad ingredients in a big serving bowl and mix together really well.

Combine the dressing ingredients in a small bowl. Pour the dressing over the salad and season with salt and pepper, then give everything a gentle toss. Enjoy!

TIP Try to keep some of the white pith on your oranges – it's where all the bioflavonoids are that help to make the fruit's vitamin C goodness absorbable and available for your body.

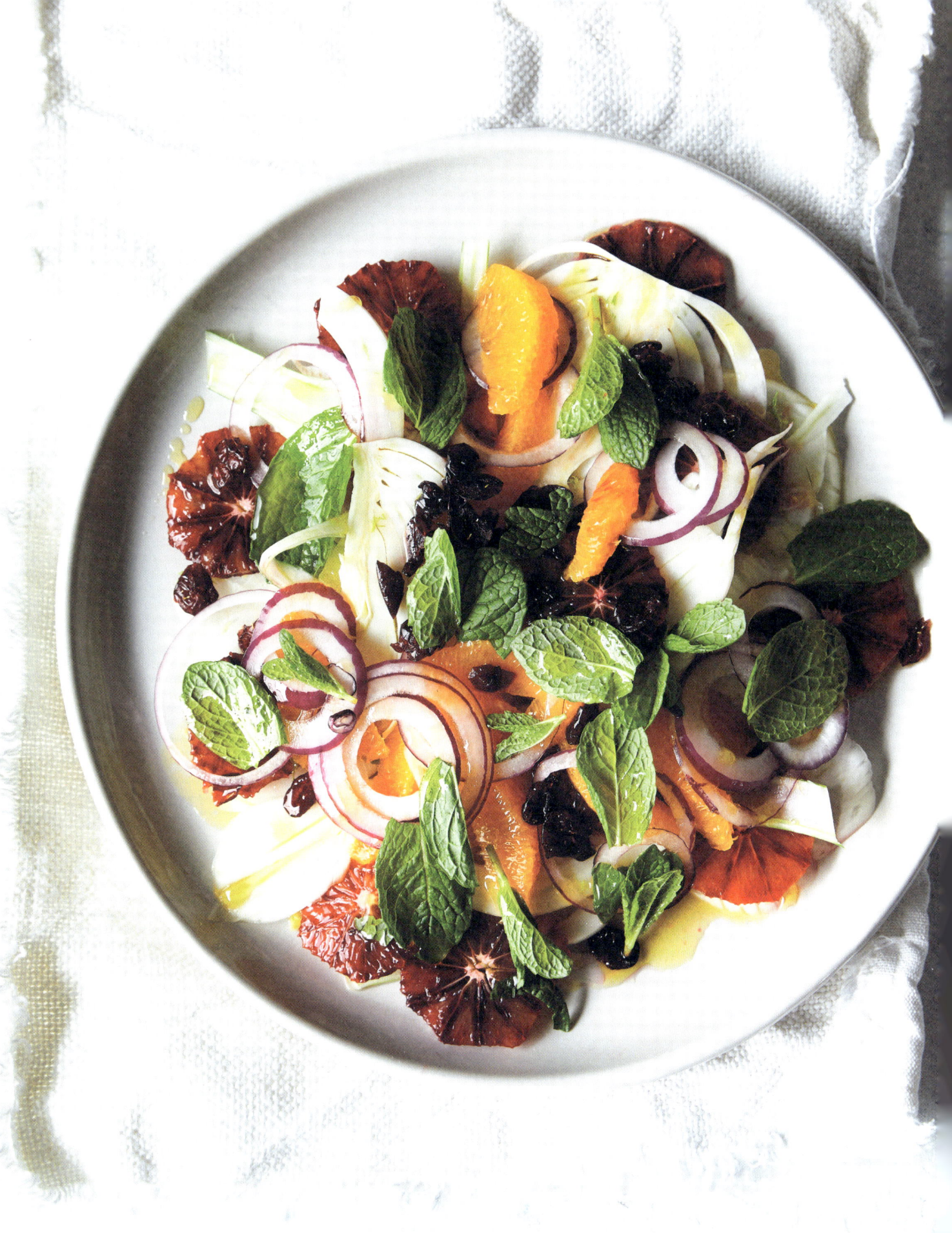

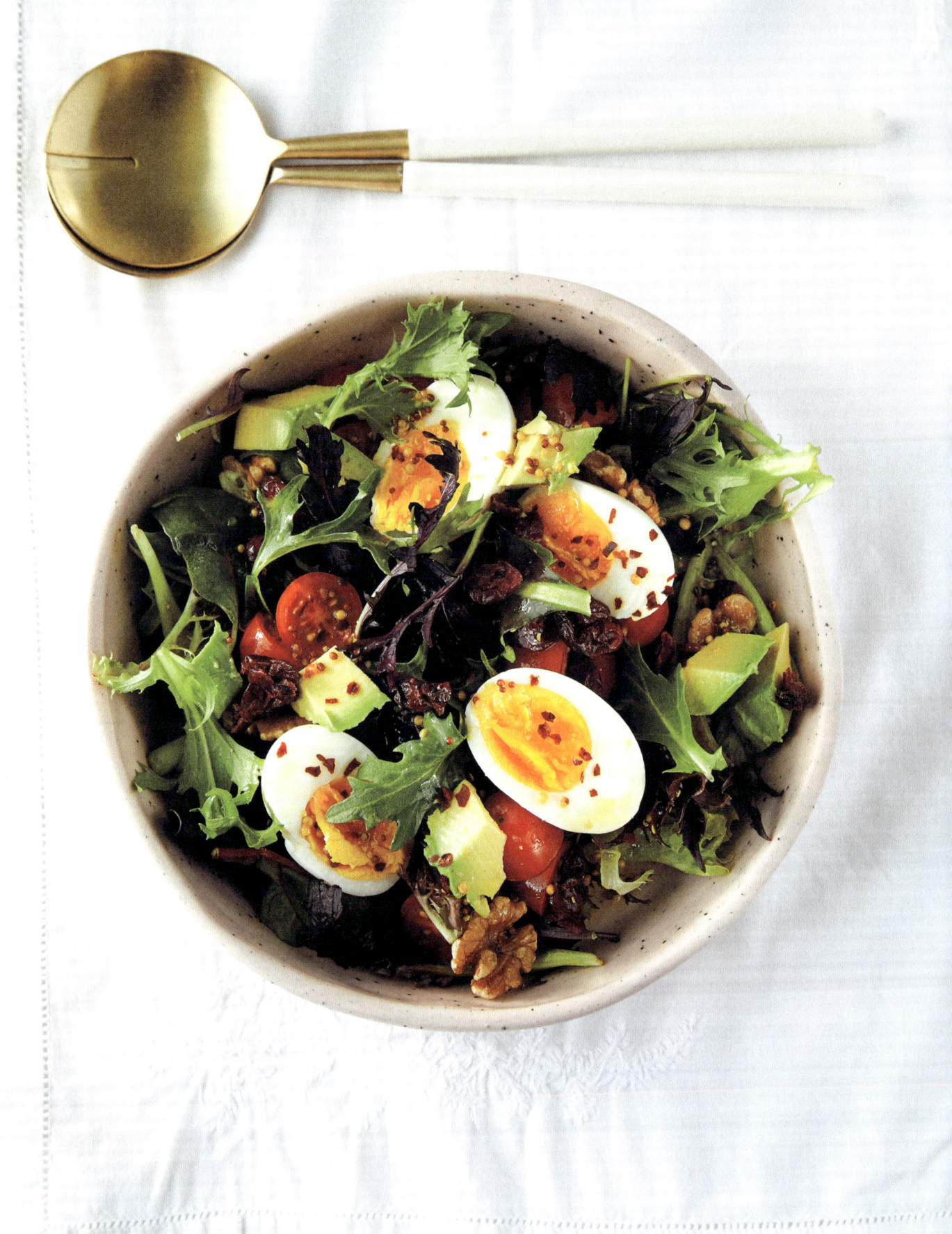

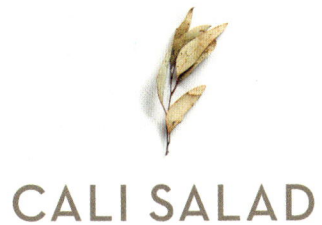

CALI SALAD

I wrote this recipe while staying at a sweet little place in West Hollywood – the perfect spot to come up with a delicious Cali salad. To me, the perfect LA salad is nutrient-dense and vibrant, and this one definitely ticks all the boxes. It's full of good fats for brain health (our brains are 60 per cent fat, so good fats help them thrive) along with protein to keep us feeling full, strong and clear in the mind, as well as fibre and antioxidants, plus almost every vitamin and mineral. They call California the land of dreams, and this is the perfect salad to help you feel on track with any goal.

SERVES 2

2 handfuls of baby salad leaves

1 avocado, diced

½ punnet (125 g) cherry tomatoes, halved

½ cup (60 g) walnuts (activated if possible, see page 108)

3 tablespoons dried cranberries

2 eggs, hard-boiled and halved

salt flakes and freshly ground black pepper

pinch of chilli flakes (optional)

DRESSING

2 tablespoons extra-virgin olive oil

1 tablespoon apple cider vinegar

1 teaspoon wholegrain mustard

This is just so simple to make. First up, combine the dressing ingredients in a small bowl, then pop the salad leaves, avocado, tomatoes, walnuts and cranberries into a large bowl, pour over the dressing and give everything a good mix. Finally, pile the halved eggs on top and season with a little salt and pepper. Serve this up as is, or top it with a sprinkling of chilli flakes if you like things hot!

TIP I think it's nice to set a little intention – a goal, or a dream – before you enjoy a healthy meal like this. We often do this at the start of a yoga class (it's called a sankalpa) and I think little things like this really help you to manifest your dreams.

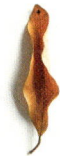

CINNAMON-HONEY CARROTS

These sweet little morsels make the perfect side dish. The cinnamon helps to balance blood-sugar levels and the carrots are a brilliant source of vitamin A, which really does aid eyesight and help us to see in dimly lit rooms.

SERVES 2

60 g butter or coconut oil, melted

3 tablespoons honey

½ teaspoon ground cinnamon

1 bunch of baby carrots, trimmed

Preheat the oven to 180°C and line a baking tray with baking paper.

Mix the melted butter or coconut oil, honey and cinnamon together in a small bowl to make a lovely glaze.

Arrange the carrots on the prepared baking tray in an even layer. Drizzle the honey glaze evenly over the carrots and bake for 10–15 minutes, or until nice and golden.

Serve with some poached chicken, baked fish fillets or pretty much any protein you like (these little gems go great guns with practically everything). Any leftovers will taste pretty delish the next day, too.

TIP Save the green tops of your carrots – they are super versatile and can be added to soups, stews, green juices or even salads (though they can be quite bitter so I think they're a bit tastier cooked). I also love them simply sautéed with some kale in a little olive oil, with some lemon juice squeezed over after cooking. Yum.

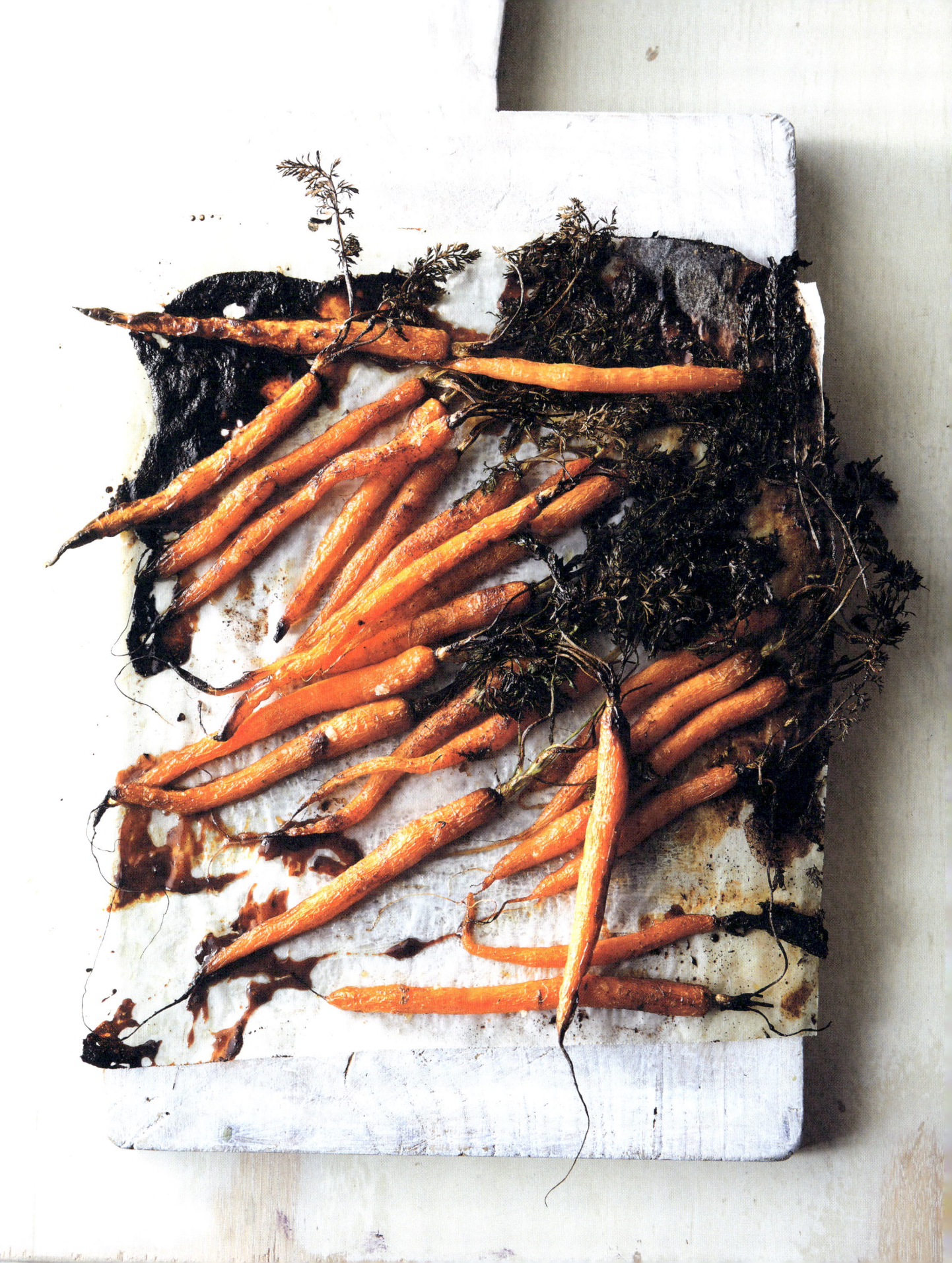

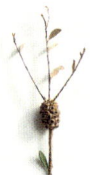

ZENNED-OUT VEGGIES

This dish is super easy to make. It's a combo of three of my favourite foods – kale, sweet potato and goat's cheese – and is something that I'll often whip up for dinner after an evening yoga class. I find that when I have complex carbohydrates at dinnertime I tend to sleep really well, so that's why this recipe is called 'zenned-out veggies'.

SERVES 2

1 sweet potato, scrubbed and cut into small chunks

3 tablespoons extra-virgin olive oil

pinch of paprika

salt flakes and freshly ground black pepper

½ bunch of kale, stalks removed and leaves finely sliced

½ cup (120 g) soft goat's cheese

3 tablespoons sunflower seeds (activated if possible, see page 108)

Preheat the oven to 180°C and line a baking tray with baking paper.

Scatter the sweet spud pieces over the prepared tray in an even layer. Drizzle over the olive oil, sprinkle with the paprika and season with salt and pepper, then bake for 20–30 minutes until slightly softened, moving the spud pieces around with a fork at the halfway stage to make sure they're cooked evenly.

Add the kale to the tray and bake for a further 10–15 minutes, or until the kale is nice and crispy and the sweet potato is cooked through. Divide the veggies between bowls, crumble over the goat's cheese, scatter over the sunflower seeds and enjoy the most delicious bowl of zenned-out veggie goodness.

TIP If you like a bit of sweetness, you can add a few sultanas, raisins or currants at the end with the sunflower seeds and goat's cheese. I've preferred to keep it more on the savoury side of late, but both versions taste great!

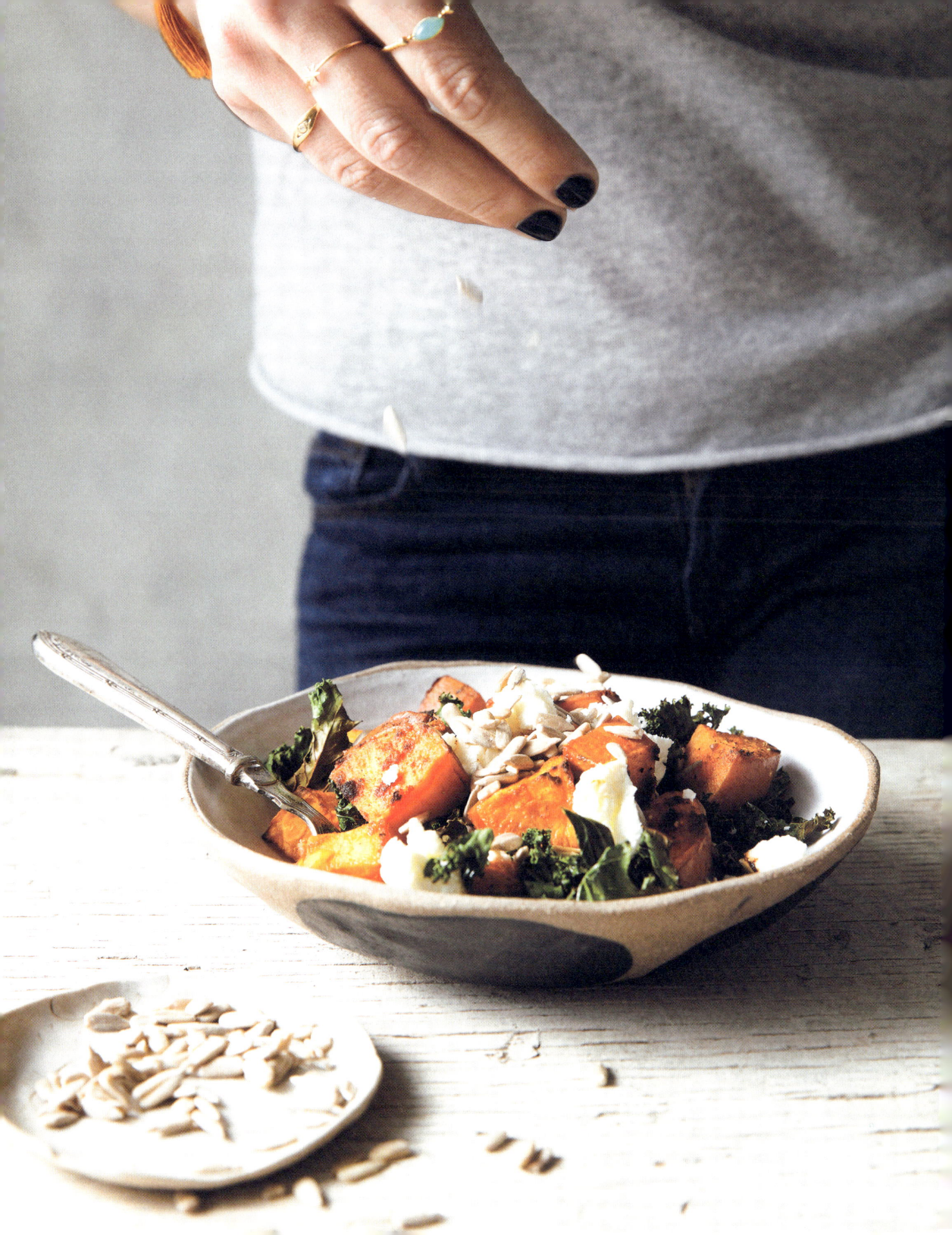

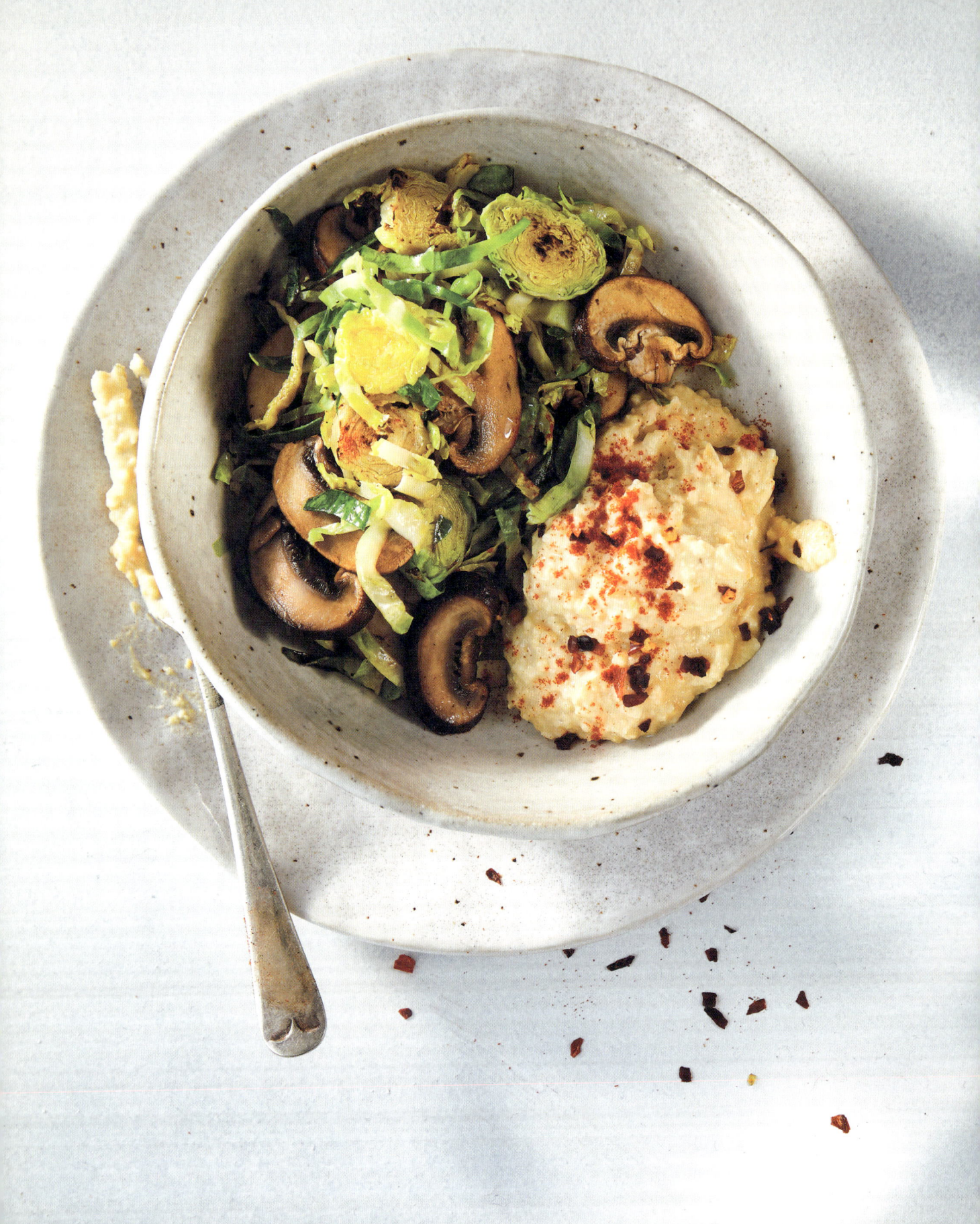

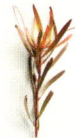

VEGAN DREAM BOWL

When I'm practising a lot of yoga, I find myself leaning towards my vegan and vegetarian recipes, and this is one of my all-time favourites. It honestly takes about 5 minutes to make and I swear I could live off it – it's high in fibre thanks to the chickpeas and brussels sprouts and is a great vegan source of protein thanks to the mushies. Most importantly, though, it tastes spot on!

SERVES 2

1 tablespoon coconut oil

large handful of brussels sprouts, finely sliced

1 cup (90 g) swiss brown mushrooms, finely sliced

salt flakes and freshly ground black pepper

pinch of chilli flakes

pinch of paprika

HUMMUS

1 x 400 g can chickpeas, drained and rinsed

2 tablespoons tahini

3 tablespoons extra-virgin olive oil

juice of 1 lemon, plus zest of ½

salt flakes and freshly ground black pepper

For the hummus, pop everything into a blender and whiz to your desired consistency. (I like mine really rustic and chunky so I just give it a few pulses, but if you like yours really smooth all you need to do is blend it for a tad longer). Set aside.

Melt the coconut oil in a frying pan set over a medium heat. Add the sliced sprouts and wait for them to turn a really bright green (this should only take 30 seconds or so), then add the mushies and cook for 3 minutes until they start to soften and release their juices.

Whip the veggies off the heat, then divide them evenly between bowls, tipping the bowls to push the veggies to one side. Add a large dollop or two of hummus to the empty sides of the bowls, season with salt and pepper, then sprinkle the chilli flakes and paprika over the lot. Now get stuck in!

TIP This hummus is an awesome staple to have in the fridge – whip it up in advance (it will keep for up to 3 days) and use it in salads, as an addition to any veggie creation or as the main event slathered over gluten-free toast and topped with sliced avo and tomato.

**FRUCTOSE FRIENDLY GLUTEN FREE
GRAIN FREE PALEO VEGAN VEGETARIAN**

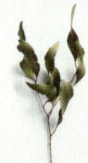

SPIRITUAL GANGSTER WRAPS

These delicious 'Spiritual Gangster' wraps are inspired by the awesome yoga gear of the same name. They are super speedy to whip up and are little nutritional powerhouses, with the actual wrap being nori seaweed – a brilliant source of iodine, which we need for healthy thyroid function to help regulate our metabolism.

SERVES 2

4 nori sheets

½ cup (130 g) hummus (see page 163 for a recipe)

1 avocado, sliced

1 large carrot, grated

1 large beetroot, grated

3 tablespoons pumpkin seeds (activated if possible, see page 108)

3 tablespoons dried cranberries

½ cup (70 g) cherry tomatoes, halved

½ cup (30 g) alfalfa sprouts

pinch of chilli flakes (optional)

salt flakes and freshly ground black pepper

Grab your first nori sheet and spoon a layer of hummus in a rough line 1 cm away from the edge closest to you. Top the hummus with a quarter of the avocado slices, a layer of the grated carrot and beetroot and a quarter of the pumpkin seeds (for crunch) and cranberries (for sweetness). Lay over enough cherry tomato halves to cover, then top with some alfalfa sprouts and a sprinkling of chilli flakes if that's your jam. Season with salt and pepper, then wrap your roll up nice and tight – I roll it away from myself but keep hugging it in tightly with each turn, which helps it hold together really well.

Dampen the edge of the nori sheet to seal, then cut the roll in half with a sharp knife. Repeat the filling and rolling with the remaining wraps and enjoy!

TIP If you're not a fan of alfalfa sprouts, try using mung bean sprouts here instead – they work really nicely, too.

DAIRY FREE GLUTEN FREE GRAIN FREE PALEO RAW VEGAN VEGETARIAN

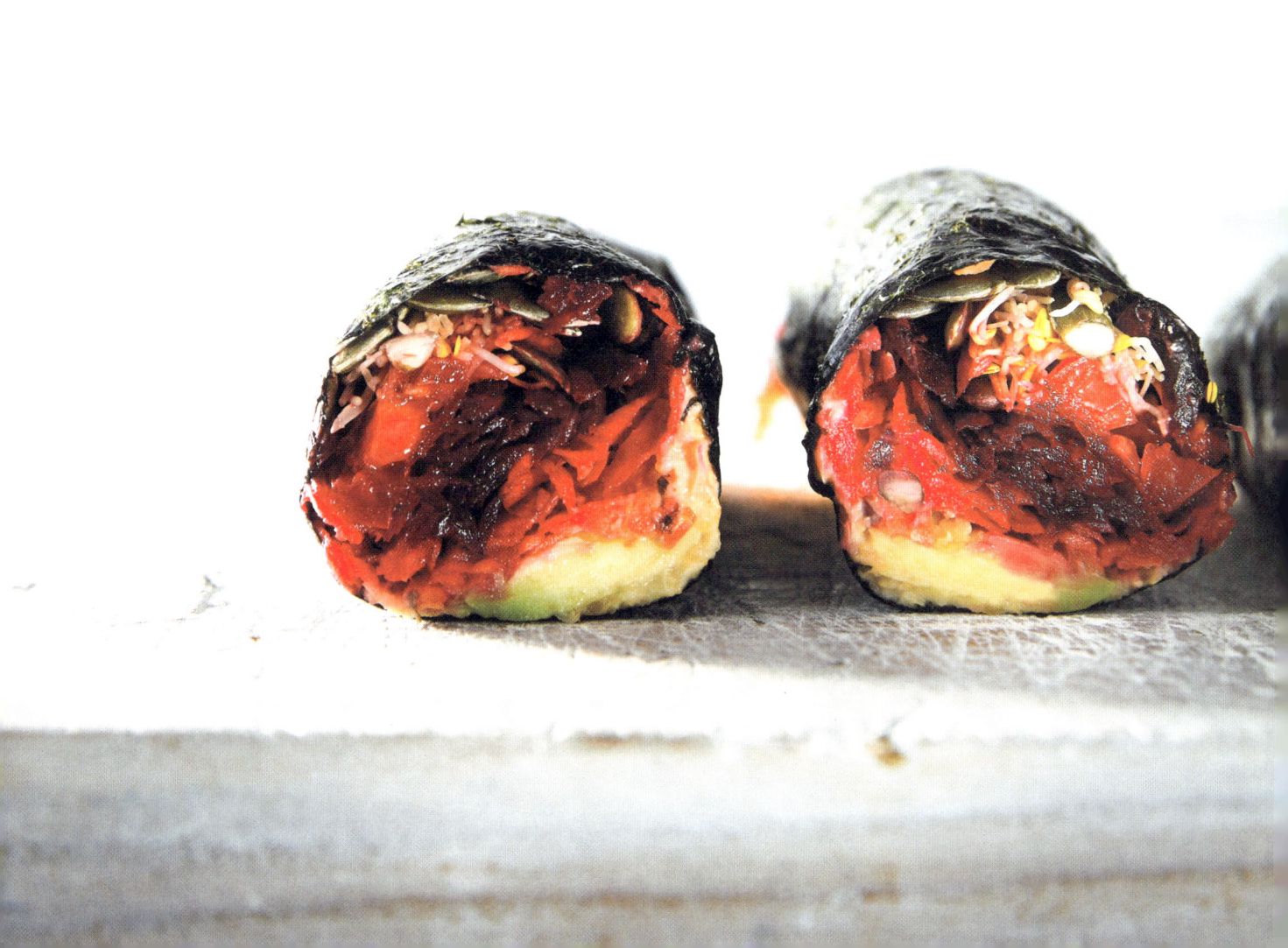

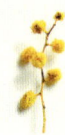

BAKED BROCCOLI BITES

I love these spice-filled flavour bombs because they're super versatile. They're great dipped in almond butter for the perfect little arvo pick me up, but they're also awesome crumbled through a salad, cut into quarters and popped in a wrap or added to a poke bowl in place of fish. These little gems contain almond meal so they're also a great source of fibre and good fats, while the ricotta adds complete protein.

SERVES 4

1 head of broccoli, broken into florets

1 cup (100 g) almond meal

½ cup (125 g) ricotta

1 teaspoon garam masala

½ teaspoon ground cumin

1 garlic clove, finely diced

2 tablespoons extra-virgin olive oil

juice of 1 lemon

salt flakes and freshly ground black pepper

3 tablespoons almond butter, to serve

handful of dill fronds, to serve

Preheat the oven to 180°C and line a baking tray with baking paper.

Add the broccoli to a saucepan set over a medium heat and pour over just enough water to cover. Bring to a simmer and cook for 4-6 minutes, or until the broccoli turns a lovely bright green. Strain, then pulse briefly in a food processor to break down into small pieces. Transfer to a bowl.

Add the almond meal, ricotta, spices, garlic, olive oil and lemon juice to the bowl, season with salt and pepper and mix everything together really well. Spoon dollops of the mixture onto the prepared tray and bake for 20-25 minutes, or until lightly golden. Remove from the oven and leave to cool slightly, then serve warm with the almond butter for dipping and a sprinkle of dill.

TIP These freeze really well, too, so make them in bulk, stash them away and you'll be set for work lunches.

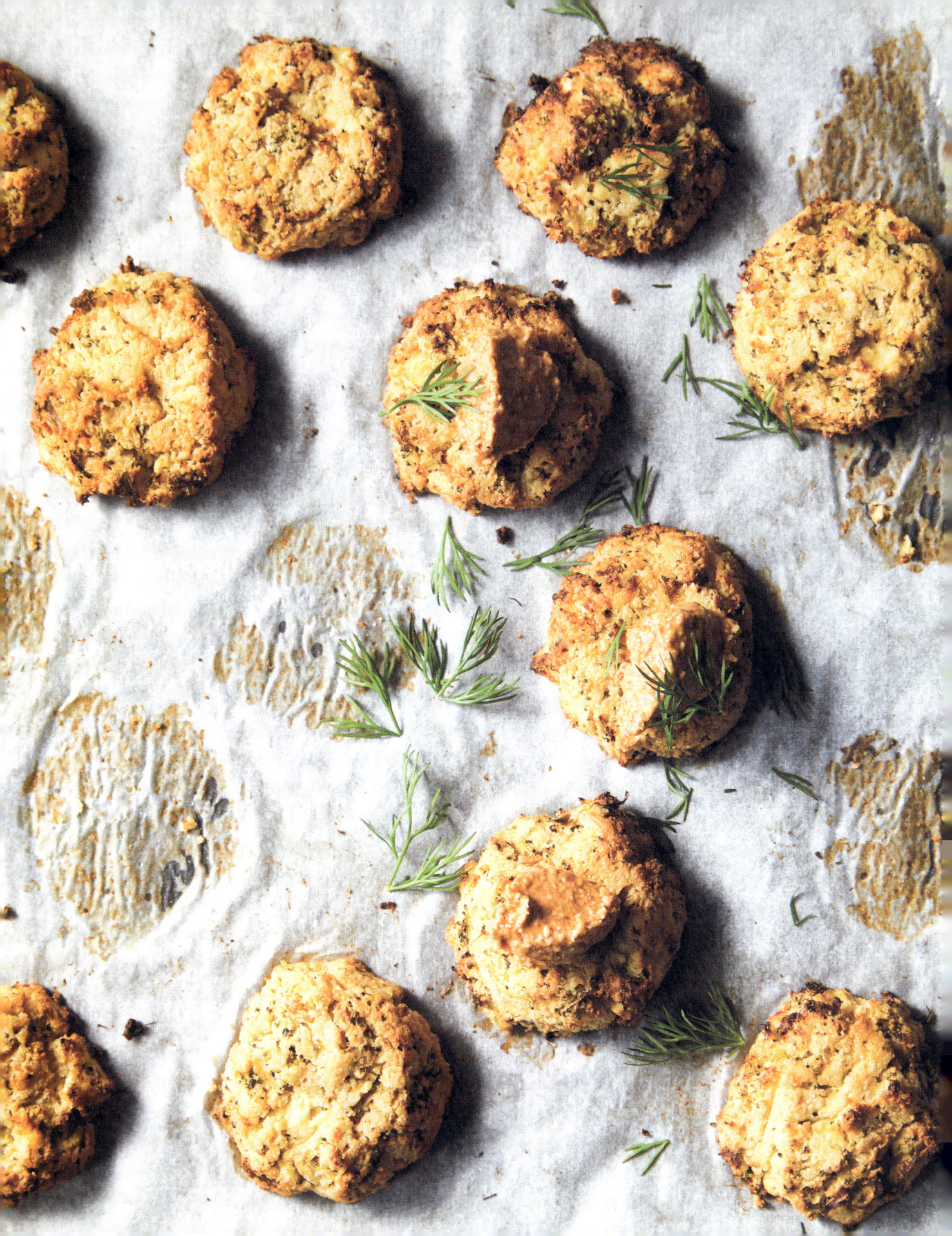

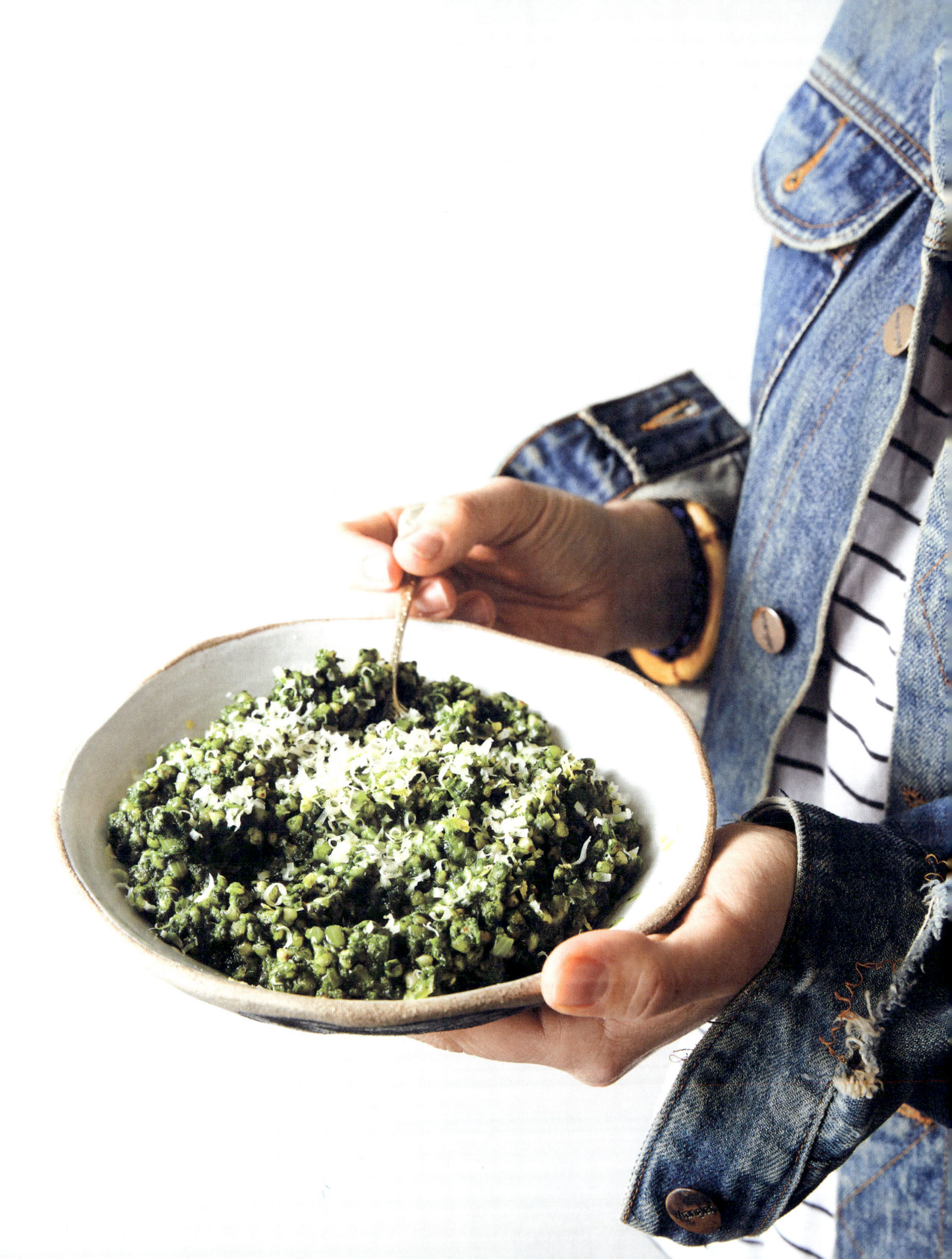

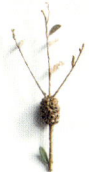

CREAMY SPINACH BUCKWHEAT RISOTTO

This creation is awesome for kids because you can call it 'monster risotto' or dinosaur food – kids love that! Not to mention it's so healthy. Buckwheat groats are not just a great source of fibre but also contain the bioflavonoid rutin, which is said to have anti-inflammatory properties. If you want to keep this recipe vegetarian, just switch the chicken stock for veggie stock.

SERVES 4

1 large bunch of spinach, finely chopped

1 cup (250 ml) coconut milk

2 tablespoons butter or coconut oil

1 onion, finely diced

2 garlic cloves, finely chopped

1 cup (160 g) buckwheat groats, soaked for 2-3 hours and rinsed

2 cups (500 ml) chicken or vegetable stock

½ cup (45 g) grated pecorino or parmesan, plus extra to serve

salt flakes and freshly ground black pepper

zest of ½ lemon, to serve

Whiz the spinach and coconut milk together in a blender (you'll end up with a lovely vibrant green liquid). Set aside.

Melt the butter or coconut oil in a large saucepan over a medium heat, add the onion and garlic and cook for 2-3 minutes until translucent. Add the buckwheat and give everything a good mix together, then pour over the stock and bring to a simmer.

Pour the spinach and coconut milk mixture into the pan and cook, stirring, for 10-15 minutes, or until almost all of the liquid has been absorbed and the risotto is looking lovely and green. Reduce the heat to low, stir through the grated pecorino or parmesan and season with salt and pepper to taste (the cheese will be salty, so you might not need much salt).

To serve, spoon the risotto into bowls and sprinkle over the lemon zest and a tad more cheese.

<u>TIPS</u> Buckwheat is actually a seed closely related to the rhubarb family and contains no gluten or wheat at all, so don't let the name scare you off this delish recipe! Being a sheep's milk cheese, pecorino can often be much easier on the stomach for people (including me) who have difficulties digesting cow's milk.

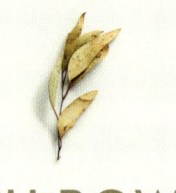

EARTH BOWLS

Earth bowls are super versatile and you can add whatever you like to them, really – they're a walk in the park to make and are a really bright, fun way of getting loads of nutrition in. You can switch out the mushrooms and mix up your protein here, adding poached chicken, salmon or even a couple of hard-boiled eggs if you'd rather. The veg, nuts and fruit can all be changed for your favourites, but this is the magic combo I love best.

SERVES 2

¼ red cabbage, grated or very finely sliced

¼ green cabbage, grated or very finely sliced

1 avocado, sliced

½ punnet (125 g) cherry tomatoes, halved

½ punnet (60 g) blueberries

handful of swiss brown mushrooms, finely sliced

1 carrot, grated

1 beetroot, grated

½ cup (80 g) macadamia nuts (activated if possible, see page 108), roughly chopped

3 tablespoons roughly chopped brazil nuts (activated if possible, see page 108)

½ cup (60 g) dried blueberries

2 tablespoons almond butter

salt flakes and freshly ground black pepper

juice of 1 lemon

The trick here is to get everything all ready on your chopping board and neatly separated out into little mounds. Then it's time to start building your bowls – I like to start with the grated cabbage as a base, then I add the rest of the ingredients one by one (apart from the lemon juice), keeping them separate so that it all looks really pretty. Season with salt and pepper (and take a quick snap, if you like), then squeeze over the lemon juice and mix everything together really well. Now tuck on in.

TIP Quinoa, sweet spud and any of your favourite nuts, seeds and fruit will all taste great in these bowls, so feel free to mix things up.

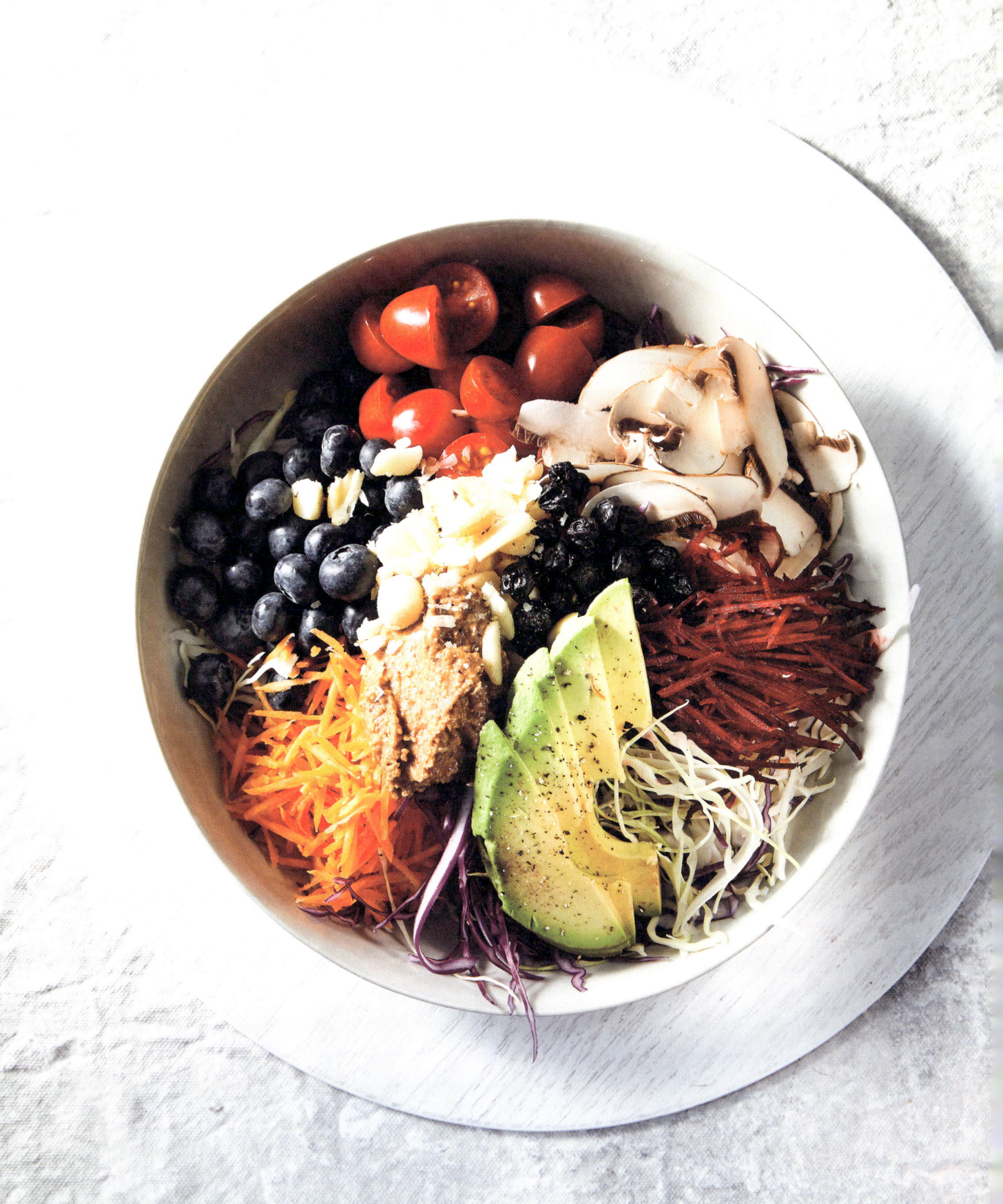

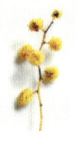

WISH NOODLES

I love using zucchini noodles in place of regular pasta – they are much higher in nutritional value and fibre, without any of the gluten and carbs. Plus, when cooked, the texture is similar to regular pasta, so you don't feel like you are missing out, and you can add pretty much anything you like to them! Together with this lovely kale and macadamia pesto they make the perfect cleansing vegan meal.

SERVES 2

1 large zucchini (or 2 medium)

½ punnet (125 g) cherry tomatoes, halved (I like to use multi-coloured)

8 green olives, pitted and sliced

3 tablespoons sunflower seeds (activated if possible, see page 108)

SUPERFOOD PESTO

1 cup (160 g) macadamia nuts (activated if possible, see page 108)

zest and juice of 1 lime or lemon

1 garlic clove

2 tablespoons extra-virgin olive oil, plus extra if needed

handful of baby spinach

handful of kale, washed and stalks removed

large handful of basil leaves, plus extra to serve

salt flakes and freshly ground black pepper

For the noodles, slice the zucchini into noodles using either a mandoline, a veggie spiraliser or a green papaya grater. Transfer to a large bowl.

To make the pesto, place all the ingredients in a food processor or blender and blitz until you have the texture you like (you may need to add a little more oil to get your desired consistency). Season to taste with salt and pepper.

Tip the pesto over the noodles, add the cherry tomatoes and green olives and mix together well. Divide between serving bowls and top with the sunflower seeds and a few extra basil leaves.

<u>**TIP**</u> If you like your zucchini noodles warm, all you have to do is dunk them in simmering water for about 1 minute, then strain and place them in a big mixing bowl. (I personally love them cold, but both work and warm is more pasta-like.)

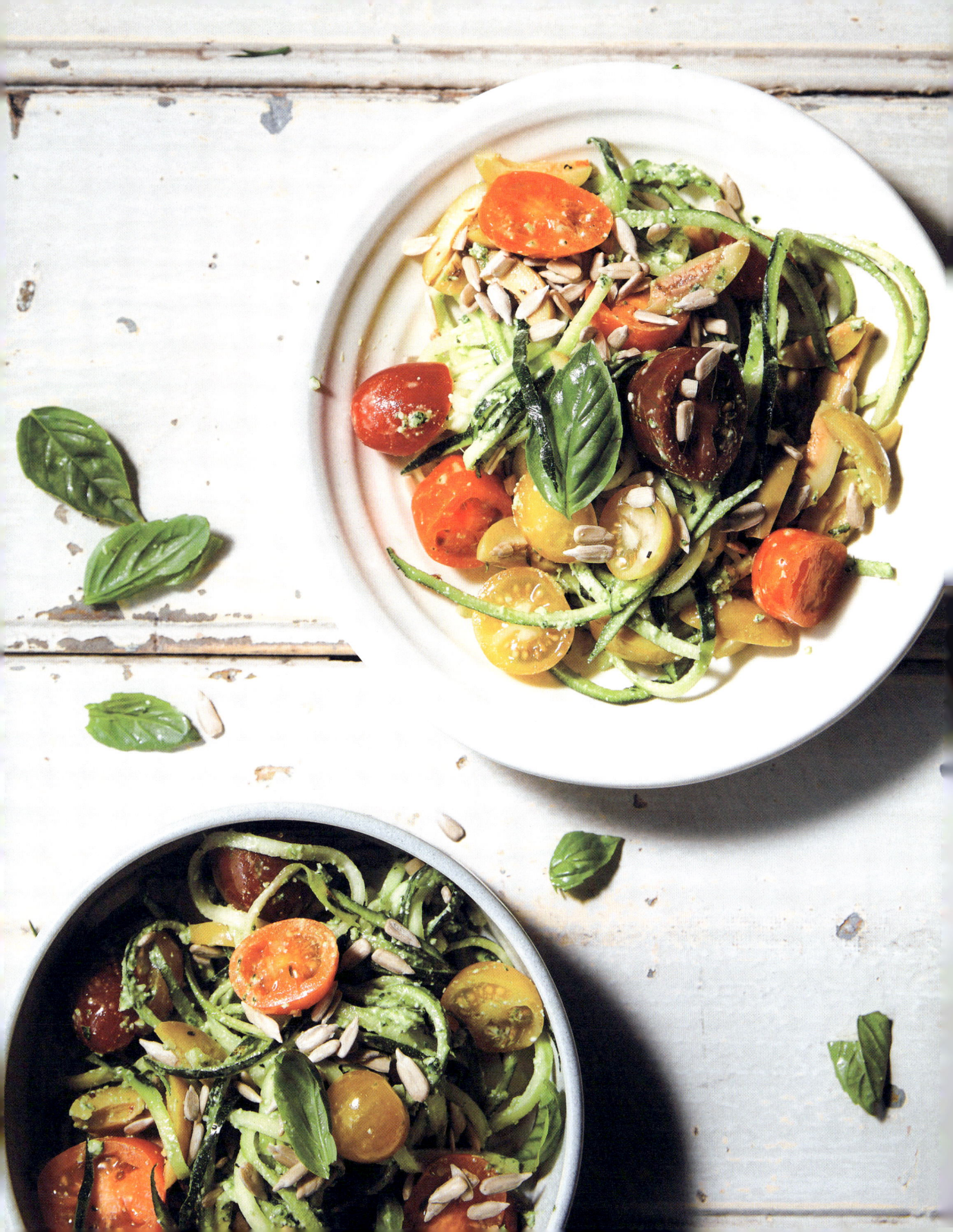

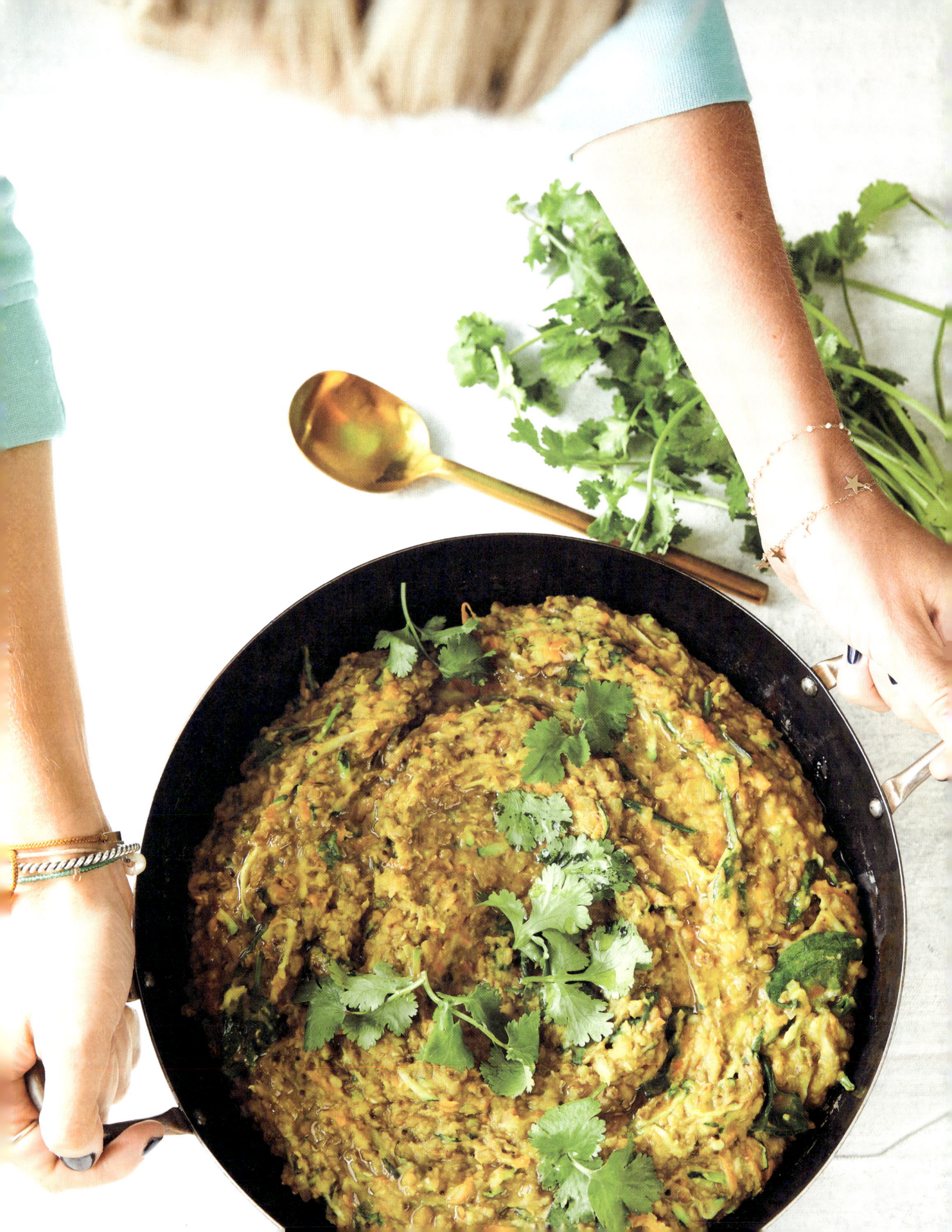

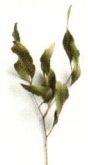

MUNG BEAN DHAL

Dhal has been used for thousands of years in traditional Indian medicine for its healing qualities – it's said to balance all three of the doshas (see page 76) and help to remove toxins (ama) from the body. People have been known to cleanse on this meal alone for a week, so it must be pretty nourishing! It's also said to aid digestion and, thanks to the spices, has beneficial anti-inflammatory properties.

SERVES 4

1 litre chicken stock, plus extra if needed

2 cups (400 g) green mung beans, soaked overnight and rinsed

½ teaspoon mustard seeds

½ teaspoon cumin seeds

2 tablespoons ghee, coconut oil or butter

1 onion, finely diced

2 garlic cloves, diced

2 cm piece of ginger, grated

2 cm piece of fresh turmeric, grated

2 carrots, grated

1 zucchini, grated

100 g baby spinach

salt flakes and freshly ground black pepper

½ bunch of coriander, leaves picked

Bring the stock to the boil in a large saucepan. Reduce the heat to a simmer, add the mung beans and cook, stirring occasionally, for 15–20 minutes, or until tender.

Meanwhile, set a frying pan over a medium heat, add the mustard and cumin seeds and dry fry until the mustard seeds begin to pop. Add the ghee, coconut oil or butter, the onion, garlic, ginger and turmeric to the pan and cook for 3 minutes (the room should smell pretty amazing at this point).

Tip the spice mixture into the mung beans and give everything a good stir, then cook for a further 5 minutes, stirring occasionally and adding a touch more stock or a splash of water if it looks as though the dhal is sticking to the bottom of the pan. Add the carrot, zucchini and baby spinach and cook, stirring, for a final 5 minutes, then remove from the heat and spoon into bowls.

Season with salt and pepper and serve topped with loads of coriander leaves.

<u>**TIPS**</u> I like my dhal nice and thick, but if you prefer yours soupy then add another 1 cup (250 ml) of stock before serving. And if you want to keep this one vegetarian, switch the chicken stock for veggie. Also, be sure to give your soaked mung beans a good rinse before using them as this makes them easier to digest.

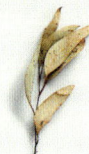

BANANA CURRY WITH COCONUT QUINOA

It may sound unusual, but this dish is both delicious and full of health benefits. I love adding bananas to meals because they're full of fibre, contain truckloads of potassium – which is an important electrolyte – and are a great source of slow-release complex carbohydrates.

SERVES 4

1 tablespoon coconut oil

½ onion, diced

½ teaspoon cumin seeds

½ teaspoon ground turmeric

1 cm piece of ginger, grated

1 green chilli, finely chopped

3 bananas, peeled and roughly chopped

½ cup (125 ml) coconut milk

salt flakes and freshly ground black pepper

juice of ½ lemon

handful of coriander leaves

COCONUT QUINOA

1 x 400 ml can coconut cream

2 tablespoons desiccated coconut

½ teaspoon coriander seeds

2 cups (400 g) mixed quinoa, rinsed

To make the coconut quinoa, combine everything in a saucepan with 2 cups (500 ml) of water and bring to the boil. Reduce the heat, cover and simmer for 15 minutes, or until the quinoa has expanded to about three times its size. Set aside and keep warm.

Melt the coconut oil in a frying pan over a medium heat, add the onion, cumin seeds, turmeric, ginger and chilli and cook for 1–2 minutes, or until everything smells delish. Add the bananas and coconut milk and cook, stirring occasionally, for 4 minutes, or until the bananas have broken down a bit and everything has come together to form a lovely thick curry. Season with a little salt and pepper, remove from the heat and stir through the coriander, then spoon onto plates. Serve with the coconut quinoa, squeezing over the lemon juice and scattering over the coriander to finish. Enjoy!

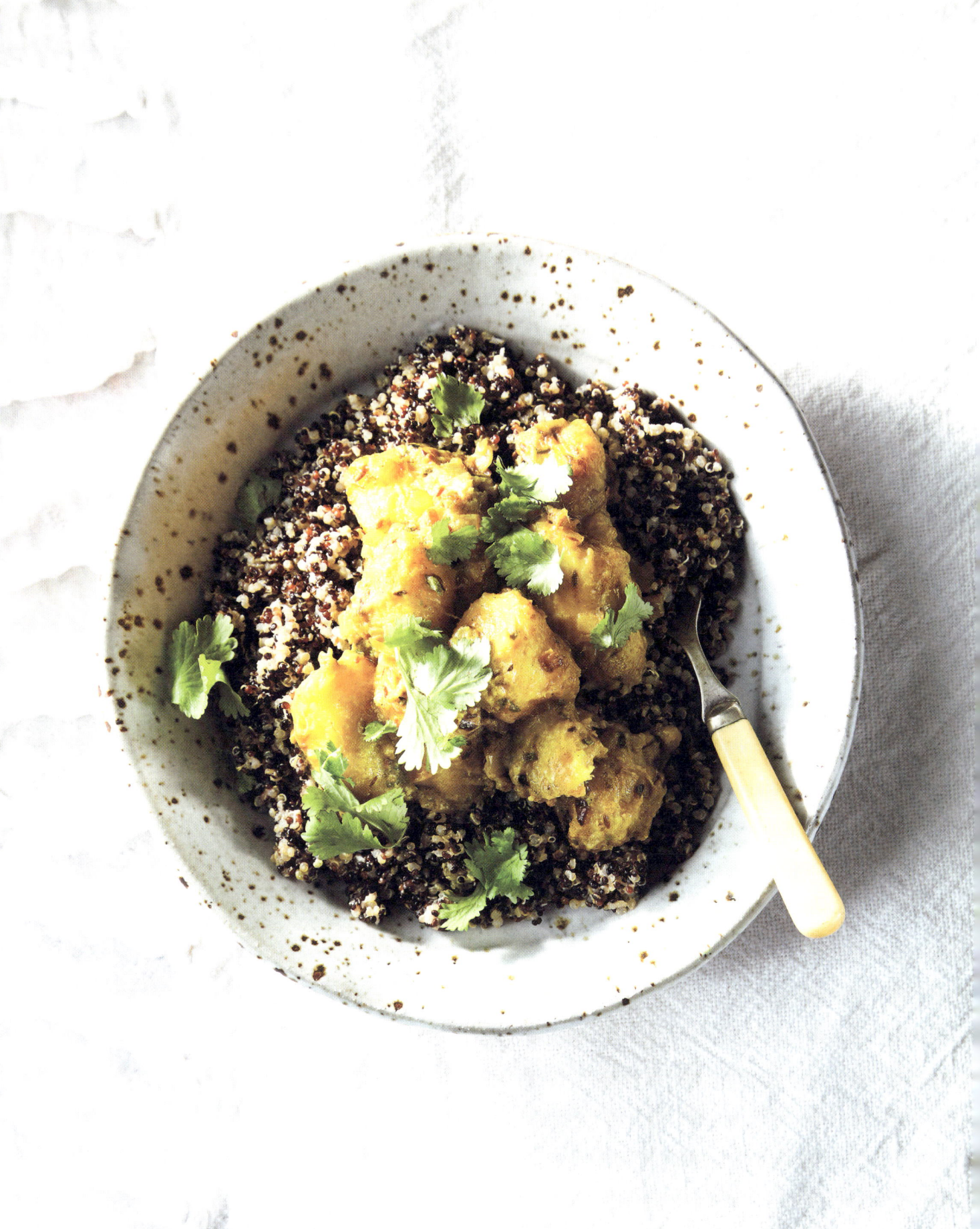

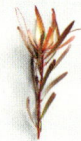

PERFECT SUPER PLATTER

This dish is inspired by some amazing food I had at a talk I gave recently. It looked so pretty – like an incredible Instagram photo – that I almost didn't want to eat it. I did, of course, and everything tasted brilliant! This is less of a set recipe and more of an assembly of simple, cute things that are really easy to prep. It's great for a party or event.

SERVES 6

1 x pink hummus (see Tip)

1 x Superfood Pesto (see page 172)

1 punnet (250 g) strawberries, halved (keep the green bits on for extra colour)

2 punnets (250 g) blueberries

4 Lebanese cucumbers, cut into sticks

2 red capsicums, cut into sticks

1 big bunch of green grapes, broken into smaller bunches

1 big bunch of red grapes, broken into smaller bunches

Cookie Dough Balls (see page 202)

Raw, Vegan Hawaiian 'Doughnuts' (see page 207)

1 cup (160 g) macadamia nuts

1 cup (130 g) dried cranberries

1 cup (125 g) sunflower seeds

150 g honeycomb, broken into large chunks

OPTIONAL TABLE DRESSING

cinnamon sticks

whole cloves

star anise

whole nutmeg

edible flowers

Start by laying one huge platter or wooden chopping board (or a few smaller ones) down the centre of the table. Then arrange all the ingredients in lots of little bowls of different shapes and heights and place them around the board, starting with the dips in the middle of the table. Place the table dressing bits and pieces around the bowls to finish things off and get everything looking great. Then step back and let everyone get stuck in – the idea is that they all make up their own little plates of goodies.

<u>TIPS</u> This is all about the height and layers so do have a good play around with everything on your platter. My mate Guy from Bondi Harvest, who's an amazing chef, taught me that food should look like edible art, and having all these colours and different layers certainly makes this spread a real beauty to look at. To make your hummus pink, add 1 chopped beetroot to my usual recipe (see page 163) in the blender before whizzing everything together. If you can, try to use activated nuts and seeds (see page 108).

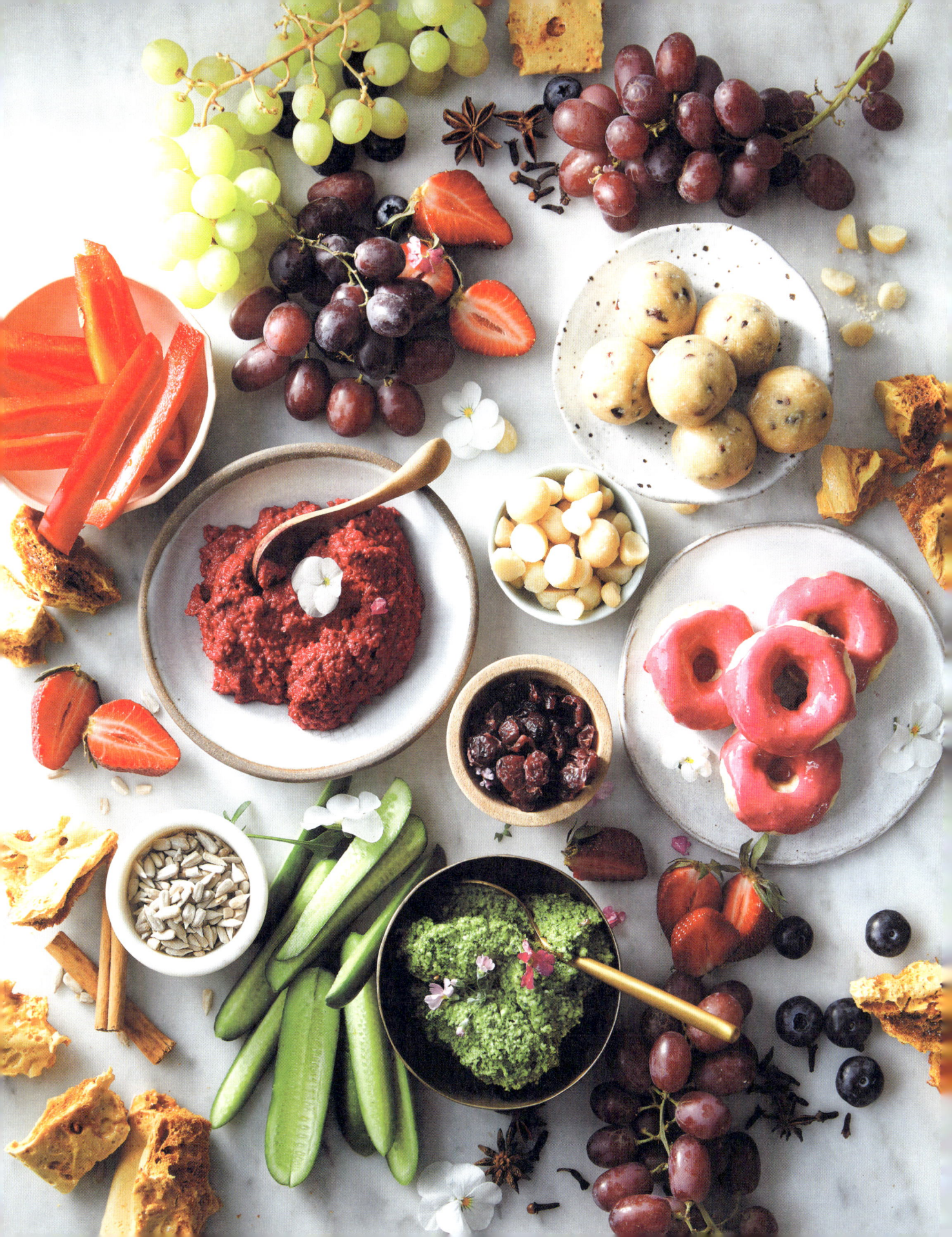

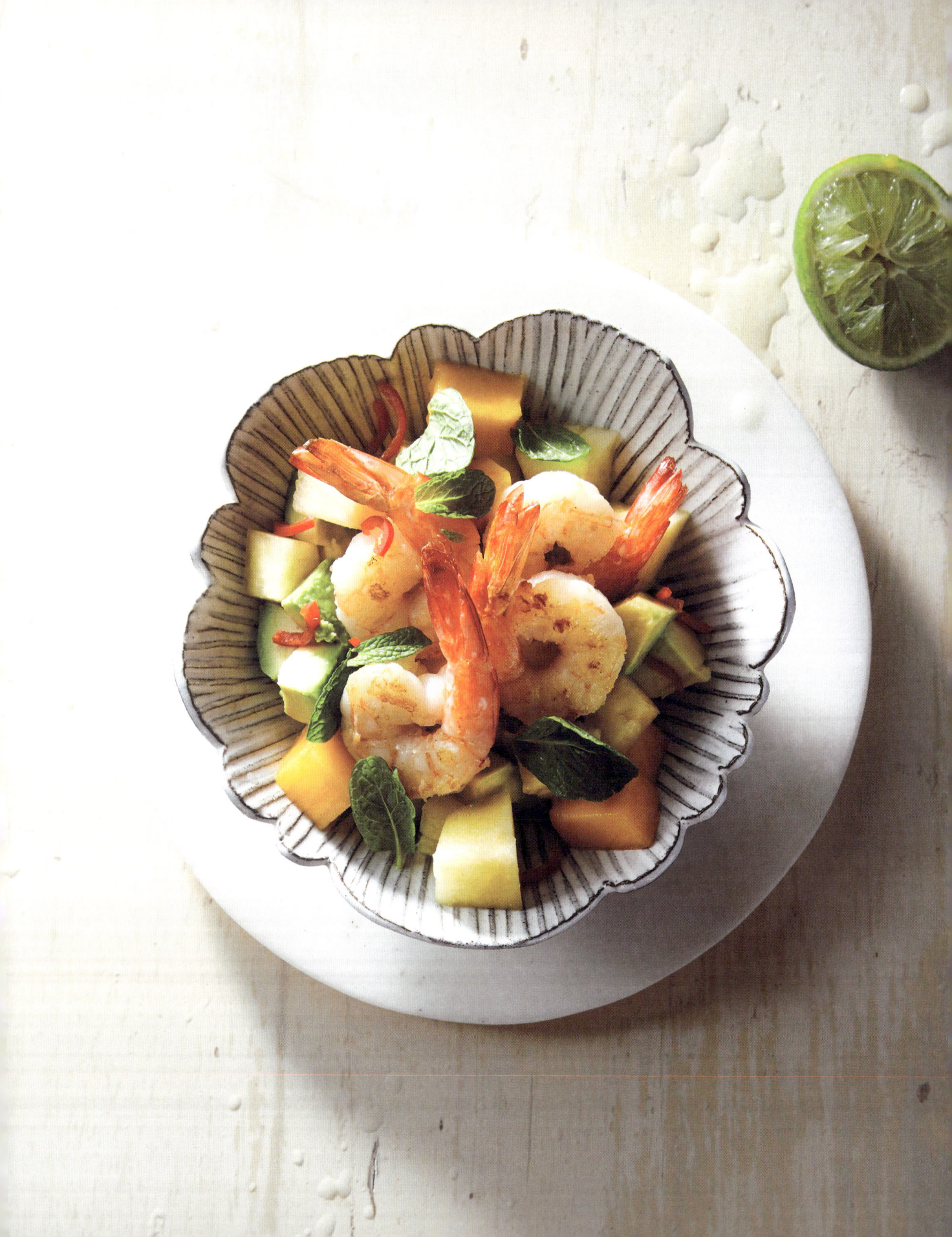

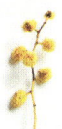

PINEAPPLE PRAWN COCKTAILS

These might seem really retro, but they're a nice, light way of getting a good whack of protein on board. The pineapple is high in bromelain – a proteolytic enzyme (that's just a fancy way of saying that it helps to digest protein) that also has anti-inflammatory properties – while the avos are a great source of fibre, potassium, vitamin C and good fats. To give these that full-on cheesy 1980s vibe, serve them up in glasses, if you prefer.

SERVES 2

½ pineapple, cubed (use the core too)

1 mango, cubed

1 avocado, diced

2 tablespoons coconut oil

200 g (about 6) raw prawns, shelled and deveined

juice of 1 lime

1 red chilli, finely chopped (optional)

mint leaves, to serve

Combine the pineapple, mango and avocado in a large bowl, then spoon the mixture into individual serving bowls.

Melt the coconut oil in a frying pan over a medium heat. Add the prawns and cook for 2 minutes, then turn over and cook for a further 1 minute, or until cooked through and nicely coloured.

Divide the prawns between the bowls, squeeze over the lime juice and scatter over the chopped chilli, if using. Top with a few mint leaves, grab a fork and get stuck in.

TIP Don't be tempted to leave out the pineapple core here, as this is where a lot of that lovely bromelain can be found.

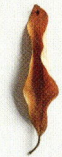

SIMPLE FLATHEAD WITH GREENS

This is a staple in my world and is exactly the sort of simple, light dinner that I love having when I'm on some kind of cleanse (and one I've been known to eat up to four times a week). White fish is such a great source of lean, complete protein, which the body works harder to process than when it's burning off carbs or fat, keeping you feeling fuller for longer. Flathead is one of my favourite white fish – it takes no time at all to cook and has a lovely, delicate flavour.

SERVES 2

1 zucchini

1 cup (90 g) broccoli florets

2 tablespoons coconut oil

4 x 80 g flathead fillets

1 avocado, sliced

1–2 tablespoons extra-virgin olive oil

salt flakes and freshly ground black pepper

juice of 1 lemon, plus zest of ½

Slice the zucchini into noodles using a mandoline, veggie spiraliser or green papaya grater.

Bring a saucepan of water to a simmer. Add the broccoli and zucchini together with 1 tablespoon of the coconut oil (I used to date a chef and he taught me this trick – it stops the veggies sticking together and makes them taste creamy) and cook for 2–3 minutes, or until they turn a nice, bright green.

Meanwhile, melt the remaining tablespoon of coconut oil in a frying pan over a medium heat. Add the flathead fillets to the pan and cook for 2 minutes, then flip them over and cook for a further 1 minute, or until cooked through.

Strain the veggies and divide them between plates along with the flathead fillets and avocado slices. Drizzle the olive oil over the veggies, season everything with a little salt and pepper and sprinkle over the lemon zest, then squeeze over the lemon juice and tuck on in. So good!

<u>TIPS</u> You can use any greens you like here – asparagus and bok choy work well, too. You can pick up a spiraliser from health-food stores or online, though a green papaya grater will also do the trick and can be bought from Asian supermarkets.

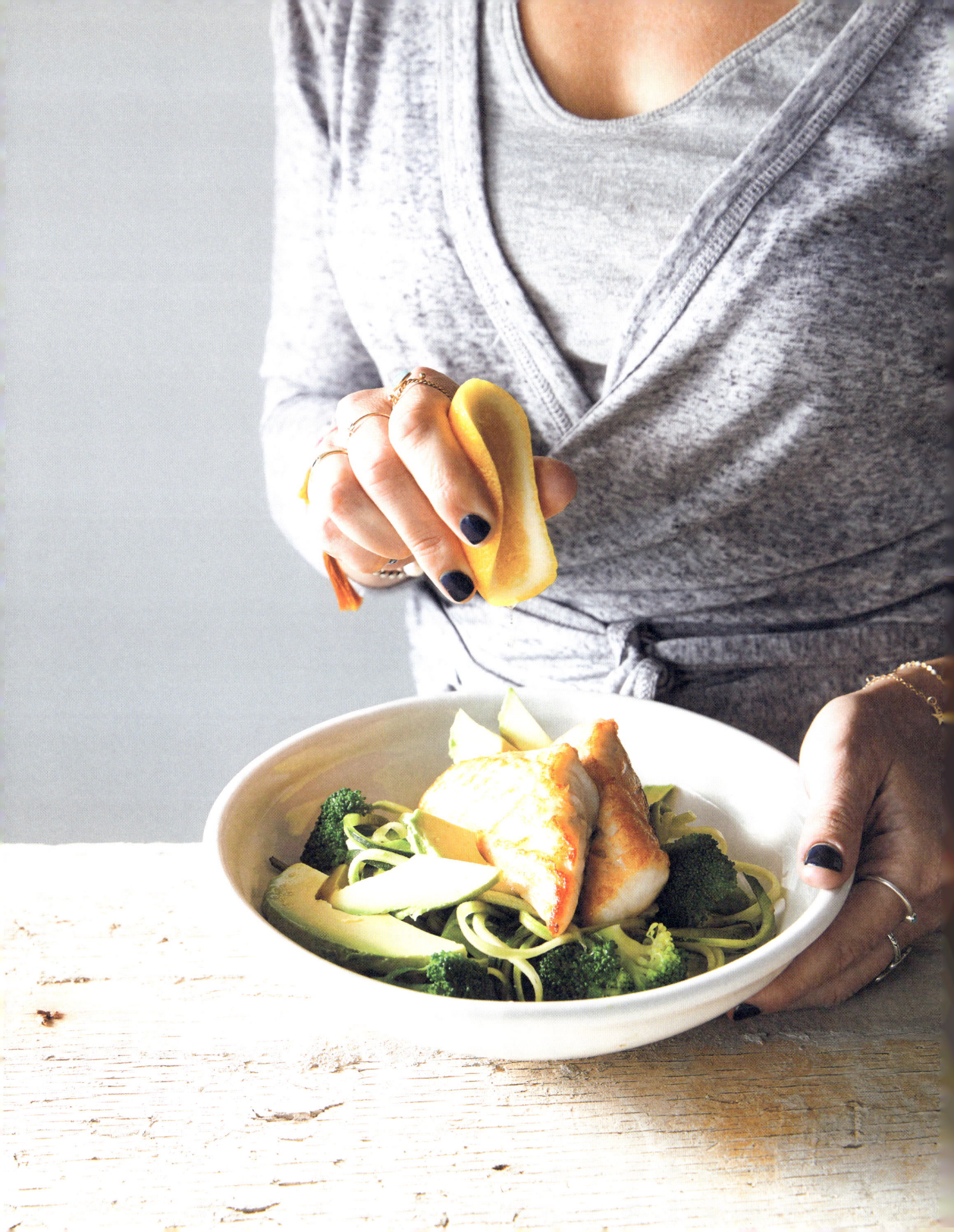

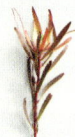

FIVE-MINUTE HEALING SUPERFOOD SALAD

This recipe is awesome because it's a nutritional bomb that is so easy to make in bulk. I've taken it on plane trips and road trips, I've taken it to events where I know there won't be healthy food available ... it's honestly such a great go-to recipe and it's easy-as to whip up. You can tweak it to suit your tastes, too; sometimes I add chopped olives, goat's cheese or jalapeños, and it works well with pretty much any protein (I love it with two soft-boiled eggs). It also tastes even better the next day, so make a big batch to give yourself enough for a few extra lunches. Side note: it's also super bright, so looks great at a dinner party or Chrissy feast.

SERVES 4

¼ bunch of kale, finely chopped

½ punnet (125 g) cherry tomatoes, halved

8 radishes, finely chopped

1 large avocado, diced

1 cup (90 g) swiss brown mushrooms, very finely diced

1 zucchini, grated

¼ red cabbage, very finely chopped

¼ green cabbage, very finely chopped

½ cup (80 g) roasted almonds (activated if possible, see page 108), roughly chopped

3 tablespoons raisins, sultanas or dried cranberries

salt flakes and freshly ground black pepper

3 tablespoons extra-virgin olive oil

juice of ½ lemon

1 x 95 g can flavoured tuna (olive oil and chilli is my fave)

This one is so simple. Just pop all the ingredients together in a bowl and give them a good old toss together, then divide the salad among bowls and dig in.

TIP You can also just throw everything into a container and shake it all about to mix it together, which, to be honest, is very practical and super handy if you're planning on taking it to uni or work for a healthy lunch. If you fancy doing that I'd suggest packing the tin of tuna separately and adding it nice and fresh just as you eat it.

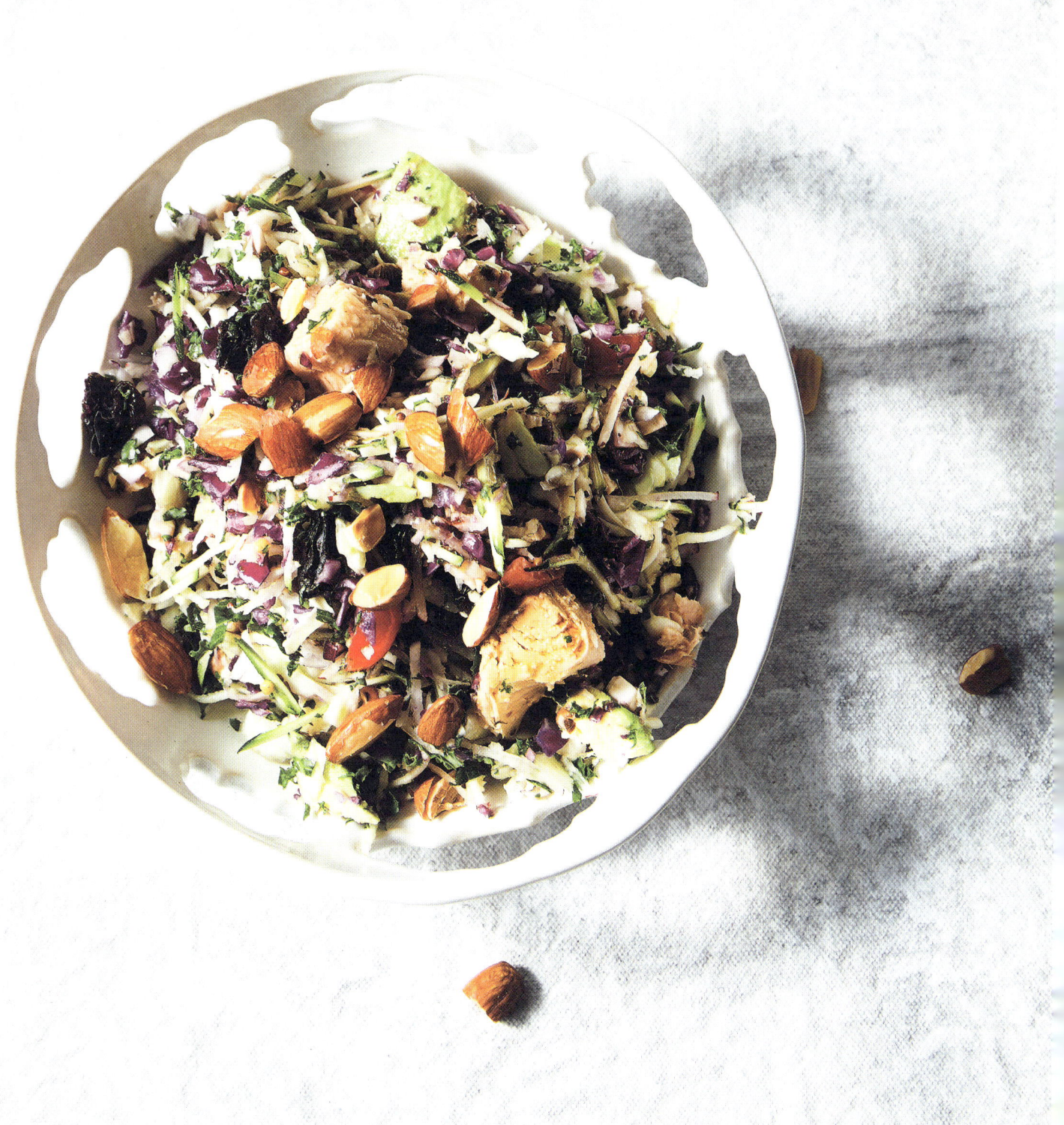

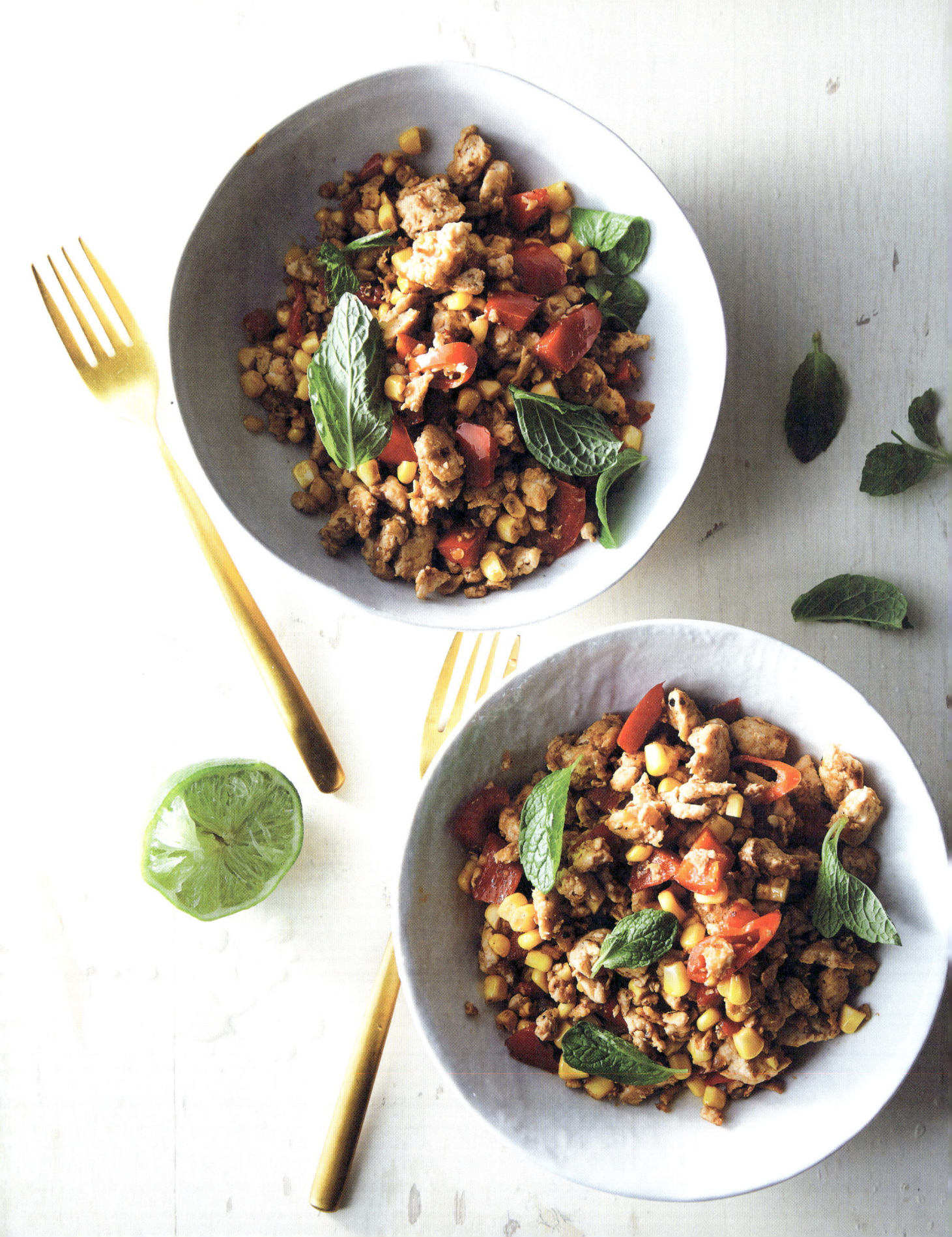

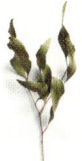

THAI MINCED CHICKEN SALAD

I was first introduced to this dish in Mauritius, and it was so amazing that I knew I had to remember as much of it as I could so that I could re-create it at home. This version, inspired by that sunset dinner, makes a lovely light post-yoga dinner or lunch, with the spicy minced chicken delivering all the essential amino acids needed to help provide a sustained energy release, as well as helping to repair the body's muscles.

SERVES 2

1 tablespoon extra-virgin olive oil

2 garlic cloves, finely chopped

¼ red onion, finely chopped

2 cm piece of ginger, finely grated

400 g chicken mince

1 red capsicum, finely chopped

1 sweetcorn cob, kernels removed

1 red chilli, finely chopped (optional)

2 teaspoons tamari

2 teaspoons fish sauce

2 limes, halved

¼ bunch of mint, leaves picked

salt flakes and freshly ground black pepper

Heat the olive oil in a frying pan over a medium heat, add the garlic and onion and sauté for 2–3 minutes, or until they begin to soften up and go translucent. Add the ginger and sauté for 30 seconds, then add the chicken mince and sauté for 5–7 minutes, or until nicely coloured and cooked through. Stir in the capsicum, corn kernels, chilli (if using), tamari and fish sauce and cook for a further 3 minutes, then remove from the heat.

Divide the mixture between bowls, squeeze over one of the limes and scatter over the mint leaves. Season generously with salt and pepper, serve with the remaining lime halves and enjoy with a mate!

GLUTEN FREE GRAIN FREE PALEO

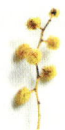

JETLAG-BE-GONE BONE BROTH

This recipe was inspired by my mate Emma Warren, who is not only a phenomenal chef but was also a lifesaver when we were on a shoot together and I had just flown in from overseas. At the time I just couldn't kick the jetlag or deal with cold Melbourne temperatures, so I was constantly sipping on bone broth. Being jam-packed full of minerals along with the powerful healers collagen and glutamine, bone broth is looked upon as a bit of an elixir these days, and Emma would add extra herbs and her magic twist to make it even tastier.

MAKES 1.3–1.5 LITRES

2 kg beef bones (a mixture of knuckle, tail, marrow and neck bones)

3 tablespoons apple cider vinegar

1 tablespoon coriander seeds

1 nutmeg, crushed using a mortar and pestle

1 star anise

1 tablespoon white peppercorns

2 teaspoons (10–12) black peppercorns

4 shallots, halved

2 cm piece of ginger, cut into thick slices

½ bunch of fresh coriander, stalks and leaves separated

Preheat the oven to 250ºC (or as hot as your oven goes). You will need a very large (8–10 litre) stockpot for this recipe.

Start by giving the bones a good wash. Place them in the stockpot and cover with cold water, then strain and repeat.

Tip the washed bones into a large roasting tin and roast them in the oven for 45–50 minutes, or until caramelised and well browned but not burnt, stirring and scraping them every 15 minutes or so.

Pop the roasted bones back in the stockpot together with the apple cider vinegar, spices, shallots, ginger and coriander stalks. Pour over enough water to cover the bones and other ingredients by about 10 cm (about 5–6 litres).

Pour a few cups of hot water into the roasting tin to lift off any remaining goodness and add this to the broth pot. Bring everything to a gentle simmer and leave to cook over a very low heat for a minimum of 12 hours (or up to 48 hours if your stove can handle cooking over super-low heat), skimming off the frothy grey foam that rises to the surface with a slotted spoon as you go and adding the coriander leaves for the final 15 minutes of cooking.

To serve, strain through a fine sieve (or through a layer of muslin for super-clear results) into a mug and sip up. Extra broth should be refrigerated straight away or frozen for later use (see Tip below). A layer of fat will solidify on top – you can either discard this or store it in the fridge to use in cooking.

<u>TIP</u> This freezes brilliantly, so make a big batch and have it ready to go in ice-cube trays. You can use it as a stock for adding to other recipes – it's so handy to have on hand. I often change up what I add to my broth, sometimes adding an egg, spring onions, spinach or grated veggies to make it more of a meal.

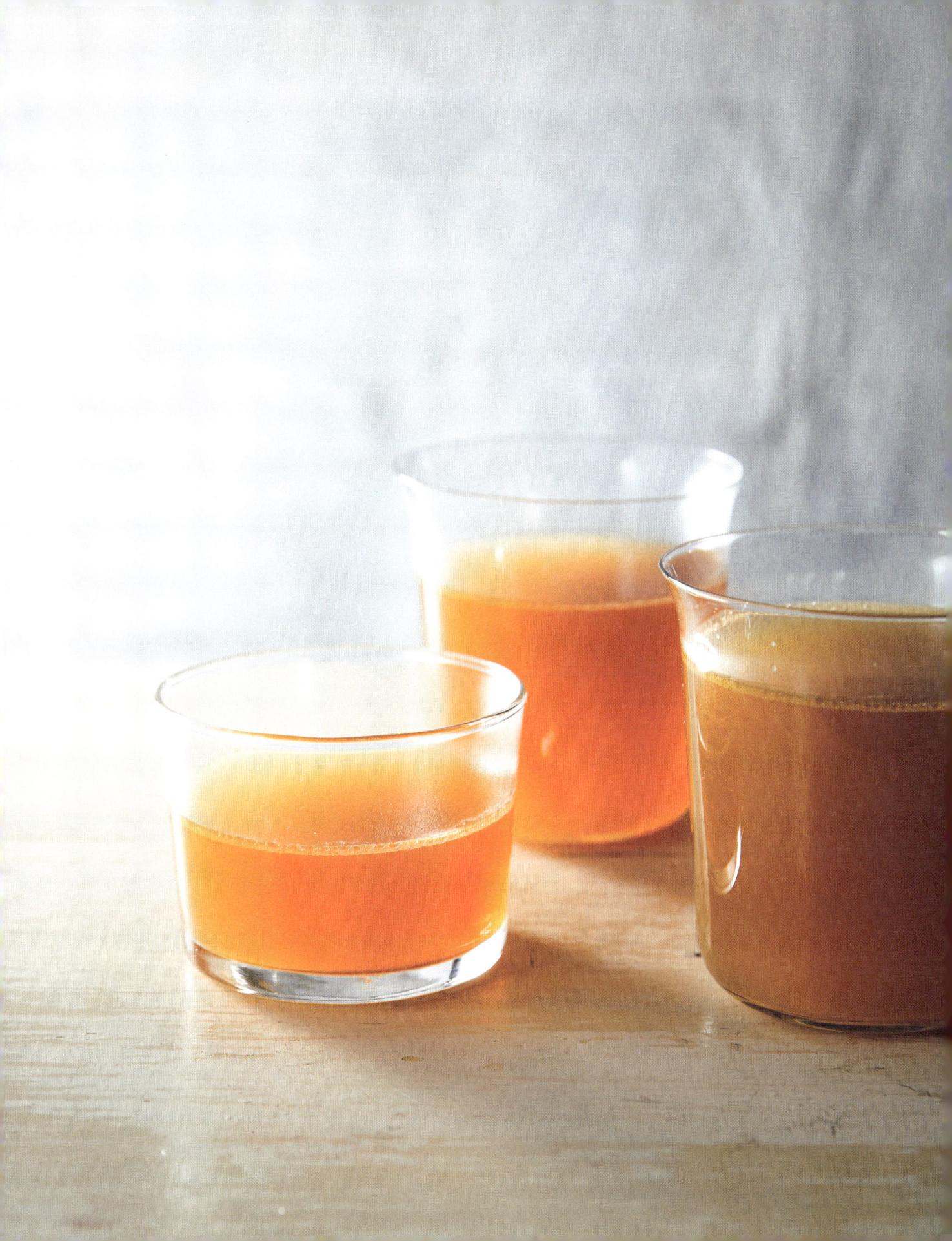

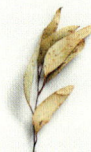

LUSCIOUS LAMB CURRY

One thing I've learnt on my travels is that we in Australia are so lucky to have access to such awesome fresh produce, and that includes our meat. Lamb is an awesome source of iron – which we need for energy and healthy metabolism function – while brown rice is chock full of fibre. This nourishing and hearty meal is perfect for when you've had a big day at work and come home starving.

SERVES 2–4

2 tablespoons extra-virgin olive oil

1 onion, finely chopped

2 garlic cloves, finely chopped

1 chilli, finely chopped (optional)

1 teaspoon ground coriander

2 teaspoons garam masala

500 g lean diced lamb

2 cups (500 ml) coconut milk

1 cup (250 ml) beef stock (or any stock you have)

2 carrots, roughly chopped

salt flakes and freshly ground black pepper

COCONUTTY BANANAS

2 bananas, sliced

juice of ½ lemon

2 tablespoons desiccated coconut

TO SERVE

steamed brown rice

coconut yoghurt

coriander leaves

Heat the oil in a large saucepan over a medium heat, add the onion, garlic and chilli and cook for 2–3 minutes until softened. Pop in the spices and cook, stirring, for another minute (it'll smell great!), then add the lamb, coconut milk, stock and carrots and season with salt and pepper. Bring to a simmer, cover with a lid and cook for 1 hour, then remove the lid and cook for a further 30 minutes, or until the meat is tender and the curry has thickened up nicely.

For the coconutty bananas, toss the banana discs together with the lemon juice and desiccated coconut in a small bowl.

Serve the curry on a bed of steamed brown rice. Top with the banana slices, dollop on a little coconut yoghurt and scatter over plenty of coriander leaves to finish. Tuck on in, and hopefully you'll have enough for leftovers the next day!

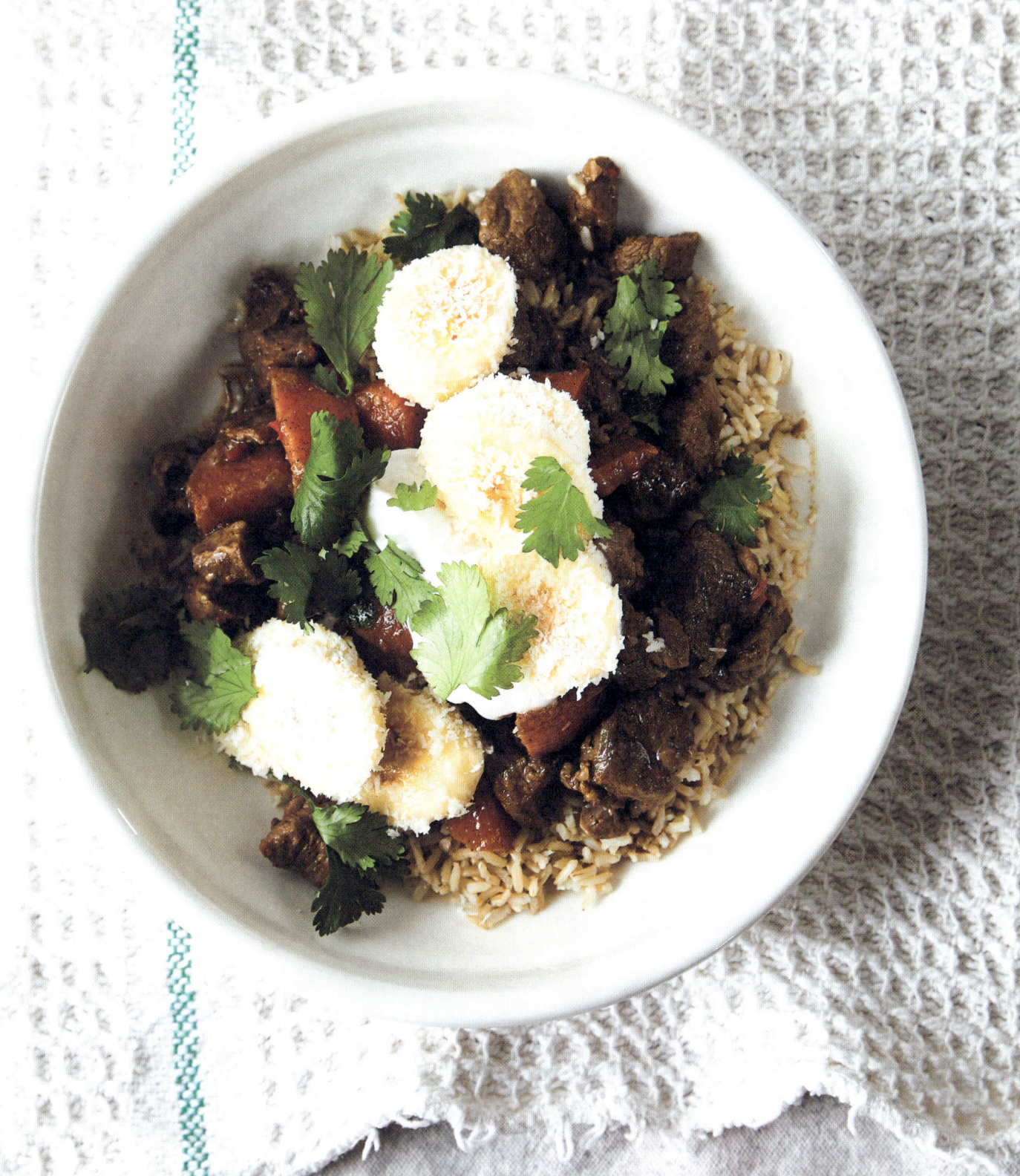

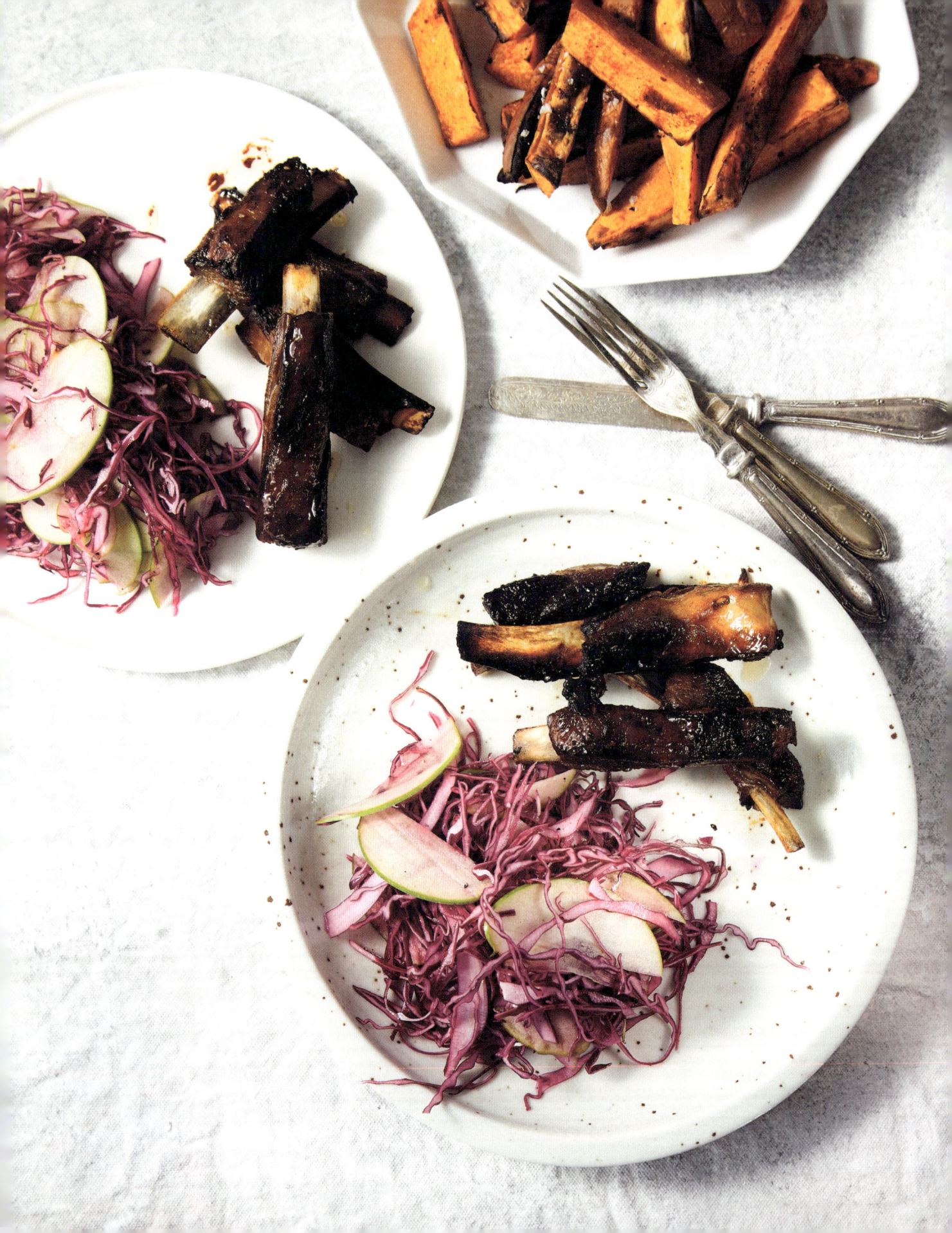

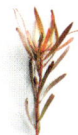

JULES' LAMB RIBLETS WITH PIPPA'S SLAW

This simple recipe was created by two very inspiring humans: Pippa, who trains me, and Jules, a weight-lifting and strength coach. They both live and breathe health, and I'm really grateful for everything that I have learned from them. I'd never had lamb ribs before tasting this creation and this salad is now up there in my all-time favourites, so I owe them big time! I love to dip sweet potatoes into the leftover juices, so feel free to serve some on the side.

SERVES 4

18–20 lamb riblets (spare ribs), at room temperature

3 tablespoons honey

3 tablespoons coconut oil

1 teaspoon salt

PIPPA'S SLAW

½ red cabbage, finely sliced

2 granny smith apples, finely sliced

⅓ cup (80 ml) apple cider vinegar

3 tablespoons extra-virgin olive oil

salt flakes and freshly ground black pepper

Preheat the oven to 160°C.

Place the riblets in a large frying pan over a high heat and cook, turning, for 1–2 minutes until sealed all over. Remove from the heat and set the riblets aside on a baking tray.

Warm the honey and coconut oil in a small saucepan until the coconut oil has melted. Drizzle the honey and coconut mixture over the riblets, sprinkle generously with salt and cover with foil. Bake for 1½ hours, then remove the foil, turn the riblets over and cook for a further 30–50 minutes, until the riblets are nice and crispy and the coconut–honey mixture is sticky and oozy.

Meanwhile, make the slaw. Grab yourself a big bowl, add the red cabbage, apples and apple cider vinegar and give everything a good mix together. Drizzle over the olive oil, season with salt and pepper and toss together. Enjoy!

TIPS You can speed things up a bit here by slicing the cabbage and apple in a food processor, if you like. The slaw tastes amazing when just made, but is even better served the following day, as this gives the cabbage the chance to pickle slightly in the vinegar – delishimo!

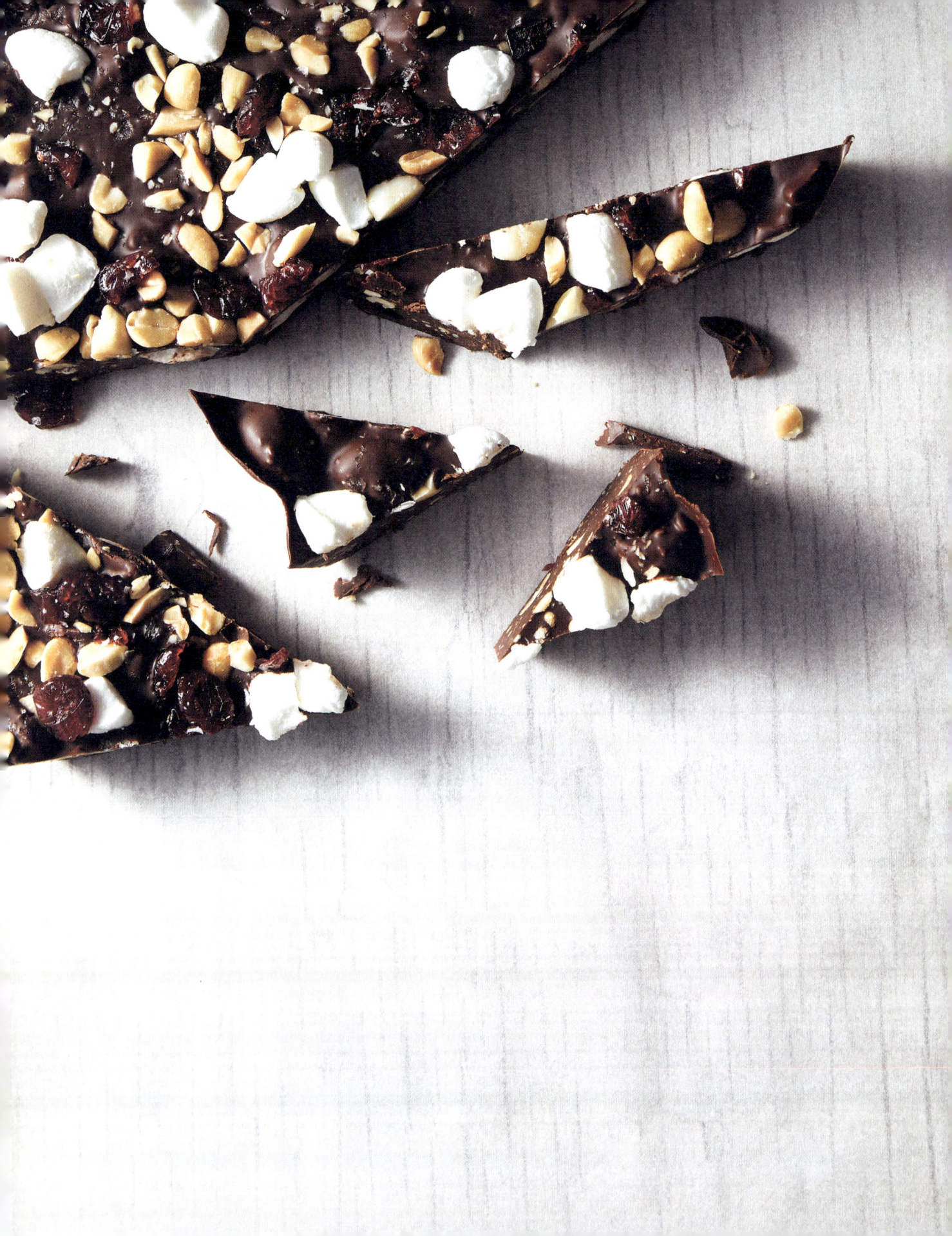

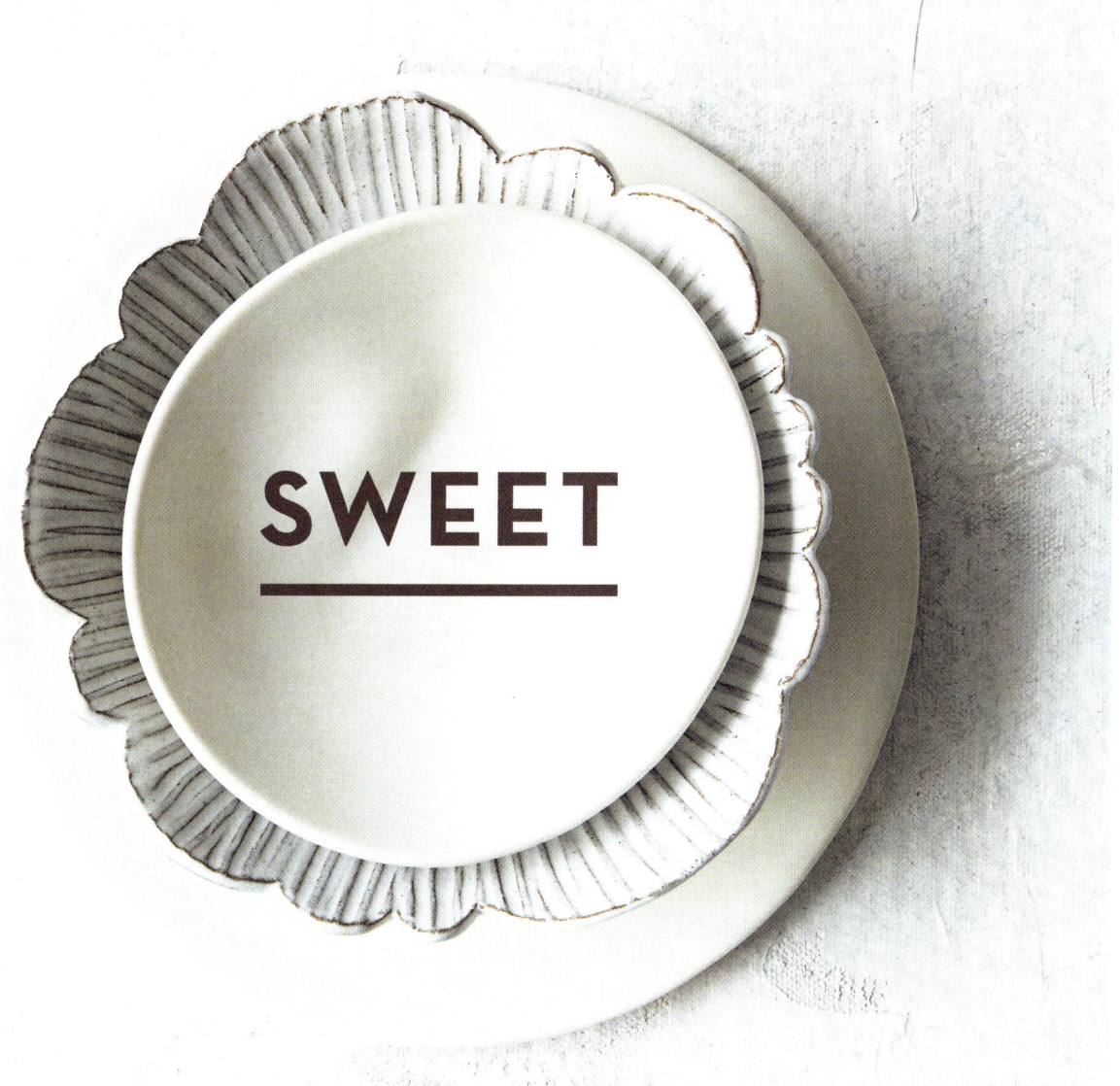

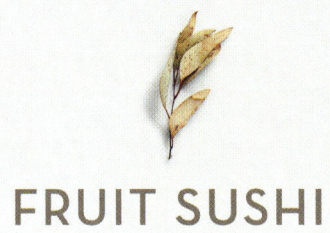

FRUIT SUSHI

I first tried fruit sushi while I was travelling in Mauritius. I'd never seen it before, but it looked so cute and was so very delicious that I just had to figure out how to create it myself! Unlike the original, this super-healthy version includes no refined sugar, but I think it's come up a real treat and makes a lovely dessert or brunch.

SERVES 2

2 tablespoons coconut sugar

½ cup (125 ml) coconut milk

1½ cups (300 g) sushi rice

1 kiwifruit, cut into wedges

1 banana, cut into wedges

4 strawberries, cut into wedges

Warm the coconut sugar and milk in a saucepan over a low heat for 3 minutes, stirring, until the sugar has fully dissolved. Set aside.

Add the sushi rice and 2 cups (500 ml) water to a saucepan set over a high heat. Cover with a lid and bring to the boil, then reduce the heat to a simmer and cook for 5 minutes. Stir in the coconut milk mixture and cook for a further 10 minutes, stirring occasionally. Tip the rice into a bowl and leave to cool.

Once cool, divide the rice into four equal parts. Spread one portion of the rice over a plastic wrap–lined bamboo sushi mat in an even layer. Arrange a line of the fruit pieces over the rice down one side of the mat, then roll the mat up from that side, keeping everything as tight as possible. Gently place the rolled sushi log in the fridge to cool and set. Repeat with the remaining rice and fruit. When ready to serve, cut each roll into 6–8 pieces, then … well, what are you waiting for? Dig in!

TIPS I like to use the bamboo sushi-rolling mats that you can pick up from the supermarket – they only cost a few dollars and they really do the trick. Also, be sure to use sushi rice here as it will definitely give you the best results. Trust me on this one.

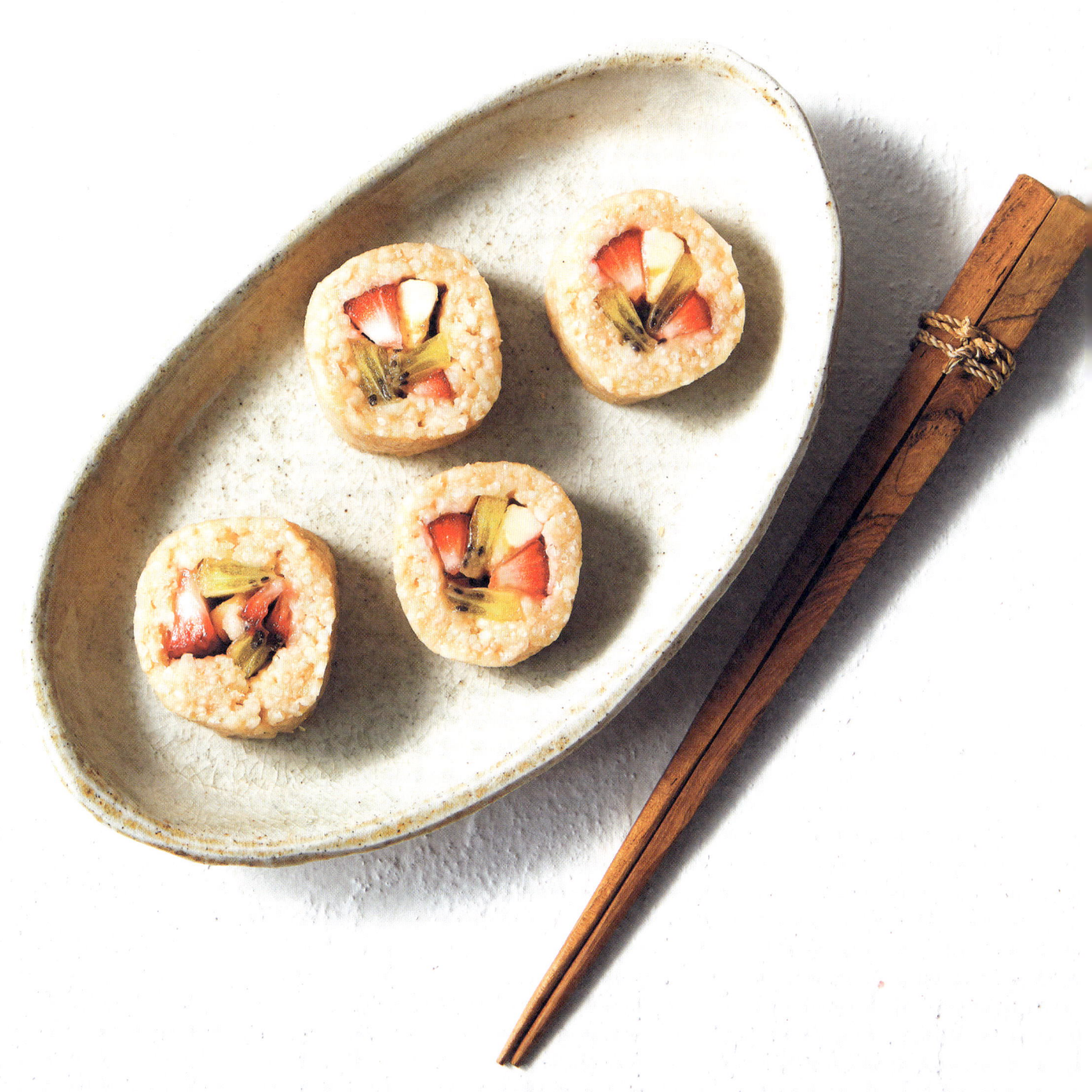

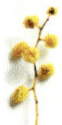

TURMERIC NICE CREAM

This is really speedy to make, tastes super delicious and has a lovely golden colour thanks to the fresh turmeric. Turmeric supports the digestive system and also has anti-inflammatory and wound-healing properties (in India you can even get turmeric-infused bandaids to help with healing). On top of all that, it's now used as a bit of a youth elixir as it's said to help promote glowing, healthy skin. I love the creaminess of this nice cream – sometimes I even like to have it as a brekkie bowl topped with paleo granola. It's just too yummy!

SERVES 2

- 2 cups (300 g) cashew nuts, (activated if possible, see page 108), plus extra to serve (optional)
- 1 frozen banana (peel it before you freeze it)
- 2 cm piece of ginger, grated
- 2 cm piece of turmeric, grated
- 2 tablespoons maple syrup
- 1 vanilla pod, split and seeds scraped (or ½ teaspoon vanilla powder)
- ½ teaspoon ground cardamom
- 3 tablespoons almond milk, plus extra if needed
- pinch of salt flakes
- ground turmeric, to serve

Pop everything in a food processor and blitz it up until you have a lovely smooth, creamy texture, adding a little extra almond milk if you need. Spoon the nice cream into bowls and top with a few extra cashews, if you like, and a sprinkling of ground turmeric to make it pretty.

<u>**TIPS**</u> This will last for 3–4 days in the fridge (though the texture will change and become more mousse-like) and even longer in the freezer – just be mindful that it will need a while to defrost as it sets pretty hard. If you can't get hold of fresh turmeric or ginger, just use ½ teaspoon each of the ground stuff instead.

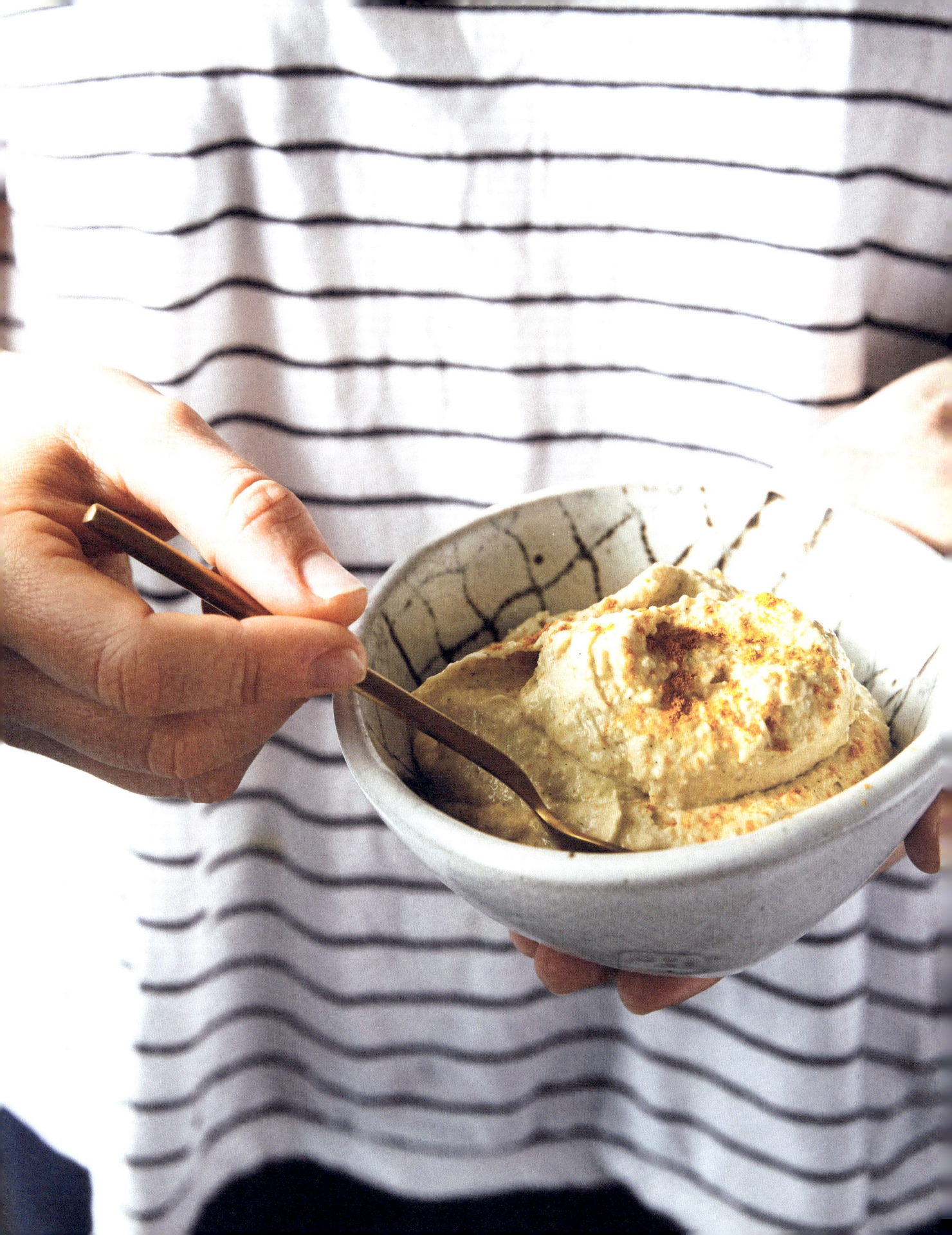

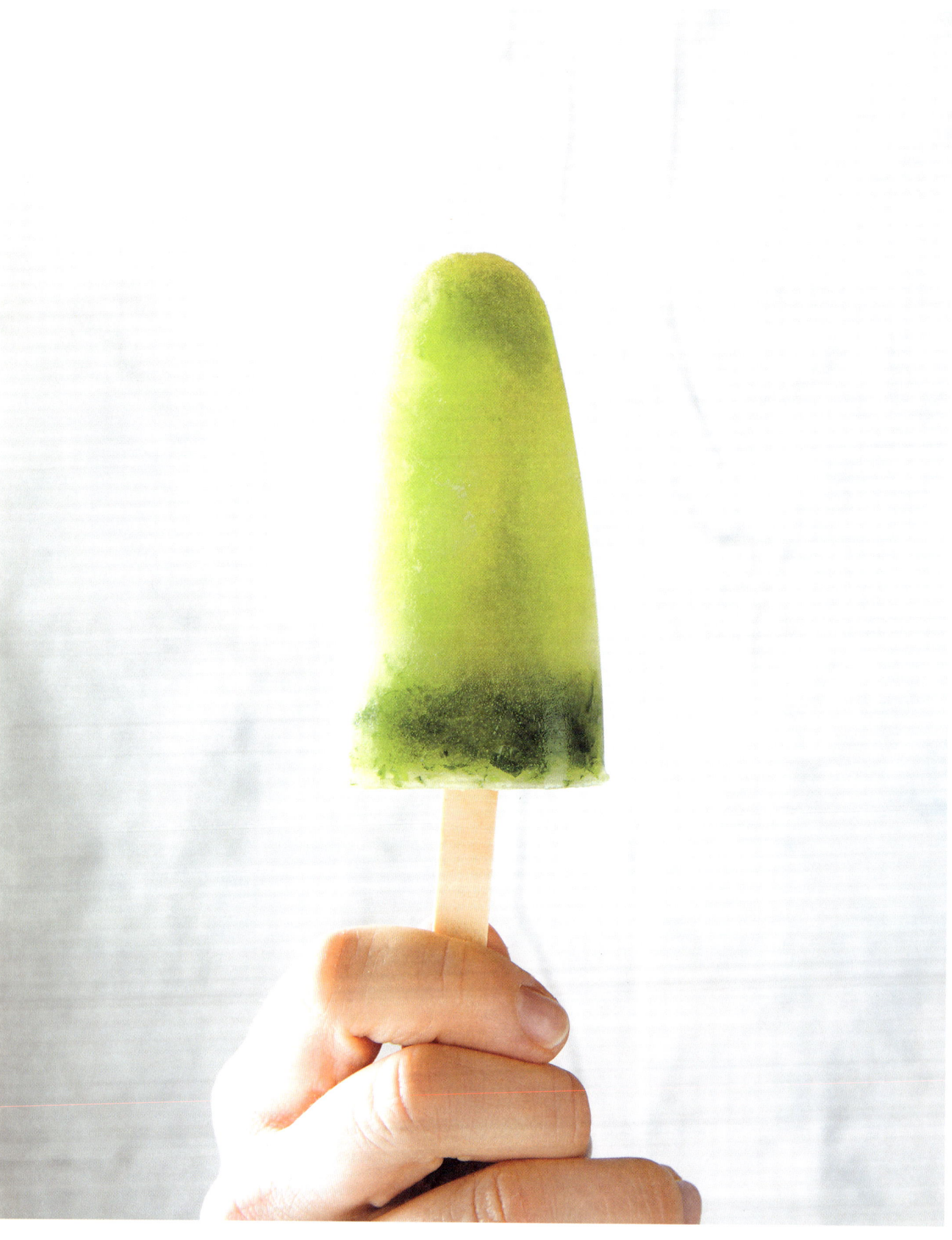

PINEAPPLE AND CUCUMBER ICY POLES

This recipe was inspired by a trip I took to the Maldives, where I swear I tasted some of the most amazing icy poles ever invented. I'm pretty sure the ones there had sugar in them, so here's my healthy but no less delicious take.

MAKES 4

1 pineapple, cubed

1 continental cucumber

juice and zest of 1 lime

¼ bunch of mint, leaves picked and very finely chopped

Pop the pineapple through a juicer and measure out 1½ cups (375 ml) of the juice. Push the cucumber through the juicer, add the juice to the pineapple together with the rest of the ingredients and give everything a good stir together. Pour the mixture into four icy-pole moulds and freeze for 6 hours. Delish, fresh and uber healthy.

DAIRY FREE GLUTEN FREE GRAIN FREE PALEO RAW VEGAN VEGETARIAN

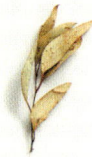

COOKIE DOUGH BALLS

I discovered raw, vegan cookie dough balls while shopping at Wholefoods in LA. Now, we're all friends here, so I can say I bought a packet of them and ate them all in one go. They were that good! Here's my version – they are my newest addiction, so I just have to share them with you.

MAKES 12

2½ cups (250 g) almond meal

½ cup (125 ml) maple syrup

½ cup (45 g) desiccated coconut

½ cup (125 ml) coconut oil, melted

1 vanilla pod, split and seeds scraped (or ½ teaspoon vanilla powder)

pinch of salt flakes

3 tablespoons almond milk (optional)

3 tablespoons cacao nibs

In a food processor or in a bowl using a stick blender, whiz together the almond meal, maple syrup, desiccated coconut, coconut oil, vanilla and salt until the mixture reaches a cookie dough–like consistency, adding a few splashes of almond milk only if the mix is too thick and not clumping together nicely.

Add the cacao nibs and give everything a last quick mix (I don't like them too finely blended), then carve out hunks of the dough with a dessert spoon and start rolling into balls.

Store the balls in an airtight container in the fridge for snacking on later – they will keep for up to 2 weeks, though they usually last just a few minutes in my house. Trust me, these are amazing!

<u>**TIPS**</u> If you want to make this into double chocolate chip cookie dough, add 1 tablespoon of cacao powder to the mixture before whizzing everything together. When buying desiccated coconut, try to get the sulphate-free stuff if you can – check the label to see if they have used sulphates in the processing.

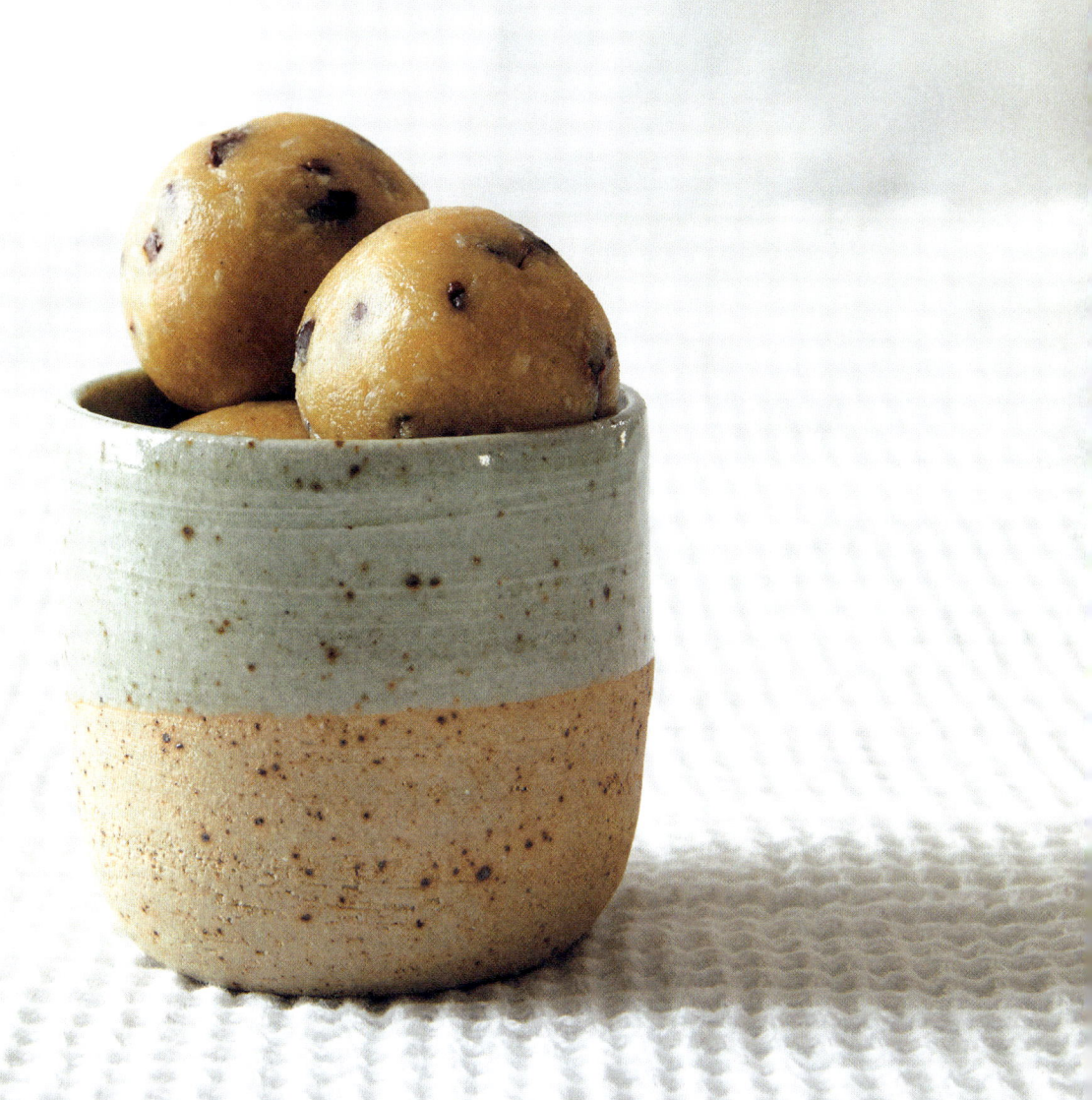

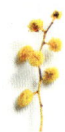

CHICKPEA CHOC-CHIP COOKIES

These sound weird, I know, but legumes such as chickpeas and other beans can make great, tasty additions to sweet recipes. I love this vegan creation because it's a great way of getting your sweet fix in while you're on a cleanse or detox. Plus, you're getting a nice whack of vegan protein from the chickpeas. If you want, you can use cacao nibs instead of the chocolate chips to make these super healthy, though the cookies won't be quite so sweet.

MAKES 16–18

1 x 400 g can chickpeas, rinsed twice and drained

3 tablespoons coconut oil, melted

3 tablespoons quinoa flour

3 tablespoons almond meal

2 tablespoons maple syrup

3 tablespoons almond butter

½ cup (100 g) coconut sugar

1 vanilla pod, split and seeds scraped

pinch of salt flakes

½ cup (85 g) vegan chocolate chips

Preheat the oven to 180°C. Line a large baking tray with baking paper.

Add the chickpeas, coconut oil, quinoa flour, almond meal, maple syrup, almond butter, coconut sugar, vanilla and salt to a food processor and blitz together to form a dough. Add the chocolate chips to the mixture and give everything one very quick pulse to mix together, then roll the mixture into little balls and place them on the prepared baking tray, leaving a little room between each cookie. Use the back of a fork to press the cookies down slightly (this is my grandma's trick, which helps flatten them into the right shape) and cook for 15–20 minutes until golden. Remove from the oven and enjoy a few hot, leaving the rest to cool. The cookies will keep in an airtight container for up to 1 week.

<u>TIPS</u> You can use dried chickpeas here and cook them from scratch if you'd rather, but I find the canned ones make things much easier. If you can't get hold of quinoa flour – or if you'd like a slightly lighter-textured cookie – then try using rice flour instead.

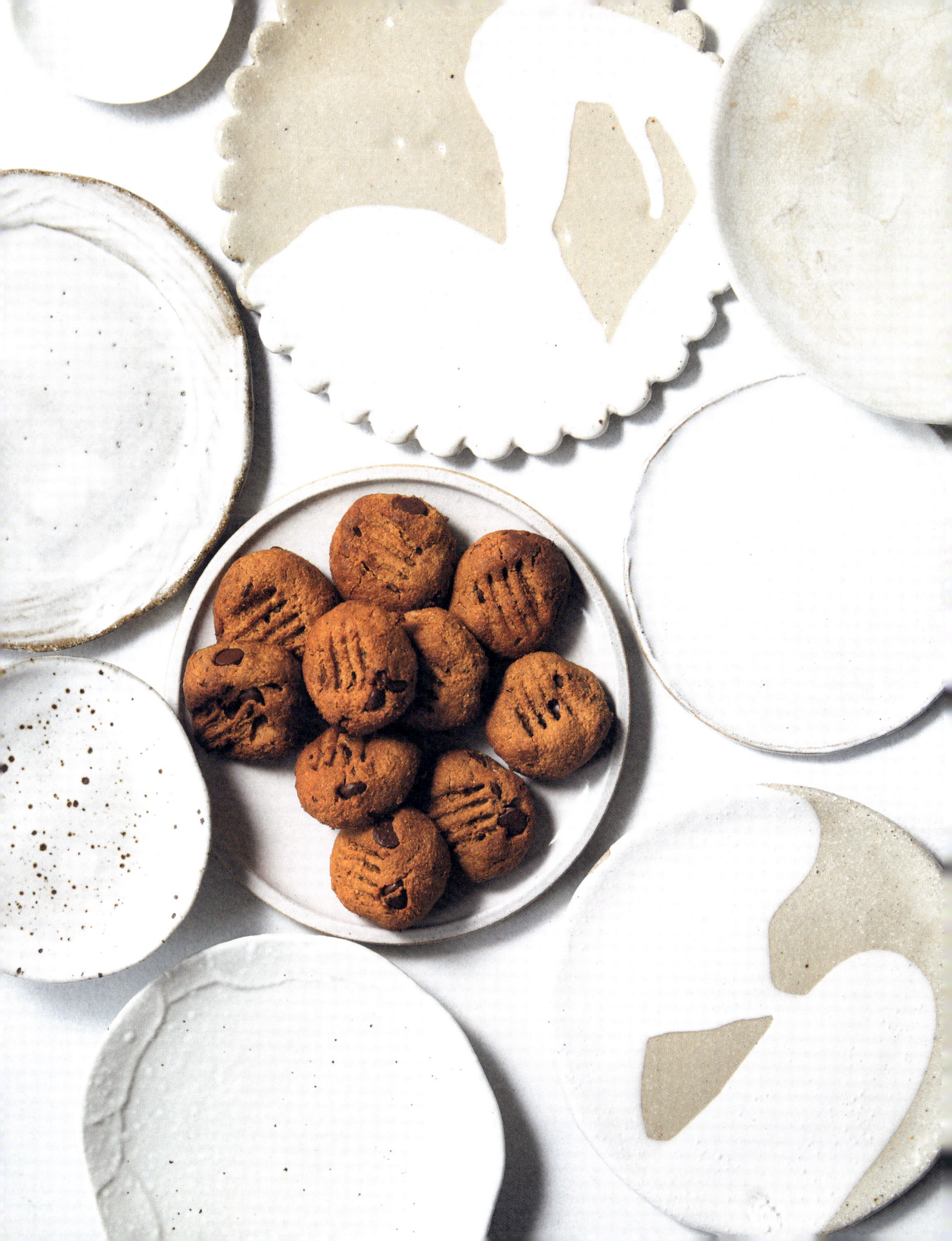

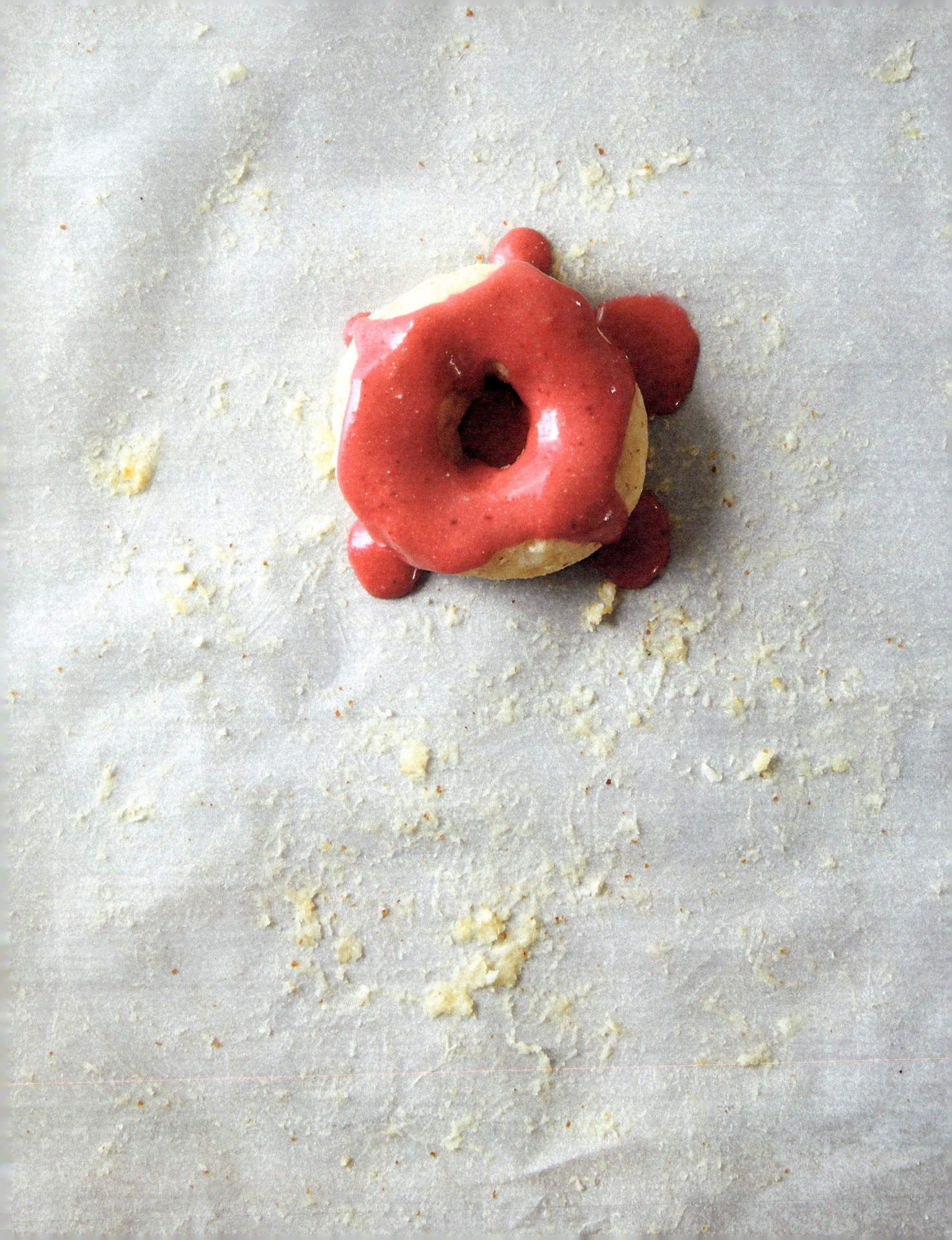

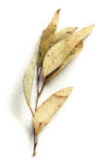

RAW, VEGAN HAWAIIAN 'DOUGHNUTS'

This recipe is my healthy take on the amazing steamed and air-baked doughnuts I have enjoyed in LA. Now, this raw, vegan version of my hands-down favourite flavour – 'the Hawaiian' – might not be quite as fluffy as the original, but it is very cute and super tasty!

MAKES ABOUT 18

1 cup (100 g) almond meal

1 cup (160 g) macadamia nuts (activated if possible, see page 108)

½ cup (45 g) desiccated coconut

3 tablespoons maple syrup

3 tablespoons almond butter

1 cup (160 g) roughly chopped pineapple chunks

½ cup (125 ml) coconut oil, melted

desiccated coconut, for sprinkling (optional)

PINK ICING

½ cup (125 ml) coconut milk

3 tablespoons maple syrup

½ cup (80 g) cashew nuts (activated if possible, see page 108)

1 teaspoon beetroot juice

Place all of the doughnut ingredients in a food processor and blitz everything together to form a wet, sticky dough. Refrigerate for 10 minutes to firm up.

Take heaped tablespoonfuls of the dough and shape them into doughnut shapes, then arrange them on a wire rack set over a baking tray lined with baking paper. Transfer to the fridge for 1 hour to chill.

For the icing, pop all of the ingredients in a blender or food processor and whiz together until smooth. Pour over the chilled doughnut bases (thanks to the baking tray, the icing won't make a mess of your kitchen) and pop back in the fridge for another 30 minutes to set.

Once the icing has set, you can sprinkle a little desiccated coconut over the doughnuts, if you like. Yum!

TIP You can skip the icing and make this mixture into simple bliss balls – there really are no rules here! Also, almost any raw bliss ball creation can become the base for these raw doughnuts, so try some of your favourites to mix up the flavours.

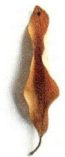

ICED BANANA CHOCOLATES

I love this little treat when I'm craving something sweet at night – it really hits the spot and stops me reaching for something naughty. And the best bit is that it only takes about 5 minutes to make!

SERVES 2

2 bananas, sliced and frozen for 20–30 minutes

crushed almonds (activated if possible, see page 108), to serve (optional)

CHOCOLATE SAUCE

½ cup (125 ml) coconut oil, melted

1 tablespoon cacao powder

2 tablespoons maple syrup

pinch of ground cinnamon

This recipe is so, so easy – just mix together the sauce ingredients in a bowl, then pop a skewer through the centre of the frozen banana slices and dunk them into the sauce. Set them aside for a minute or two to let the sauce harden a tad before enjoying (or, if you're anything like me, tuck straight in). Alternatively, you can throw all the banana slices in a bowl and drizzle the sauce over the top, sprinkling the lot with a few crushed almonds to finish, if you like. Either way, this is truly delicious.

TIP This sauce is also great over other fruit – I love drizzling it over a mix of strawberries and blueberries before topping the lot off with a sprinkling of chia seeds. Yum!

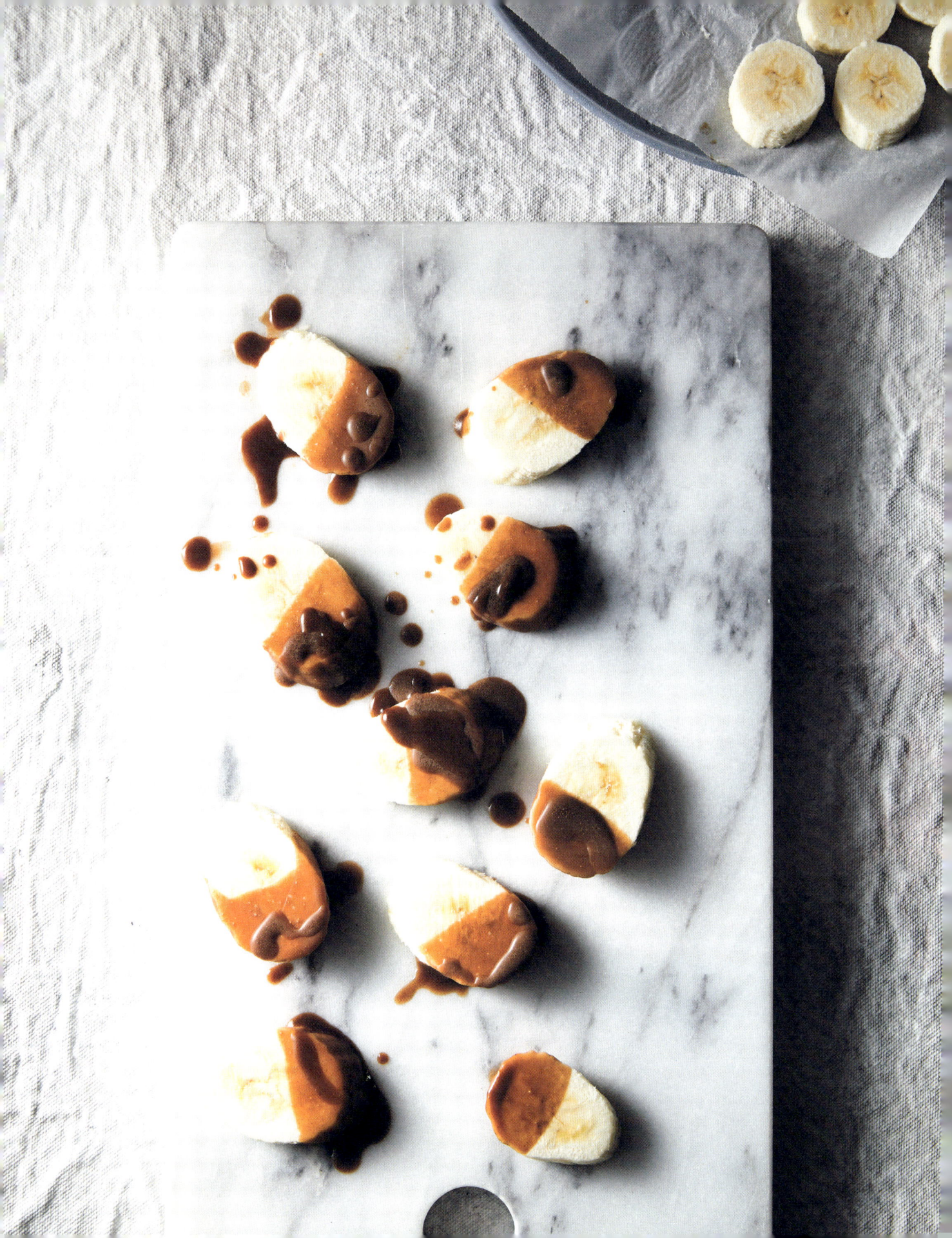

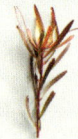

VEDIC VEGAN ROCKY ROAD

This recipe is ridiculously speedy to make, tastes like a naughty treat and makes a perfect present. In Ayurvedic medicine, ginger is used to aid digestion and boost the respiratory and immune systems. I've added it here along with the turmeric to make this into a nourishing, healing treat.

SERVES 12

- 2 cups (340 g) vegan chocolate chips
- ½ cup (140 g) peanut butter
- ½ teaspoon ground ginger
- ¼ teaspoon ground turmeric
- 3 tablespoons dried cranberries
- 3 tablespoons roughly chopped macadamia nuts (activated if possible, see page 108)
- 3 tablespoons roughly chopped peanuts (reserve a few for the topping)
- 1 cup (90 g) vegan marshmallows, roughly chopped (reserve a few for the topping)
- pinch of salt flakes

Line a baking tray with baking paper.

Melt the chocolate chips in a bowl set over a saucepan of lightly simmering water (or use a double boiler if you have one), then remove from the heat and stir through the peanut butter, ginger and turmeric. Now add the cranberries, macadamia nuts and peanuts, reserving a few peanuts for decorating later, then leave the chocolate to cool a bit before folding through most of the marshmallows (you don't want to do this while the chocolate is too hot or they will melt).

Give everything a last lucky stir or two to make sure it's all mixed together evenly, then spoon the mixture out onto your lined baking tray. Scatter over the reserved peanuts and marshmallows, sprinkle over the salt flakes and pop in the fridge for 2 hours to set before cutting into 12 squares. Enjoy these little gems with a few mates.

TIP You can use regular chocolate chips and marshmallows if you're not vegan.

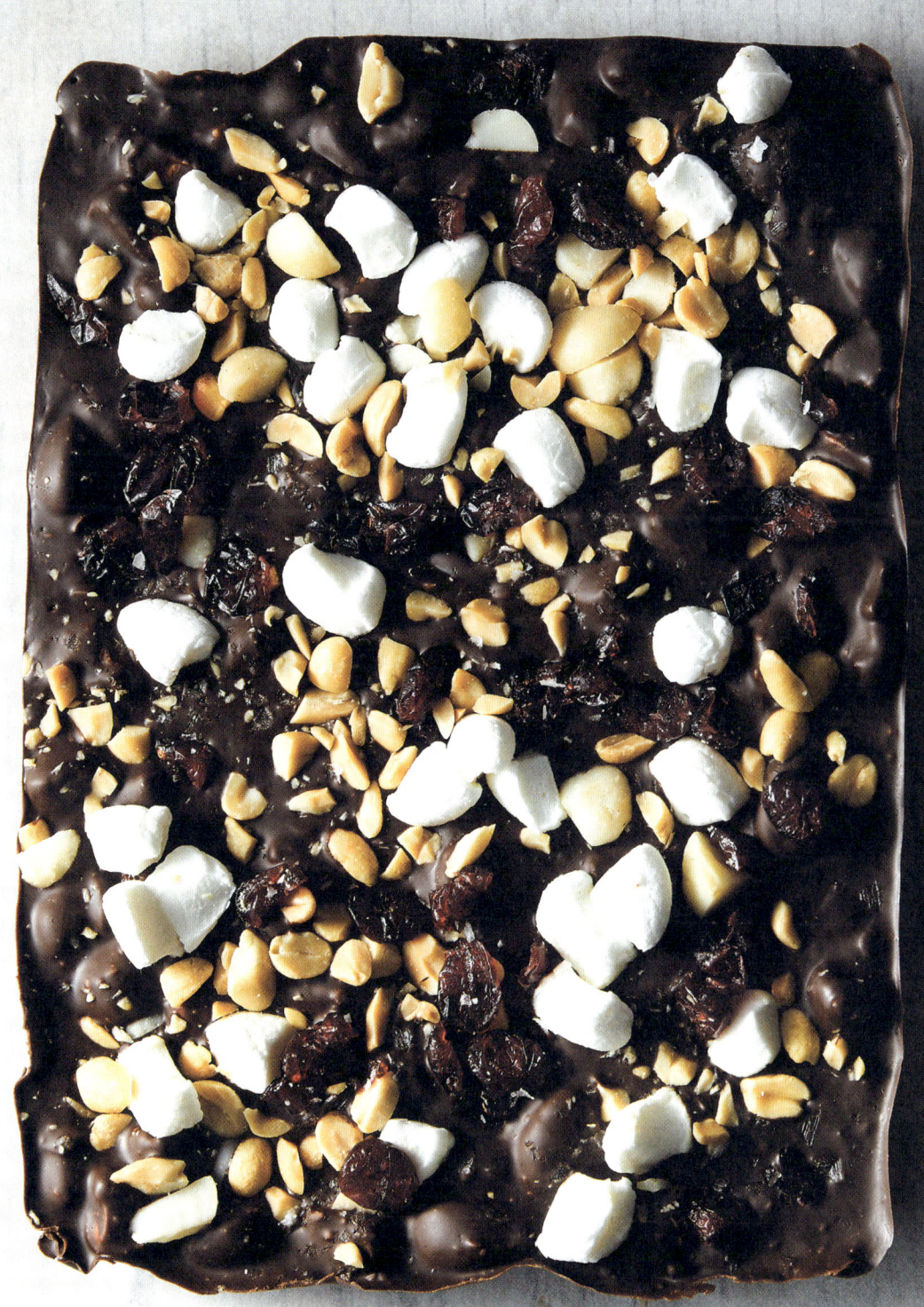

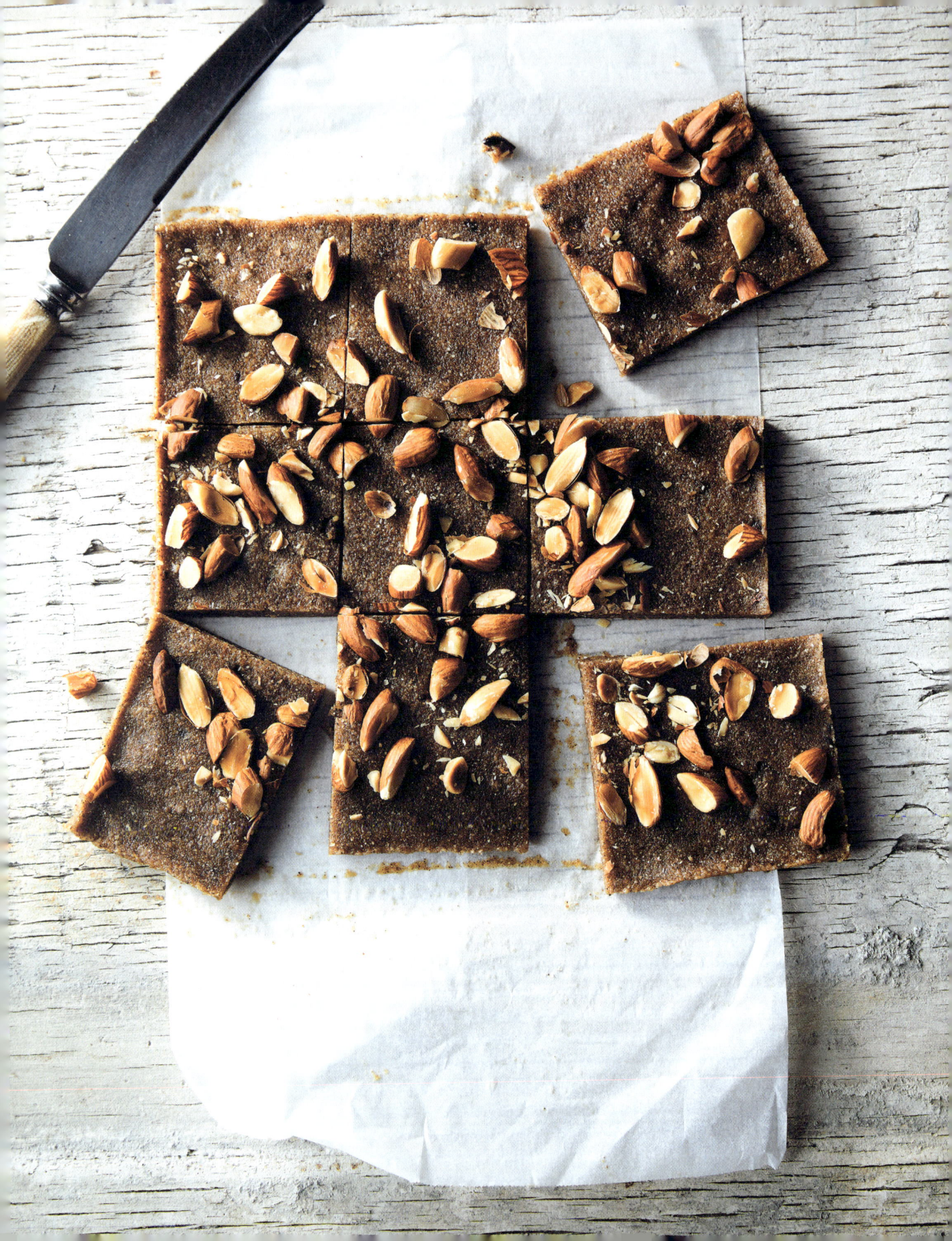

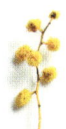

RAW CHOC, COFFEE AND ALMOND SLICE

I love having this as a mid-morning snack when I'm getting peckish and it's also my go-to post-yoga kick-starter. The caffeine boost from the coffee and cacao nibs should have you on a nice high all morning, while the fats and protein in the nuts will help to keep you feeling full right up until lunch.

SERVES 9

1 cup (100 g) almond meal

3 tablespoons coconut flour

½ cup (140 g) almond butter

1 tablespoon cacao butter, melted

½ cup (125 ml) maple syrup

1 tablespoon ground coffee

pinch of salt flakes, plus extra for topping

1 tablespoon cacao nibs

3 tablespoons chopped almonds (activated if possible, see page 108)

Grease a 20 cm square baking tin and line with baking paper.

In a food processor, blitz together the almond meal, coconut flour, almond butter, cacao butter, maple syrup, coffee and salt to form a dough-like mixture. Stir through the cacao nibs, then spoon the mixture into the prepared baking tin, spreading it out evenly and pressing it down with damp hands to cover the base completely.

Top with the chopped almonds and another pinch of salt flakes, then pop the tin in the freezer for 1 hour to chill and firm. Slice into nine squares and serve straight from the freezer.

TIP If you're not a coffee fan then just leave it out and make this a choc-almond slice instead – it'll still be delish and the kids will love it!

DAIRY FREE GLUTEN FREE GRAIN FREE
PALEO RAW VEGAN VEGETARIAN

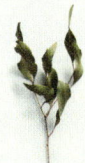

SNICKERDOODLE COOKIES

I first discovered snickerdoodle cookies in LA. They're an amazing soft, chewy cinnamon cookie and they're mighty addictive. So good, in fact, that I just had to put a gluten-free version of them in this book.

MAKES 12

250 g butter, softened

1½ cups (300 g) coconut sugar

3 eggs

1 vanilla pod, split and seeds scraped (or ½ teaspoon vanilla powder)

2½ cups (250 g) almond meal (or other gluten-free flour such as buckwheat or quinoa flour)

1 teaspoon baking powder

½ teaspoon ground cinnamon

pinch of salt flakes

COATING

3 tablespoons coconut sugar

½ teaspoon ground cinnamon

Preheat the oven to 180°C. Line a large baking tray with baking paper.

Beat the butter and sugar together in a bowl with a wooden spoon (or using a stand mixer) until pale and creamy. Continuing to beat, add the eggs one at a time followed by the vanilla, then gently fold through the almond meal, baking powder, cinnamon and salt and give everything a good stir together to form a dough. Pop the dough into a bowl and transfer to the fridge for 20–30 minutes to chill and firm.

Meanwhile, to make the coating, mix the coconut sugar and cinnamon together in a bowl.

Once chilled, divide the cookie dough into 12 equal-sized pieces, then roll each into a big ball. Roll the balls in the coating and lay them on the baking tray, flattened to about 1 cm thick, leaving about 5 cm between each ball. Bake for 10–15 minutes, or until nice and golden, then remove the cookies from the oven, sprinkle with the remaining coating and leave them to cool on the tray. And there you have it – your very own healthy version of an American snickerdoodle!

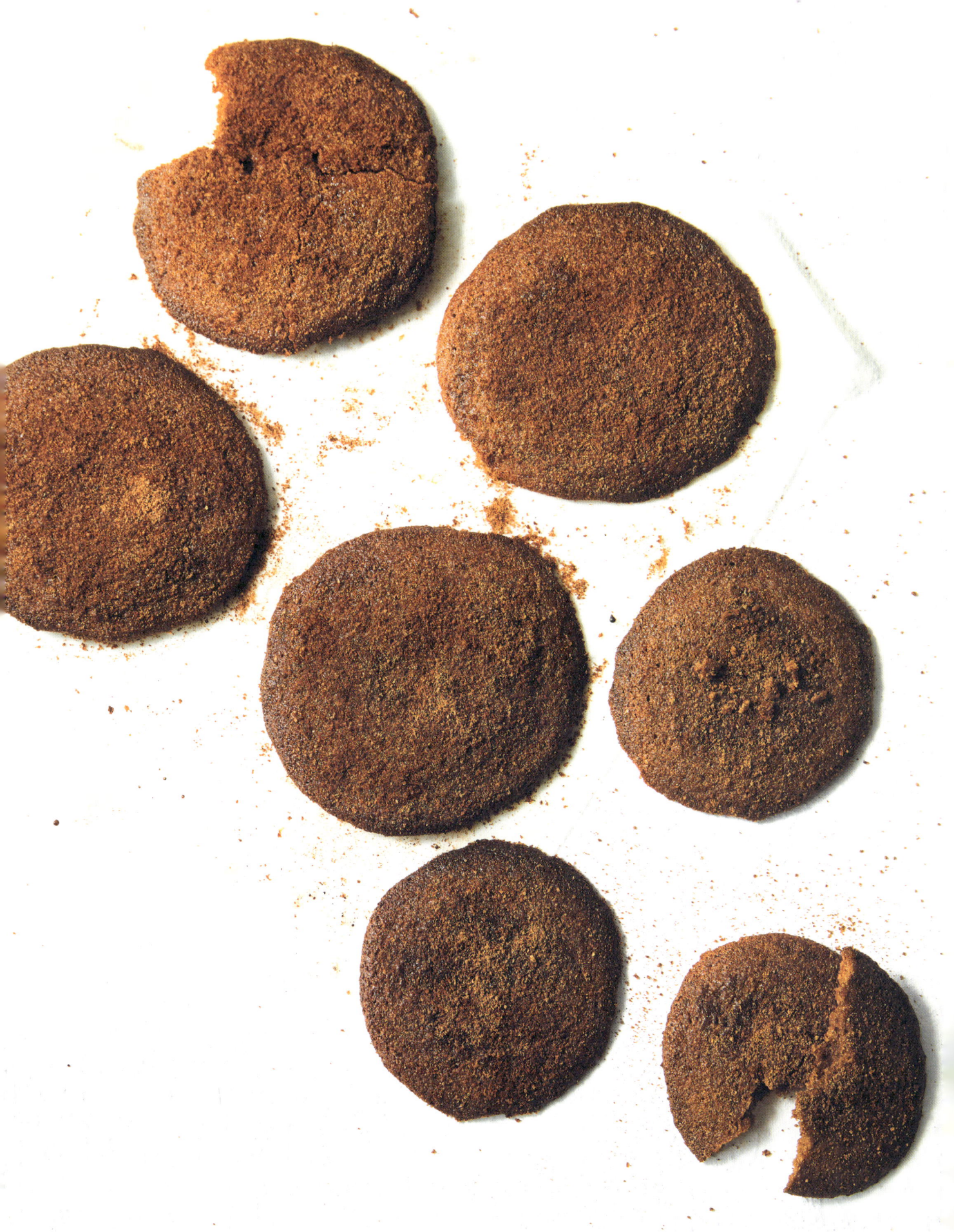

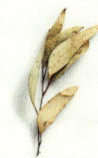

TEACUP TIRAMISU

I just love the idea of something this cute and delicious! Unlike the usual tiramisu, this isn't fiddly to make – I wanted to keep things as healthy, quick and simple as possible, so there are no ladyfinger biscuits in here. Instead, you have a simple, clean little treat that will give you a nice burst of energy as well as being high in fibre, thanks to the avocado.

SERVES 4

BASE

1½ cups (150 g) almond meal

3 tablespoons melted coconut oil

1 tablespoon almond milk

6 pitted medjool dates

MOUSSE

1 avocado

1 tablespoon cacao powder

1½ teaspoons ground coffee

1 tablespoon coconut oil

1 frozen banana

3 tablespoons coconut milk

CREAMY TOPPING

1 cup (150 g) cashew nuts (activated if possible, see page 108)

3 tablespoons maple syrup

3 tablespoons coconut milk

½ teaspoon vanilla extract or ½ vanilla pod, split and seeds scraped (or ½ teaspoon vanilla powder)

desiccated coconut or ground coffee, to serve

First up, grab four teacups (or glasses, whatever floats your boat) and place them on the kitchen bench.

Pop the base ingredients in a food processor and give them a good whiz together, then scoop out the mixture and divide it among the teacups to form a nice, even layer in each. Transfer the cups to the fridge to chill for a few minutes.

Meanwhile, throw all the mousse ingredients into the food processor and blend them together until nice and smooth (I personally don't bother cleaning out the processor before I make the mousse part). Spoon the mousse into the teacups over the base, then pop them straight back into the fridge.

Give your food processor a wipe out at this stage (you need to do this now because you want the creamy topping to taste clean and vanilla-like, rather than of chocolate and coffee). Add the cashews, maple syrup, coconut milk and vanilla and blend until nice and creamy. Top the mousse with the creamy topping and decorate with a sprinkling of desiccated coconut or ground coffee, then store in the fridge to set for at least 30 minutes, or until you're ready to enjoy this cute dessert.

TIP If you're not a coffee fiend, just hold the coffee here – it'll still taste brilliant without it.

YOGA FOOD   DAIRY FREE GLUTEN FREE GRAIN FREE PALEO RAW VEGAN VEGETARIAN

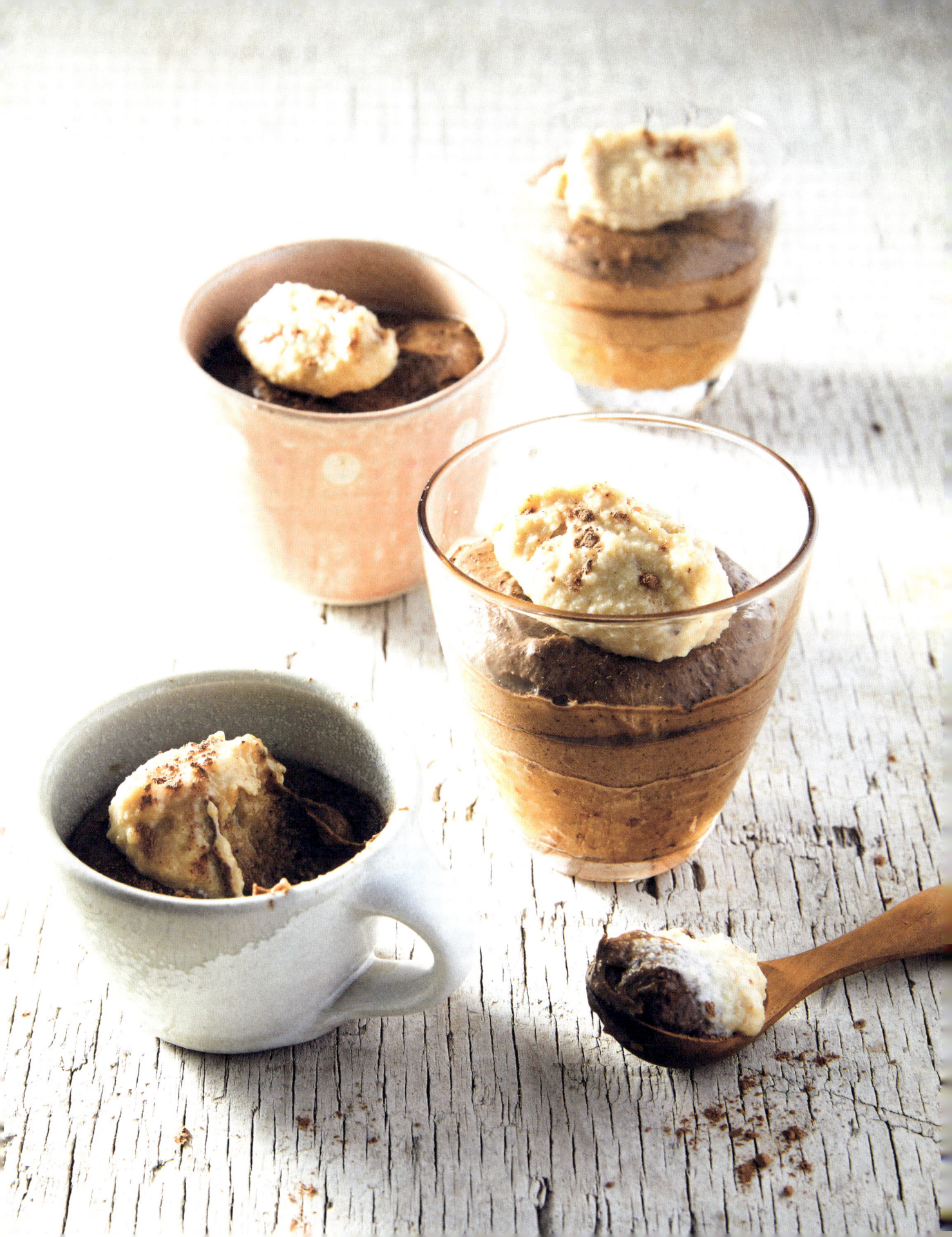

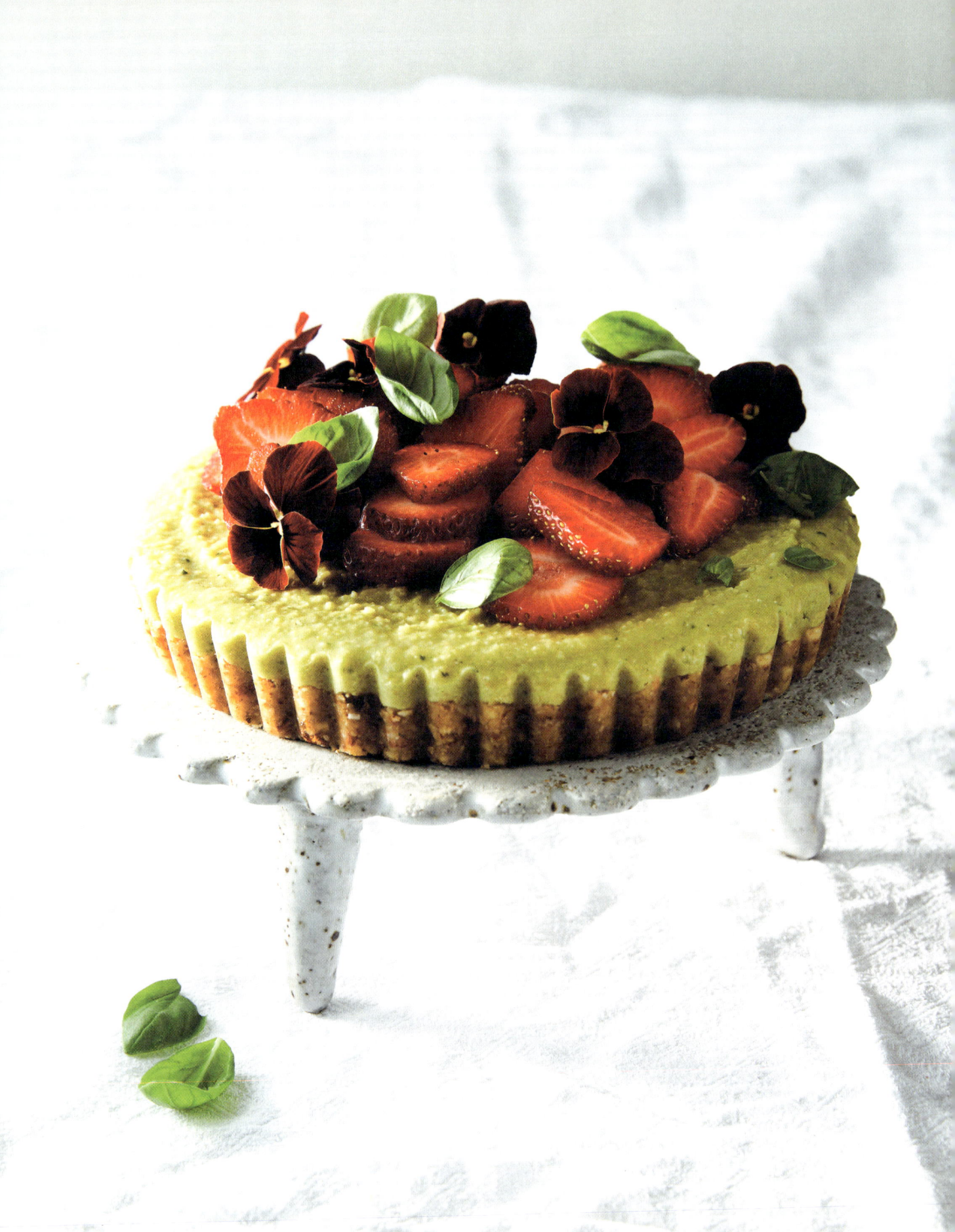

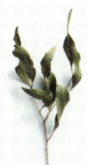

RAW BASIL AND STRAWBERRY TART

If you have any of my other cookbooks, you'll know that I'm a sucker for an amazing tart. You know, the kind you can take to a dinner party and everyone is blown away that it is raw and vegan. I like mine super pretty and topped with some kind of edible flower. The combination of strawberries and basil here might be new to a few, but trust me, it's a flavour-match made in heaven.

SERVES 8

BASE

1½ cups (240 g) almonds (activated if possible, see page 108)

½ cup (45 g) desiccated coconut

6 pitted medjool dates

1 tablespoon coconut oil, melted

2 tablespoons almond butter

3 tablespoons almond milk

FILLING

2 cups (300 g) cashew nuts (activated if possible, see page 108)

zest and juice of 1 lemon

8–10 basil leaves

½ cup (125 ml) coconut oil, melted

½ cup (125 ml) maple syrup (or sweetener of your choice)

TOPPING

1 punnet (250 g) strawberries, sliced

a few small basil leaves

handful of edible flowers

Pop all the base ingredients in a food processor and whiz them together to form a crumbly biscuit consistency.

Add the base mixture to an 18 cm pie tin and, using damp hands, pat it down and out to the edges of the tin to form a nice, even layer. Transfer to the fridge to chill briefly.

For the filling, blitz all the ingredients together in the food processor until creamy and completely smooth.

Remove the tart tin from the fridge and spoon over the filling, then spread it out evenly with a spatula. Return the tart tin to the fridge for at least 2 hours, or until the filling has set firm.

Arrange the topping ingredients over the top of the tart in a pretty pattern before serving up and digging in.

DAIRY FREE GLUTEN FREE GRAIN FREE
PALEO RAW VEGAN VEGETARIAN

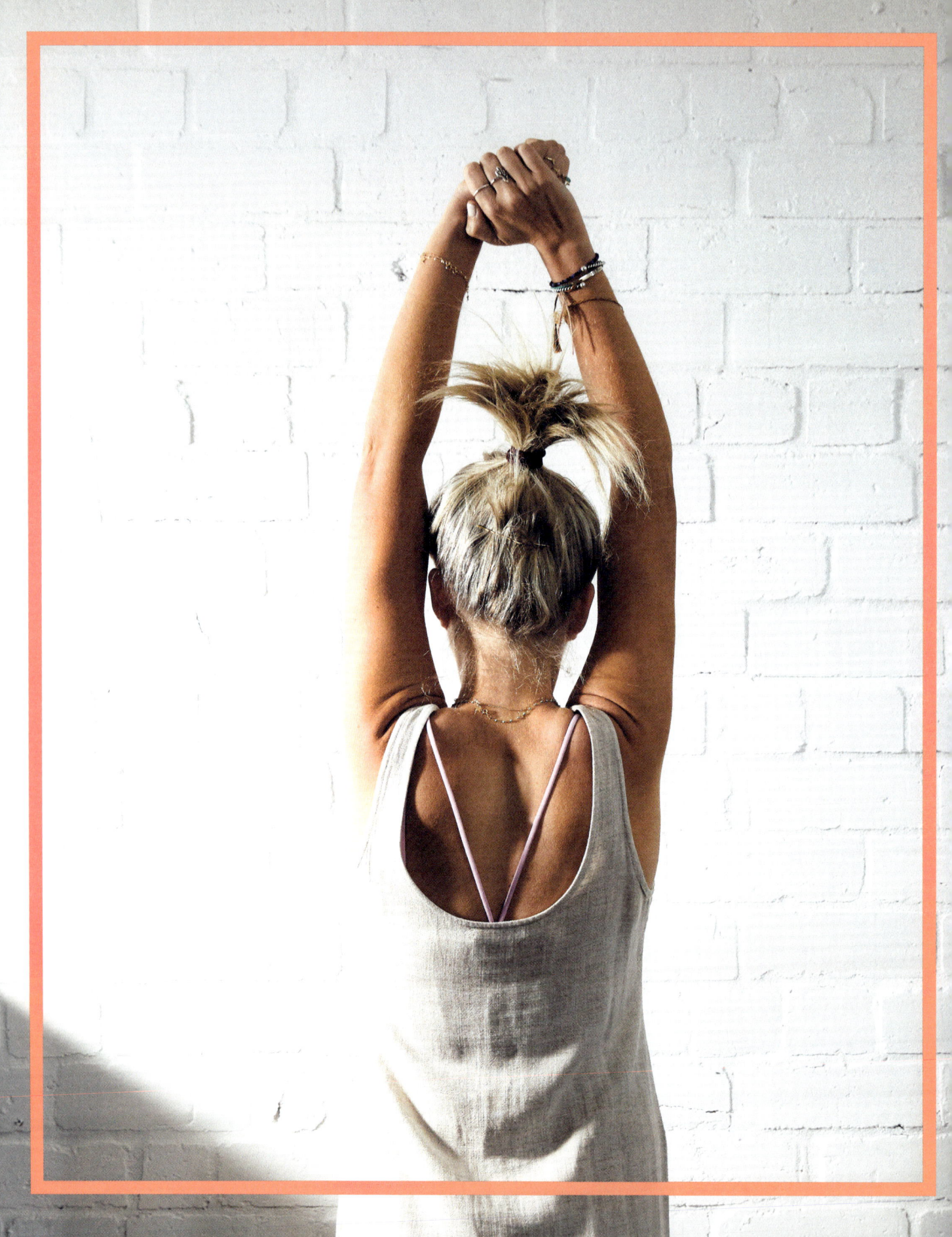

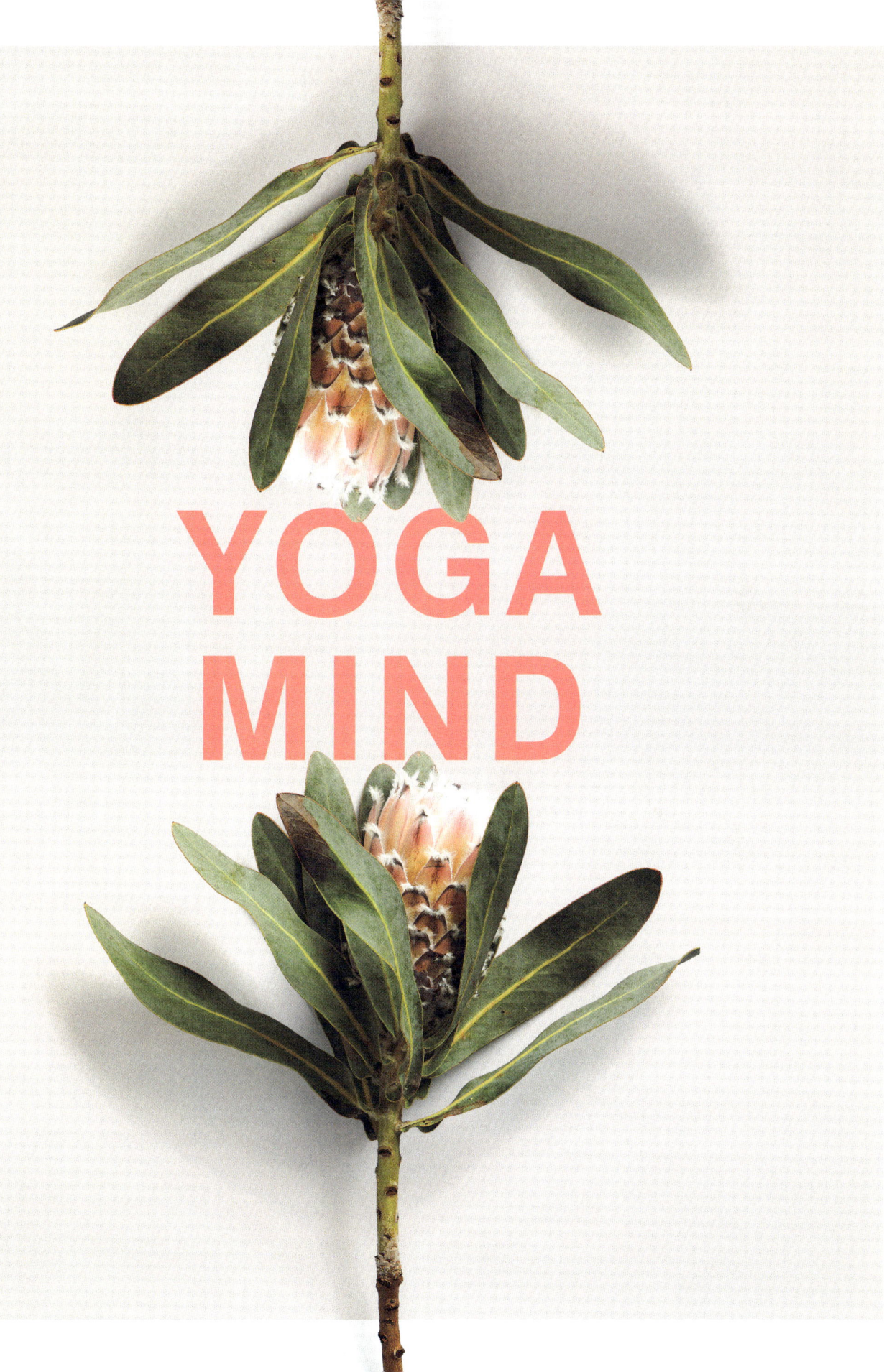

YOGA MIND

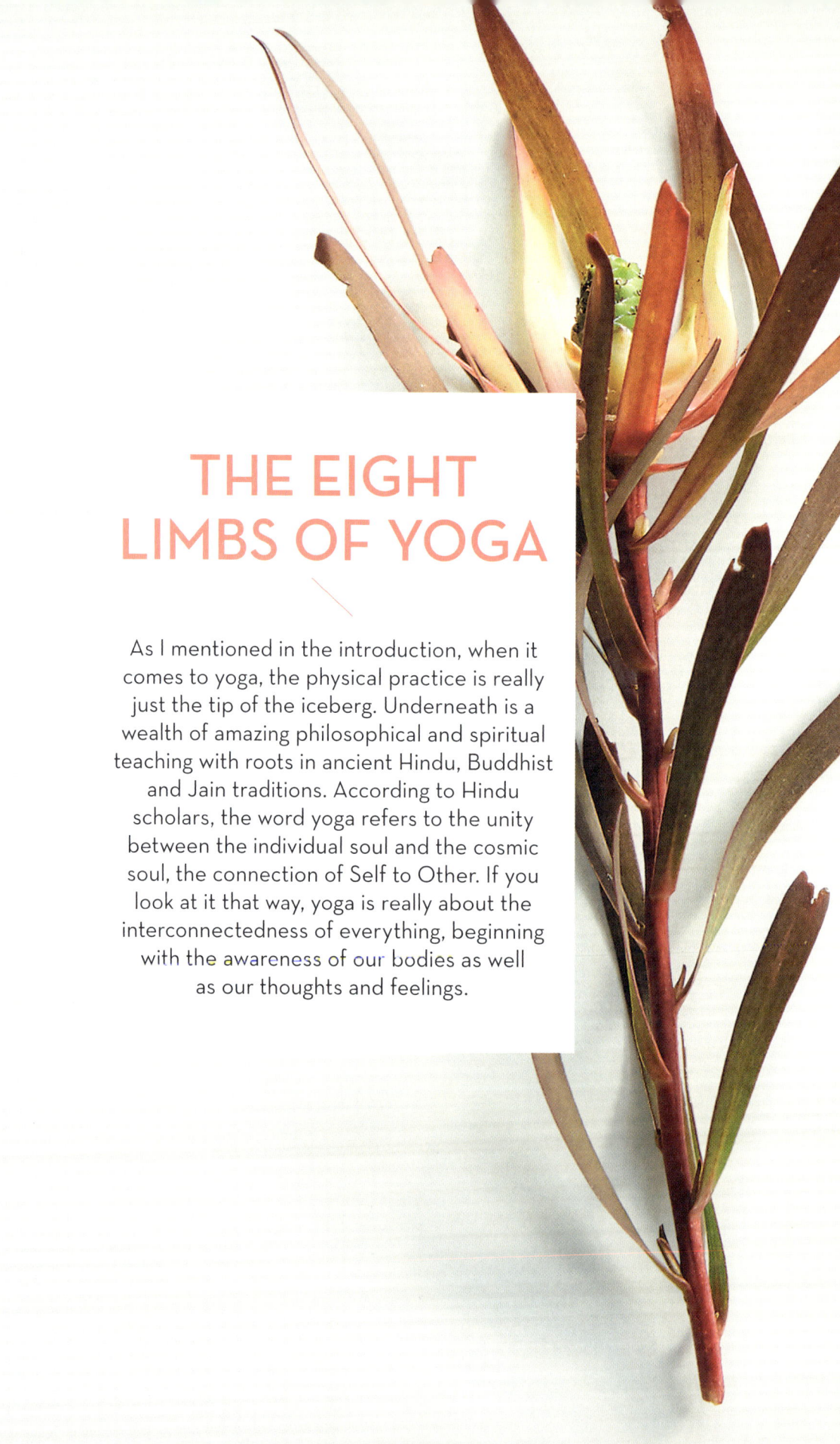

THE EIGHT LIMBS OF YOGA

As I mentioned in the introduction, when it comes to yoga, the physical practice is really just the tip of the iceberg. Underneath is a wealth of amazing philosophical and spiritual teaching with roots in ancient Hindu, Buddhist and Jain traditions. According to Hindu scholars, the word yoga refers to the unity between the individual soul and the cosmic soul, the connection of Self to Other. If you look at it that way, yoga is really about the interconnectedness of everything, beginning with the awareness of our bodies as well as our thoughts and feelings.

According to the Yoga Sutras of Patanjali, to become aware of this oneness, we must follow the 'eight limbs' of yoga.

1. The yamas

Yama means 'restraint' and includes five principles that we must follow in our relationships with others:

- **Ahimsa:** compassion and nonviolence; this guides us to share the world with other beings and to do no harm.
- **Satya:** truthfulness – in how we deal with others as well as with ourselves.
- **Asteya:** not stealing. Human beings are busy stealing from the earth and from others, and in so doing, are stealing the chance of being the best version of ourselves.
- **Brahmacharya:** literally means 'walking with god' and is believed to refer to celibacy or control in one's sex life.
- **Aparigraha:** not being covetous. Holding onto material objects and people will bring unhappiness and disappointment; letting go brings freedom.

2. The niyamas

Niyama means spiritual observance, and includes the following principles:

- **Saucha:** cleanliness in body, mind, attitude and action.
- **Santosha:** contentment. We spend so much time worrying about things that are out of our control. Santosha is acceptance and appreciation of this moment as it is.
- **Tapas:** literally means 'heat' and refers to our endurance – our ability to cope with the heat of change and of darker times.
- **Svadhyaya:** refers to both the study of the sacred scriptures and of one's self. It means knowing who you are, your values, what makes you tick.
- **Ishvara pranidhana:** surrender to god. This is about trusting the process of life, enjoying the ride with an open heart rather than fighting what happens. It means trusting in the gift that is your life.

3. The asanas

The asanas are the poses that make up your yoga practice. It is believed that showing up on the mat consistently with no attachment to the outcome not only builds discipline, but also prepares the body for long periods of sitting still in meditation. Now, I know the idea of sitting sounds easy, but it's actually *really* hard – you'll find yourself fidgeting, moving about, getting a numb-bum! The asanas are designed to open and lengthen the spine and the long muscles over the butt and hips – all of which help you to sit comfortably.

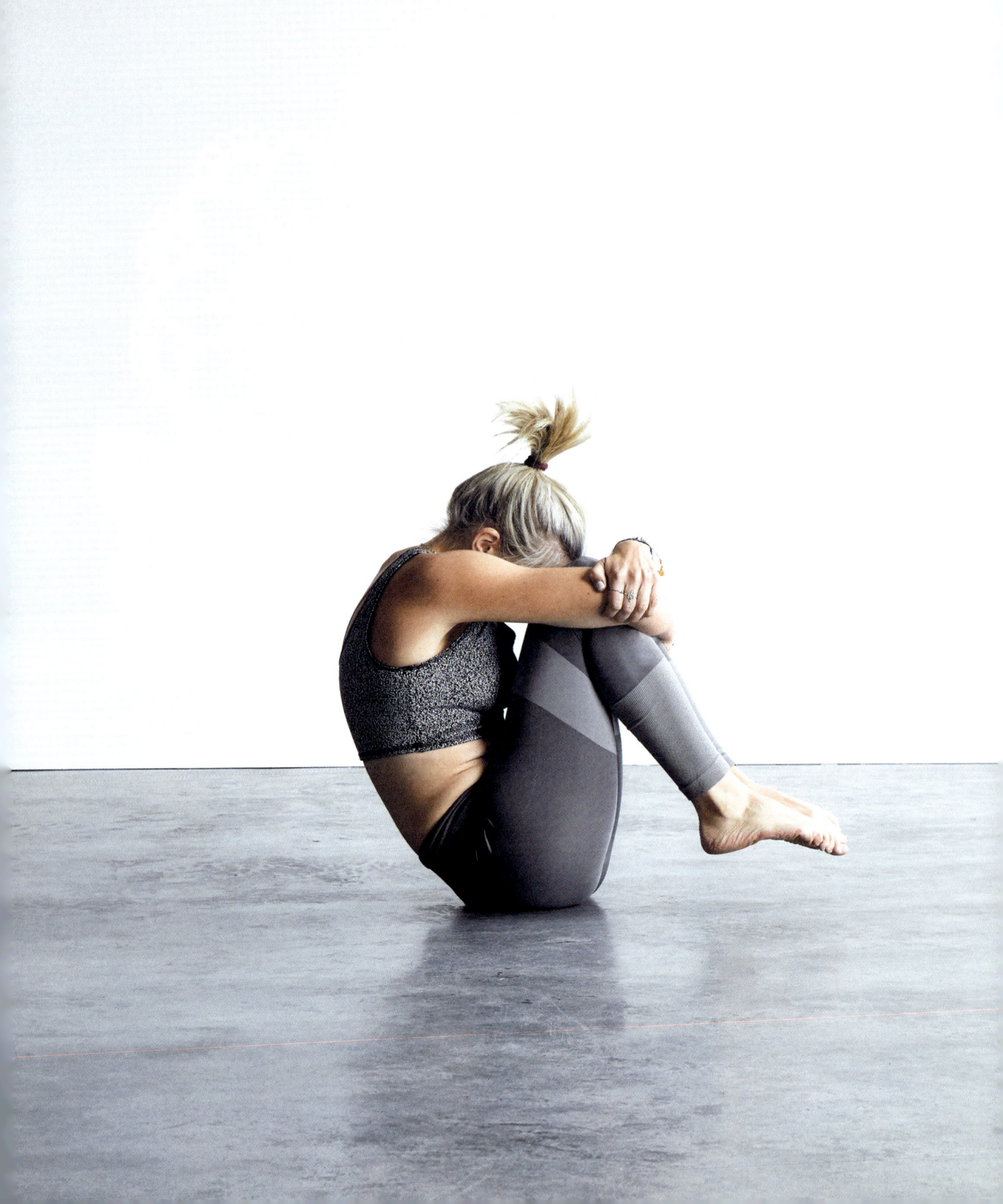

Honesty is telling other people the truth. Integrity is telling yourself the truth.

4. Pranayama

Pranayama (literally, 'life force extension') is all about breath control, which is believed to free the flow of 'prana' (life energy). There are many pranayama exercises, including alternate nostril breathing (see page 229), which is used to calm the mind and emotions, and breath of fire, which is used to raise energy and heighten awareness.

5. Pratyahara

This is the conscious withdrawal of energy from the senses. It doesn't mean withdrawing into your shell, rather it is about stepping back and creating a space around our perceptions – observing them rather than identifying with them, so that we can respond rather than react. This is a lot like mindfulness (see page 226).

6. Dharana

Dharana refers to pure concentration – the ability to focus our attention without being sidetracked or distracted. It's a bit like flow – that feeling you get when you are so completely absorbed in doing something that you lose track of time. Your mind stops chattering and you are completely in the moment.

7. Dhyana

This refers to meditation and contemplation, to awareness without attachment. In Hinduism, the yogi practises dhyana to realise his or her true self (atman, or soul).

8. Samadhi

This is what all yoga works towards: the bliss of enlightenment. The profound connection to the divine.

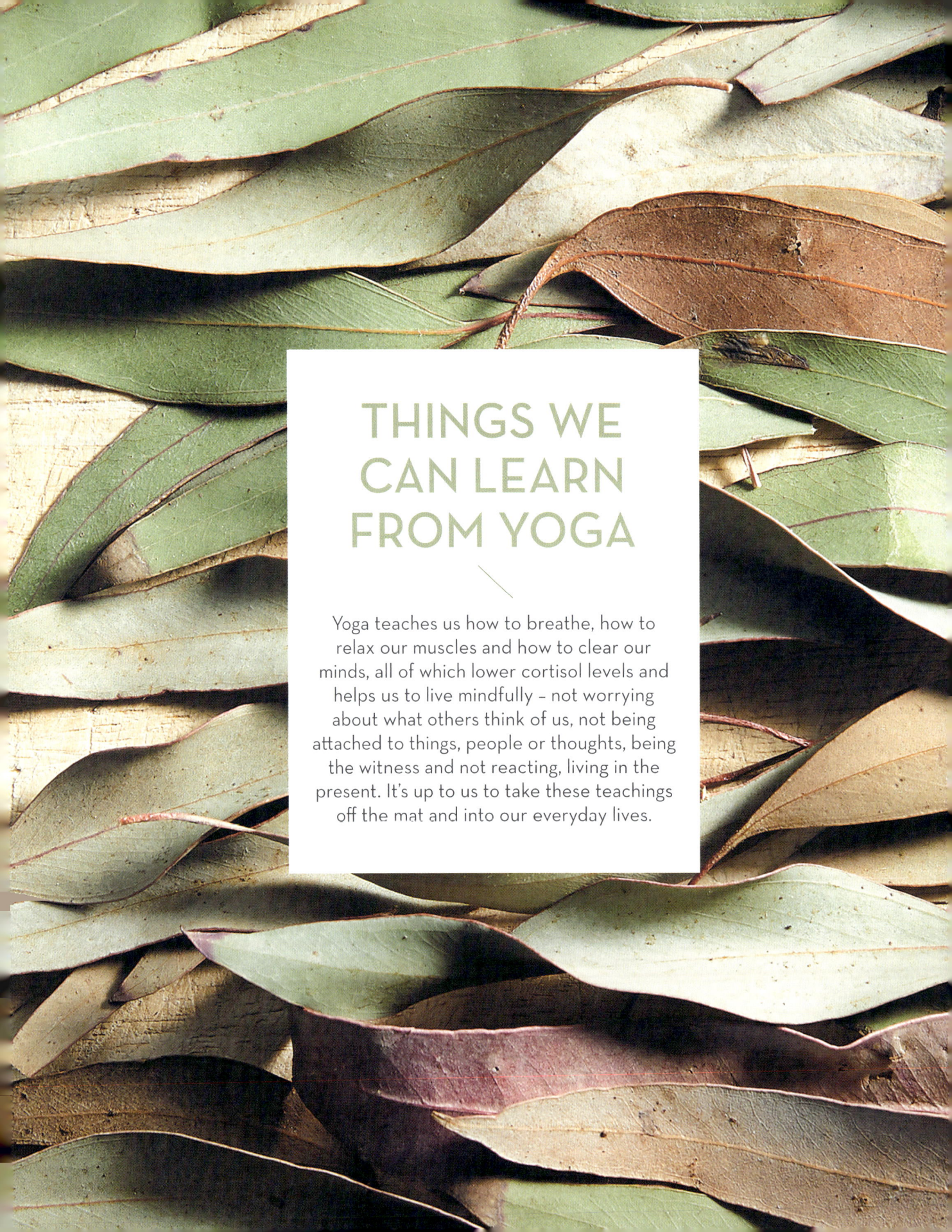

THINGS WE CAN LEARN FROM YOGA

Yoga teaches us how to breathe, how to relax our muscles and how to clear our minds, all of which lower cortisol levels and helps us to live mindfully – not worrying about what others think of us, not being attached to things, people or thoughts, being the witness and not reacting, living in the present. It's up to us to take these teachings off the mat and into our everyday lives.

When you're real and living from your heart, that's where the magic is.

Gratitude

Yoga has helped me understand how the expectations I place on myself mirror the expectations I place on others. The truth is, I've put a lot of pressure on people to try to get them to be who I want them to be. I've expected too much and taken them for granted without even realising it. It took a rough patch to figure out that I'm incredibly lucky to be living this life and to feel grateful to all the beautiful souls I am lucky enough to connect with.

Integrity

Social media makes it really hard to work out who is being real and who is faking it. But in the end, we can't know what anyone else is thinking and feeling. We can only know ourselves. And since there's only one you, why not be the best version of you? So be honest, be kind and be truthful, without apologising or feeling guilty. Chances are, most people will love that, but so what if they don't? Don't waste one second worrying about what other people will think of you – it's their business, and you can't control it anyway. Put all your energy into living from your heart. Honesty is telling other people the truth. Integrity is telling yourself the truth.

Sankalpa: to set an intention

I love walking into a yoga class where the teacher asks me to set a 'sankalpa' for my practice. Sometimes I'll set a long-term life goal or sometimes I'll just aim for a feeling, though whatever it is, I make sure it comes from the heart. If I can't think of anything for myself, I might send love to someone close to me or someone I may have seen in the street on my way to yoga who may be struggling.

So trust your sankalpa, and when the thoughts begin to creep in during your yoga class (they always do) come back to your intention, focus on it, feel it, connect to it. When you're strong and centred and your mind is clear, it's the perfect time to focus on your dreams. I often have the most wonderful epiphanies in the yoga room!

Non-attachment

As a person who loves to set goals and watch dreams unfold (and who loves nice clothes and handbags!), non-attachment is a tricky concept for me. You see, on the one hand, yogic principles teach that we must work towards our goal (intention) with determined, consistent commitment, but on the other hand, we must have no attachment to the outcome. Now, I understand why this is important – it helps us to stop worrying about the future and to accept what happens – but try telling an Olympic athlete to practise non-attachment; it's not going to go down well when they've spent their whole life training to win a gold medal! So here's how I look at it: I try to practise non-attachment in relationships, but for other stuff I just let my mind go where it needs to.

For example, say I go on a few dates with someone and I really like them, that's when I click into non-attachment and tell myself 'I'm not in charge here – what will be will be'. I figure I can't control anything or anyone, so why not just focus on being kind and having an open heart? Actually, I got to practise this while writing this book. I'd been completely in love with a guy who didn't feel the same way, so instead of torturing myself by hanging in there hoping that he might change his mind, I broke up with him. It was hard, but it was the kind thing to do – both for myself and for him.

One of my favourite forms of pranayama is alternate nostril breathing, a practice that many successful athletes and politicians use to de-stress and keep calm.

Breath awareness

Breathing is something we do so naturally that it seems weird to give it much thought, but it is actually a key aspect in most yoga practice. One of the reasons I love vinyasa is its union of movement with breath – it just feels so amazing in the body and clears my mind. Both hatha and kundalini yoga use pranayama (breath control).

One of my favourite forms of pranayama is alternate nostril breathing. Start by placing the tips of the index and middle fingers of the right hand in between the eyebrows, the ring finger and little finger on the left nostril, and the thumb on the right nostril. You will use the ring finger and little finger to open or close the left nostril and the thumb to open or close the right nostril.

Now, press your thumb down on the right nostril and breathe out gently through the left nostril. Inhale from the left nostril and then block it by gently pressing it with the ring finger and little finger.

Remove the right thumb from the right nostril, and exhale. Now, inhale from the right nostril and exhale from the left. You have now completed one round. Repeat nine times.

Meditation

Meditation is the practice of focusing attention, of quietening the mind so that we are 'aware' but not 'thinking'. It's been practised for millennia in different religious traditions, and there is strong evidence for its positive effects on physical and mental health. I've done a Vedic meditation course, but there's also Transcendental Meditation (TM) – both require 20 minutes' practice every morning and night. There are heaps of meditation apps, too, which are a great way to start your meditation journey.

The way I see it is there are no rules. Whatever gets you to sit still and turn your attention inwards will do the trick, so try a few different types of meditation and find out what works for you. You could start by going out into nature, taking your shoes off and finding a comfy spot. Sit down and close your eyes. Listen to the sounds around you. Feel the air on your face. Now focus on your breathing. In. Out. Notice thoughts, gently returning your attention to the breath. You can do this. You have the time. Just. Breathe.

Life is pretty magical.

YOGA MIND

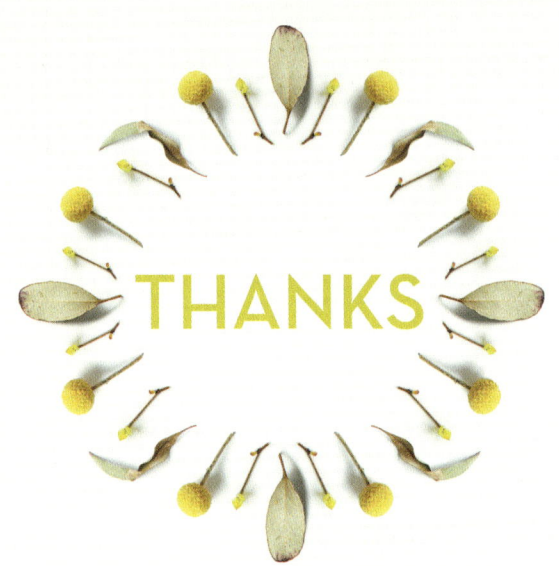

THANKS

Emma van Leest, you went too soon. I know you will live on in so many souls and hearts, especially through your husband, Hunter, and children, Koen and Saskia. Your artwork is very special.

To you, the person who holds this book in your hands. Without your support this book wouldn't even exist. I'm grateful forever. Thank you from my heart to yours!

Linda Raymond, I don't know where I'd be without you. Thank you for taking me under your wing. I will be forever grateful for your love and kindness.

Mary Small, I love your vison and I am so grateful to be so involved in the creative process. It means more to me than you know.

Clare Marshall, thank you for supporting me; it's our little baby. Thank you for being so patient with me wanting to proofread this manuscript a zillion times!

Ingrid Ohlsson, thank you for letting this fellow yogi bring her dream to life!

Armelle Habib, you see the magic even when I can't. You are, without a doubt, one of the coolest people I know.

Karina Duncan. Little hen, you are so much more than a workmate, you're someone who inspires me every single day. I'm so grateful for our friendship.

Jane Negline, you are, hands down, one of the most awesome humans I've ever had the pleasure to work with and one I call a great friend. Thank you for believing in the big dreams. It means more than you know.

Lauren Cilento Miller, thank you for helping me make this dream come true.

Michelle Mackintosh, I know how much love you put into this. Thank you so, so much.

Emma Warren. Guapa, you're not only super talented, you're kind and bloody smart, too. A very cool combo of brilliance. Working with you isn't work, it's living.

Caroline Griffiths, I love your kind and gentle energy; it's always so lovely working with you.

Simon Davis, thank you for working your magic to make this book the best it can be.

Miriam Cannell, love working with you; editing genius.

Emma Roocke, the queen of the perfect ball. Dare I say it, these ones were your best work yet!

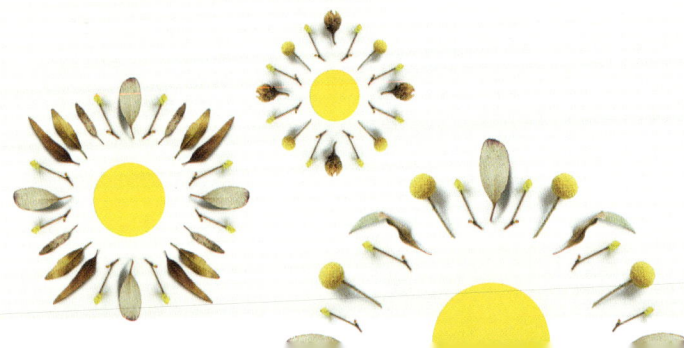

Kate Radford. For your natural glowy make up; so fun and dreamy working with you!

Steph Rooney, I always love working with you.

Clare Keighery, brill book publicist. Thank you for coming with me to talks and events, and helping the launch come together!

Philippa Whitfield Pomeranz, every time we work together makes my heart happy. Pip, let's create more magic.

Hayley Van Spanje. I love working with you; you tell it how it is, and I love that.

Lee Lee Sutherland. Thank you for being part of this from the start.

Lucy Roach, I'm forever grateful to you for giving me my first chance.

Charlotte Ree, thank you for being part of the process, even from afar. Your support means loads.

Dadio, thank you for inspiring me to chase the big dream!

Mum, you're my number-one supporter. Thank you.

Andrea Evans. A. Apple, here's to believing in the really big dreams that only we can see. So much to look forward to!

Maddie Dixson, my biophilia bud. Thank you for your kind heart; I love our spirit hangs.

Cartia Mallan, your fire-heart inspires me more than you know, beauty. Always live from that place.

Guy Turland, you are a 'salt of the earth' human. I love being around you.

Bridget Bodenham. Thank you for such magical and lovely props.

Cork Leaf. The coolest yogi mat! I didn't want to give it back, loved it!

Tristan Smith. Baby bro, we drive each other nuts, but I love you to the moon and back.

Samara Kennedy. Keep your heart open, chicken; that's where the magic happens!

Salvatore Malatesta. Sal, your vision and passion is infectious.

Lach Ward. A pleasure working with you. You are my favourite combo of human; strong but gentle.

Tayte Bale. Always a pleasure working with your talented soul, Tayters.

Happy Place dream team. Sarah and the gang, thank you for working so hard to create delish smoothies and goodies at the smoothie bar.

Tim O'Keefe. Thank you for being a friend who inspires me. We don't get to work together as much these days, but seeing you is always a joy.

Rivis Donnelly. You've been a supporter from day one and I can't thank you enough.

Rebecca Rich, thank you for your recipe testing magic.

Nick Manuell, thanks for always having my back.

Leisel Jones. Chicken, love your real heart. It's an honour to be your mate.

Dan Adair. You inspire me loads. Always have; always will.

Charlie Goldsmith. You are one of the coolest hearts I know, CG. I'll always be your number one spud.

Jamie Gonzalez. Thank you for teaching me that 'not all will love you back; love anyway'.

Loretta Carraro, for teaching me your crystal and reiki wisdom. You are a very inspiring soul, always remember that.

Julia George, your readings are very special. I feel very lucky to have crossed your path.

Celia, Evie, Kobe and Steve Jones. Your support never goes unnoticed. Thank you so much and here's to the magic of crystals! You guys inspire me.

Yoke Yoga and Chris Wilson. Thank you for not only giving me a lovely place to practice and film, but to also to teach. It's an absolute honour.

Powerliving. I travel all over the place and having both of your studios as bases is a huge help. It further helps my yoges to grow and develop so I'm really grateful for that.

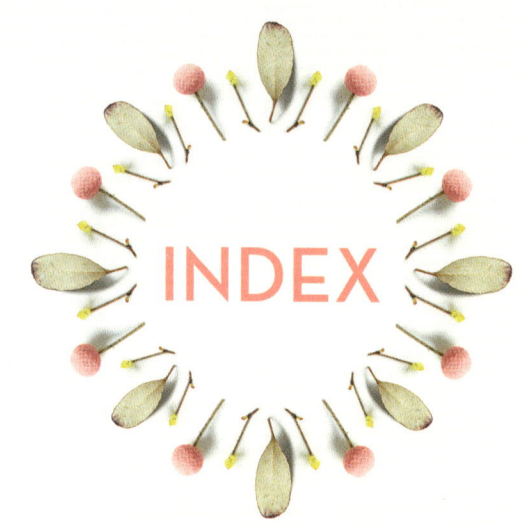

INDEX

A
acro yoga 21
activating nuts and seeds 108, 114
adho mukha svanasana 39
alanasana 56
allergies see gluten allergy, coeliac disease, pollen allergy
almonds 71
   almond butter 106
   almond meal 106
   Baked broccoli bites 166
   Banana brekkie cake 142
   Cookie dough balls 202
   nut milk 108
   Paleo chamomile and lemon loaf 136
   Raw basil and strawberry tart 219
   Raw choc, coffee and almond slice 213
   Snickerdoodle cookies 214
alpha-linolenic acid (ALA) 73
Alzheimer's disease 77
amino acids 70, 71, 187
anti-inflammatories 76, 77, 78, 169, 175, 181, 198
antioxidants 68, 76, 77, 78, 109, 114, 120
anusara yoga 21, 28
anxiety 16, 25, 75
apanasana 61
apples
   Chakra-balancing juice 112
   Jules' lamb riblets with Pippa's slaw 193
   Pippa's slaw 193
ardha anuvittasana 53
ardha chandrasana 43, 49
ardha navasana 45
ardha uttanasana 37

asafoetida 76
asanas 7, 8, 22, 223
   adho mukha svanasana 39
   alanasana 56
   apanasana 61
   ardha anuvittasana 53
   ardha chandrasana 43, 49
   ardha navasana 45
   ardha uttanasana 37
   balasana 59
   bhujangasana 39
   chapasana 57
   chaturanga dandasana 38
   dandasana 57
   eka pada chaturanga 46
   natarajasana 51
   navasana 44
   parivrtta anjaneyasana 46
   parivrtta utkatasana 61
   phalakasana variation knee to nose 45
   savasana 55
   setu bandha sarvangasana 52
   tadasana 37
   trikonasana 60
   upavistha konasana 57
   urdhva dhanurasana 53
   urdhva hastasana 37
   urdhva mukha svanasana 38
   urdhva prasarita eka padasana 42
   ustrasana 49, 55
   utkatasana 40, 43
   uttanasana 37, 51, 59
   uttihita chaturanga dandasana 38
   viparita karani 58
   viparita virabhadrasana 41

virabhadrasana 1 41
virabhadrasana 2 41
virabhadrasana 3 56
see also poses
ashtanga yoga 21, 23, 25, 28
attachment see non-attachment
avocados
Cali salad 157
Earth bowls 170
Five-minute healing superfood salad 184
Pineapple prawn cocktails 181
Simple flathead with greens 182
Simple veggie bowl 92
Spiritual gangster wraps 164
Sweet spud hash browns with haloumi 147
Ayurvedic medicine 69, 76, 77, 78, 114, 210
Ayurvedic spices 76–77

B
Baked broccoli bites 166
balance 15
balasana 59
Banana brekkie cake 142
Banana curry with coconut quinoa 176
banana jam, Mauritian 141
bananas
Banana brekkie cake 142
Banana curry with coconut quinoa 176
coconutty bananas 190
Creamy almond oats 91
Crepes with 'Nutella' and banana jam 141
Fruit sushi 196
Iced banana chocolates 208
Luscious lamb curry 190
Mauritian banana jam 141
Salted caramel bone broth smoothie 123
Spiced turmeric oats 91
Teacup tiramisu 216
Tropicana smoothie bowl 114
Turmeric nice cream 198
Warm banana-chai smoothie 120
Warm turmeric karma oats 130
Basic cooked quinoa 89
beans 11, 70, 71
see also mung beans
bee pollen 106
beetroot
Chakra-balancing juice 112
Earth bowls 170
pink hummus 178
Spiced beetroot dip with rainbow veg 152
Spiritual gangster wraps 164
bhujangasana 39

Bikram yoga 21, 22
bircher, 'Snickers' 135
blood pressure 15, 77
blueberries
Detox green smoothie 90
Earth bowls 170
Perfect super platter 178
Quinoa porridge 92
Superfood salad 93
boat pose 44
bone broth
Jetlag-be-gone bone broth 188
Salted caramel bone broth smoothie 123
bowls
Earth bowls 170
Simple veggie bowl 92
Tropicana smoothie bowl 114
Vegan dream bowl 163
brain function 15, 124
breath control 15, 19, 23, 25, 97, 225, 229
see also pranayama
bridge pose 52
broccoli
Baked broccoli bites 166
Simple flathead with greens 182
Simple veggie bowl 92
Superfood egg white scramble 144
broga yoga 22
broth see bone broth
bruschetta, Nectarine and strawberry 138
brussels sprouts: Vegan dream bowl 163
buckwheat 70, 74, 106, 169
Creamy spinach buckwheat risotto 169
Crepes with 'Nutella' and banana jam 141
butt toner sequence 42–43

C
cabbage
Earth bowls 170
Five-minute healing superfood salad 184
Jules' lamb riblets with Pippa's slaw 193
Pippa's slaw 193
Superfood salad 93
cacao 107
cake, Banana brekkie 142
Cali salad 157
camel pose 49, 55
canoe pose 45
capsicum
Perfect super platter 178
Spiced beetroot dip with rainbow veg 152
Thai minced chicken salad 187
carbohydrates 67, 147, 160, 176

carrots
   carrot tops 158
   Chakra-balancing juice 112
   Cinnamon-honey carrots 158
   Earth bowls 170
   Luscious lamb curry 190
   Mung bean dhal 175
   Spiced beetroot dip with rainbow veg 152
   Spiritual gangster wraps 164
cashew nuts 71
   Iced maple-cashew latte 117
   nut milk 108
   Raw basil and strawberry tart 219
   Spiced beetroot dip with rainbow veg 152
   Teacup tiramisu 216
   Turmeric nice cream 198
celery: Chakra-balancing juice 112
chaga 124
chair pose 40, 61
chair pose with eagle arms 43
chair twist 61
Chakra-balancing juice 112
chamomile 78
   Paleo chamomile and lemon loaf 136
chapasana 57
chaturanga dandasana 38
cheese 70, 169
   Creamy spinach buckwheat risotto 169
   Sweet spud hash browns with haloumi 147
   Zenned-out veggies 160
   see also ricotta
chia seeds 73, 85, 107
chicken: Thai minced chicken salad 187
Chickpea choc chip cookies 204
chickpeas 70, 71
   Chickpea choc chip cookies 204
   hummus 163
   pink hummus 178
   Spiritual gangster wraps 164
   Vegan dream bowl 163
child's pose 59
chilli 85, 107
chocolate 81, 107
   Chickpea choc chip cookies 204
   chocolate sauce 208
   Iced banana chocolates 208
   Raw choc, coffee and almond slice 213
   'Snickers' bircher 135
   Vedic vegan rocky road 210
chocolate sauce 208
Choudhury, Bikram 21, 22
Cinnamon-honey carrots 158

circulation 77, 78, 85, 120
clean eating 11, 65–80
cleanse
   cleansing yoga sequence 60–61
   coping with cravings 96–97
   daily itinerary 98–101
   get organised 86
   recipes 88–94
   seven-day vegan cleanse 83–101
   shopping list 87
cobra pose 39
coconut
   Banana curry with coconut quinoa 176
   coconut flour 107
   coconut milk/cream 107
   coconut oil 107
   coconut quinoa 176
   coconut sugar 107
   coconutty bananas 190
   coconut water 107
   desiccated coconut 202
   Green tea and coconut bubble tea 118
   Luscious lamb curry 190
coconut quinoa 176
coconutty bananas 190
coeliac disease 75, 108
coffee 85
   Iced maple-cashew latte 117
   Raw choc, coffee and almond slice 213
   'Shroom coffee 124
   Teacup tiramisu 216
complete protein 70, 142, 148, 166, 182
   see also protein
Cookie dough balls 202
cookies, Snickerdoodle 214
coriander 76
corn 71
   Thai minced chicken salad 187
corpse pose 55
cravings 85, 99
   coping with cravings 96–97
   sugar cravings 78, 85, 99, 208
Creamy almond oats 91
Creamy spinach buckwheat risotto 169
Crepes with 'Nutella' and banana jam 141
crescent lunge 56
crescent lunge twist 46
cucumber
   Perfect super platter 178
   Pineapple and cucumber icy poles 201
   Spiced beetroot dip with rainbow veg 152
cumin 77

curcumin 77, 130
curries
    Banana curry with coconut quinoa 176
    Luscious lamb curry 190

D

dhal, Mung bean 175
dancer pose 51
dandasana 57
dates, medjool 108
    Horchata 126
    Raw basil and strawberry tart 219
    'Snickers' bircher 135
    Teacup tiramisu 216
depression 16
detox 21, 22, 60, 77, 85, 204
    see also cleanse
Detox green smoothie 90
dharana 225
dhyana 15, 225
    see also meditation
digestion 77, 78, 97, 114, 120, 175, 210
Digestion starter 98
digestive system 61, 85, 136, 198
dip, Spiced beetroot, with rainbow veg 152
disaccharides 67
doshas 76
    see also energy
'doughnuts', Raw, vegan Hawaiian 207
down dog 39
downward facing dog 39

E

Earth bowls 170
egg of the universe pose 61
eggs 70
    Cali salad 157
    Salmon and kale omelette 148
    Superfood egg white scramble 144
eight limbs of yoga 21, 222–225
    see also ashtanga
eight-fold path 8
eka pada chaturanga 46
energy 39, 66, 67, 70, 72, 90, 108, 187, 190, 216, 225
    see also doshas, kundalini energy, prana
essential fatty acids 72, 73

F

fats, healthy 72
fatty acids, essential 72, 73
fennel 77, 78
    Fennel and orange salad 154
    Spiced beetroot dip with rainbow veg 152

Fennel and orange salad 154
fish 70, 73
    Five-minute healing superfood salad 184
    Salmon and kale omelette 148
    Simple flathead with greens 182
Five-minute healing superfood salad 184
flexibility 15, 16, 22, 25, 28
flow yoga 25
forward fold 37, 51
forward fold with supported elbows 59
four-limbed staff pose 38
free-radical damage 77
Friend, John 21
fructose 67, 108
fructose malabsorption 76
Fruit sushi 196

G

GABA 16
Gannon, Sharon 23
ginger 77, 78
    Ginger granola with peach 132
Ginger granola with peach 132
glucose 67
gluten 75
gluten intolerance 75
grains 71
    see also whole grains
granola, Ginger, with peach 132
grapes: Perfect super platter 178
Green tea and coconut bubble tea 118
grounding rituals 32
Gunas 69

H

half moon pose 43, 49
halfway lift 37
hash browns, Sweet spud, with haloumi 147
hatha yoga 16, 22, 25, 28, 31, 229
healthy fats 72, 74, 92, 97
herbal teas 78
high lunge 56
high plank 38
Hinduism 32, 69, 222
hing 76
hip-hop yoga 22
honey, raw 108
Horchata 126
hot yoga 22, 28, 31
hummus 163
hummus, pink 178
hydration 31, 78, 97

I

Iced banana chocolates 208
Iced maple-cashew latte 117
icing, pink 207
icy poles, Pineapple and cucumber 201
intentions 69, 157, 227, 228
Iyengar, B. K. S 23
Iyengar yoga 21, 23, 25, 28, 31

J

jetlag 48
Jetlag-be-gone bone broth 188
jivamukti yoga 23, 28
Jois, K. Pattabhi 21
juice, Chakra-balancing 112
Jules' lamb riblets with Pippa's slaw 193

K

kale
Five-minute healing superfood salad 184
Salmon and kale omelette 148
Superfood egg white scramble 144
superfood pesto 172
Wish noodles 172
Zenned-out veggies 160
kamut 71, 74, 75
kasha *see* buckwheat
kiwi: Fruit sushi 196
knees to chest pose 61
kundalini energy 23, 44
kundalini yoga 23, 28, 44, 57, 229

L

lactose 67
lamb
Jules' lamb riblets with Pippa's slaw 193
Luscious lamb curry 190
latte, Iced maple-cashew 117
latte, Turmeric 94
legumes 70, 71
Life, David 23
lion's mane 124
liquorice 78
loaf: Paleo chamomile and lemon loaf 136
low boat pose 45
low plank pose 38
Luscious lamb curry 190
lycopene 68

M

macadamia nuts
nut milk 108
Perfect super platter 178
Raw, vegan Hawaiian 'doughnuts' 207
superfood pesto 172
Wish noodles 172
Warm banana-chai smoothie 120
mangoes
Pineapple prawn cocktails 181
Tropicana smoothie bowl 114
maple syrup 108
Mauritian banana jam 141
meditation 15, 23, 25, 32, 55, 85, 223, 229
see also dhyana
mental health 16, 229
milk, non-dairy 108
milk, nut 108
millet 70, 74, 108
mindful eating 80, 97
monosaccharides 67
Mung bean dhal 175
mung beans 70
Mung bean dhal 175
Superfood salad 93
mushrooms 68
Earth bowls 170
Five-minute healing superfood salad 184
Vegan dream bowl 163
Zucchini pasta salad 93
see also chaga, lion's mane

N

natarajasana 51
nausea 77
navasana 44
Nectarine and strawberry bruschetta 138
nice cream, Turmeric 198
niyamas 8, 223
non-attachment 223, 225, 228
noodles, Wish 172
nut milks 108
'Nutella' 141
nuts and seeds 67, 71, 108
see also almonds, cashew nuts, macadamia nuts
nuts and seeds, activating 108

O

oats 74, 75, 108
Creamy almond oats 91
Ginger granola with peach 132
'Snickers' bircher 135
Spiced turmeric oats 91
Warm turmeric karma oats 130
olive oil 72, 109
omega-3 72, 73, 107

omega-6 72, 73
omelette, Salmon and kale 148
one-legged plank 46
orange: Fennel and orange salad 154

P
Paleo chamomile and lemon loaf 136
parivrtta anjaneyasana 46
parivrtta utkatasana 61
pasta salad, Zucchini 93
Perfect super platter 178
pesto, superfood 172
pesto, Vegan basil 89
phalakasana variation knee to nose 45
pineapple
   Chakra-balancing juice 112
   Pineapple and cucumber icy poles 201
   Pineapple prawn cocktails 181
   Raw, vegan Hawaiian 'doughnuts' 207
Pineapple and cucumber icy poles 201
Pineapple prawn cocktails 181
pink icing 207
Pippa's slaw 193
platter, Perfect super 178
pollen allergy 106
polyunsaturated fatty acids 73
porridge, Quinoa 92
poses
   boat pose 44
   bridge pose 52
   camel pose 49, 55
   canoe pose 45
   chair pose 40, 61
   chair pose with eagle arms 43
   chair twist 61
   child's pose 59
   cobra 39
   corpse pose 55
   crescent lunge 56
   crescent lunge twist 46
   dancer pose 51
   down dog 39
   downward facing dog 39
   egg of the universe pose 61
   forward fold 37, 51
   forward fold with supported elbows 59
   four-limbed staff pose 38
   half moon pose 43, 49
   halfway lift 37
   high lunge 56
   high plank 38
   knees to chest pose 61
   low boat pose 45
   low plank pose 38
   one-legged plank 46
   prayer pose 37
   reverse warrior 41
   shoelace pose 43
   sitting wide leg forward fold 57
   staff pose 57
   standing backbend 53
   standing mountain pose 37
   standing splits 42
   sugar cane pose 57
   tiger curls knee to nose variation 45
   triangle pose 60
   twisted roots 59
   up dog 38
   upward bow 53
   upward facing dog 38
   upward salute 37
   warrior 1 41
   warrior 2 41
   warrior 3 56
   wheel pose 53
   wide legs up the wall 58
positive thinking 19
posture 19
potassium 77
power yoga 23
prana 39, 69, 225
   see also energy
pranayama 8, 15, 55, 225, 229
   see also breath control
pratyahara 225
prayer pose 37
prawns: Pineapple prawn cocktails 181
processed carbs 67
processed foods 66, 86
protein 68, 70, 74, 75, 85, 106, 107, 108, 109, 126, 138, 163, 181, 182, 204, 213
   see also complete protein
protein combining 70–71
protein powders 123

Q
quinoa 109
   Banana curry with coconut quinoa 176
   Basic cooked quinoa 89
   coconut quinoa 176
   Horchata 126
   Quinoa porridge 92
   Quinoa salad 94
   Superfood salad 93
Quinoa porridge 92
Quinoa salad 94

R

Rajas 69
Raw basil and strawberry tart 219
Raw choc, coffee and almond slice 213
Raw, vegan Hawaiian 'doughnuts' 207
relaxation 16, 19, 22, 25, 27, 28, 58–59, 97
restorative yoga 25, 28, 31
reverse warrior 41
ricotta 70
    Baked broccoli bites 166
    Nectarine and strawberry bruschetta 138
risotto, Creamy spinach buckwheat 169
Roasted sweet potato 88
rocky road, Vedic vegan 210

S

salads
    Cali salad 157
    Fennel and orange salad 154
    Five-minute healing superfood salad 184
    Quinoa salad 94
    Superfood salad 93
    Thai minced chicken salad 187
    Zucchini pasta salad 93
Salmon and kale omelette 148
salt 109
Salted caramel bone broth smoothie 123
samadhi 225
sankalpa 157, 227
Sattva 69
Sattvic diet 69
savasana 55
sequences 36–61
    butt toner 42–43
    for cleansing 60–61
    for sadness 54–57
    for sleep 58–59
    for travelling 48–51
    pre-date 52–53
    sun A warm-up 36–39
    ten-minute work-out 40–41
    tummy toner 44–46
setu bandha sarvangasana 52
seven-day vegan cleanse 83–101
shoelace pose 43
shopping list for seven-day cleanse 87
'Shroom coffee 124
Simple flathead with greens 182
Simple veggie bowl 92
sitting wide leg forward fold 57
sleep 25, 58–59
slice, Raw choc, coffee and almond 213

smoothies
    Detox green smoothie 90
    Salted caramel bone broth smoothie 123
    Tropicana smoothie bowl 114
    Warm banana-chai smoothie 120
Snickerdoodle cookies 214
'Snickers' bircher 135
Spiced beetroot dip with rainbow veg 152
Spiced turmeric oats 91
spices, Ayurvedic 76–77
spinach
    Creamy spinach buckwheat risotto 169
    Detox green smoothie 90
    Mung bean dhal 175
Spiritual gangster wraps 164
spirituality 23, 28, 223
staff pose 57
standing backbend 53
standing mountain pose 37
standing splits 42
starches 67
stevia 109
strawberries
    Fruit sushi 196
    Nectarine and strawberry bruschetta 138
    Perfect super platter 178
    Raw basil and strawberry tart 219
strength 15, 19, 21, 22, 25, 28
stress 15, 19
sucrose 67
sugar cane pose 57
sugar cravings see cravings
sugars 67
sun A warm-up 36–39
Superfood egg white scramble 144
superfood pesto 172
Superfood salad 93
surya namaskar 36–39
sweet potato
    Roasted sweet potato 88
    Simple veggie bowl 92
    sweet spud hash browns 147
    Sweet spud hash browns with haloumi 147
    Zenned-out veggies 160
sweet spud hash browns 147
Sweet spud hash browns with haloumi 147

T

tadasana 37
tahini 109
tamari 109
Tamas 69
tart, Raw basil and strawberry 219

tea: Green tea and coconut bubble tea 118
　see also herbal tea
Teacup tiramisu 216
ten-minute work-out 40–41
Thai minced chicken salad 187
tiger curls knee to nose variation 45
tiramisu, Teacup 216
Transcendental meditation 229
triangle pose 60
triglycerides 67
trikonasana 60
Tropicana smoothie bowl 114
tulsi 78
Tummy toner sequence 44–46
turmeric 77, 78
　Mung bean dhal 175
　Spiced turmeric oats 91
　Tropicana smoothie bowl 114
　Turmeric latte 94
　Turmeric nice cream 198
　Warm turmeric karma oats 130
Turmeric latte 94
Turmeric nice cream 198
twisted roots 59

U

up dog 38
upavistha konasana 57
upward bow 53
upward facing dog 38
upward salute 39
urdhva dhanurasana 53
urdhva hastasana 37
urdhva mukha svanasana 38
urdhva prasarita eka padasana 42
ustrasana 49, 55
utkatasana 40, 43
uttanasana 37, 51, 59
uttihita chaturanga dandasana 38

V

vanilla pods 109
vasodilator 77
Vedic meditation 229
Vedic vegan rocky road 210
Vegan basil pesto 89
Vegan dream bowl 163
vinyasa flow see vinyasa yoga
vinyasa yoga 15, 21, 22, 23, 25, 28, 31, 229
viparita karani 58
virabhadrasana 1 41
virabhadrasana 2 41
virabhadrasana 3 56

W

Warm banana-chai smoothie 120
Warm turmeric karma oats 130
warrior 1 41
warrior 2 41
warrior 3 56
water see hydration
wheel pose 53
whole grains 74
　see also grains
wide legs up the wall 58
Wish noodles 172
wraps, Spiritual gangster 164

Y

yamas 8, 223
yin yoga 25, 28, 31, 58, 59
yoga
　eight limbs of yoga 222–225
　evening yoga 98
　mats 31
　morning yoga 36–39, 98
　poses 36–61
　　see also asanas, poses, sequences
　props 21, 23, 25, 31
　rituals 32
　studio, choosing 26–28
　things we can learn from yoga 226–229
　to music 25, 27
　types of yoga 20–25
　typical day in yoga life 81
　　see also acro yoga, anusara yoga, ashtanga yoga, Bikram yoga, broga yoga, flow yoga, hatha yoga, hip-hop yoga, hot yoga, Iyengar yoga, jivamukti yoga, kundalini yoga, power yoga, restorative yoga, yinyasa yoga, yin yoga
yoghurt 109

Z

Zenned-out veggies 160
zucchini
　Five-minute healing superfood salad 184
　Mung bean dhal 175
　Simple flathead with greens 182
　Superfood egg white scramble 144
　Wish noodles 172
　Zucchini pasta salad 93
Zucchini pasta salad 93

A Plum book

First published in 2018 by
Pan Macmillan Australia Pty Limited
Level 25, 1 Market Street,
Sydney, NSW 2000, Australia

Level 3, 112 Wellington Parade,
East Melbourne, VIC 3002, Australia

Text copyright © Lola Berry 2018
Design Michelle Mackintosh copyright © Pan Macmillan 2018
Photography Armelle Habib copyright © Pan Macmillan 2018

The moral right of the author has been asserted.

Design by Michelle Mackintosh
Paper-cut art by Emma van Leest
Edited by Miriam Cannell and Simon Davis
Index by Helena Holmgren
Photography by Armelle Habib
Prop and food styling by Karina Duncan
Food preparation by Caroline Griffiths, Emma Roocke and
　　Emma Warren
Typeset by Pauline Haas
Colour reproduction by Splitting Image Colour Studio
Printed and bound in China by 1010 Printing International Limited

A CIP catalogue record for this book is available from the National Library of Australia.

All rights reserved. No part of this book may be reproduced or transmitted by any person or entity (including Google, Amazon or similar organisations), in any form or means, electronic or mechanical, including photocopying, recording, scanning or by any information storage and retrieval system, without prior permission in writing from the publisher.

We advise that the information contained in this book does not negate personal responsibility on the part of the reader for their own health and safety. It is recommended that individually tailored advice is sought from your healthcare or medical professional. The publishers and their respective employees, agents and authors are not liable for injuries or damage occasioned to any person as a result of reading or following the information contained in this book.

The publisher would like to thank the following for their generosity in providing props for the book: Bridget Bodenham and Cork Leaf.